Thieme

Multiorgan Resections for Cancer

Advanced Surgical Techniques

Marco P Merlini, MD, FACS, FRSM, FACA, FCCP
Professor of Surgery
Faculté de Biologie et Médecine
University of Lausanne
Head of the Department of Surgery
General Hospital
La Chaux-de-Fonds
Switzerland

Ronald F Martin, MD, FACS
Staff Surgeon
Department of Surgery
Marshfield Clinic
Marshfield, Wisconsin
Clinical Associate Professor of Surgery
University of Vermont
Burlington, Vermont
USA
Lieutenant Colonel
Medical Corps
United States Army Reserve

With contributions by
M Dusmet, AE Castellanos, C Karakousis, RF Martin,
MP Merlini, WC Meyers, M Oncel, IN Ponomarenko,
RM Quiros, FH Remzi, HL Rossi, T Saclarides, LJ Skandalakis,
JE Skandalakis, PH Sugarbaker, V Usatoff, HJ Wanebo,
RCN Williamson, O Zoras

272 illustrations

Thieme
Stuttgart · New York

Library of Congress Cataloging-in-Publication Data
Multiorgan resections for cancer : advanced surgical techniques / [edited by] M.P. Merlini, R.F. Martin.
p. ; cm.
ISBN 3-13-135611-1 (alk. paper) – ISBN 1-58890-354-0 (alk. paper)
1. Gastrointestinal system–Cancer–Surgery. I. Merlini, Marco P. II. Martin, R. F.
[DNLM: 1. Digestive System Neoplasms–surgery. WI 149 M961.2006]
RD668.M85.2006
616.99'433059–dc22
2006009251

Important note: Medicine is an ever-changing science undergoing continual development. Research and clinical experience are continually expanding our knowledge, in particular our knowledge of proper treatment and drug therapy. Insofar as this book mentions any dosage or application, readers may rest assured that the authors, editors, and publishers have made every effort to ensure that such references are in accordance with **the state of knowledge at the time of production of the book.**

Nevertheless, this does not involve, imply, or express any guarantee or responsibility on the part of the publishers in respect to any dosage instructions and forms of applications stated in the book. **Every user is requested to examine carefully** the manufacturers' leaflets accompanying each drug and to check, if necessary in consultation with a physician or specialist, whether the dosage schedules mentioned therein or the contraindications stated by the manufacturers differ from the statements made in the present book. Such examination is particularly important with drugs that are either rarely used or have been newly released on the market. Every dosage schedule or every form of application used is entirely at the user's own risk and responsibility. The authors and publishers request every user to report to the publishers any discrepancies or inaccuracies noticed. If errors in this work are found after publication, errata will be posted at www.thieme.com on the product description page.

Rüdigerstrasse 14, 70469 Stuttgart, Germany
http://www.thieme.de
Thieme New York, 333 Seventh Avenue,
New York, NY 10001, USA
http://www.thieme.com

Typesetting by primustype hurler GmbH, Notzingen
Printed in Germany by Appl, Wemding

ISBN-10: 3-13-135611-1 (GTV)
ISBN-13: 978-3-13-135611-6 (GTV)
ISBN-10: 1-58890-354-0 (TNY)
ISBN-13: 978-1-58890-354-9 (TNY)

1 2 3 4 5 6

Foreword

This book represents the ultimate challenge of a surgical oncology practice, that is to consider going beyond the ordinary surgical resection criteria to include removal of organs adjacent to the primary cancer site for the completion of an "en-bloc" resection of locally advanced cancers. As a result of their extensive training and exposure to patients with advanced cancers, the authors are very experienced in the operations they describe. Nowhere are the benefits of specialized surgical oncology training more apparent than in the subjects addressed in this book. Throughout the book, the authors emphasize the need for careful detailed preoperative work-up and evaluation of the patient, careful case selection, and acknowledgment of confidence in the surgical skill and personal experience required to undertake such advanced procedures.

A common thread discussed within the chapters of this book is that a significant proportion of patients with locally advanced cancers nevertheless have lymph nodes free of metastatic disease, indicating a reduced risk of distant metastases despite large tumor size. This biological situation increases the probability of long-term disease-free survival. The high proportion of patients with negative lymph nodes indicates that many of these advanced cancers have a unique biological behavior which, while permitting more advanced local growth even into one or more adjacent organs, may result in significant benefit from an extended operation. One justification for such extended surgery is that substantial long-term disease-free survival can be achieved with the patient exposed to a reasonable level of risk of postoperative morbidity and even mortality.

Many years ago, during a presidential address relating to the basic principles involved in surgical oncology, I described surgical oncology using the following metaphor: "biology is the king, case selection is the queen, and the technical maneuvers undertaken are the princes and princesses of the realm." Sometimes the elaborate technical features and equipment available today encourage surgeons to get carried away into thinking they can ignore the basic biology of the disease and careful patient selection for appropriate procedures. However this may lead to a situation where "the princes or princesses attempt to revolt and overthrow the regime"; by focussing on the technology they are almost always "defeated by the powerful forces of the king and queen, which represent basic oncologic biology and careful case selection." This metaphor is particularly applicable in multiorgan resection for locally advanced cancers in the presumed absence of distant metastases. Before undertaking a risky extended operation, every attempt should be made to characterize, within the knowable facts, the reasonable health of the patient and the absence of distant metastases to fit the surgery to the expectation of a reasonable result.

Some procedures proposed by authors in this volume are yet to be widely accepted or documented by long-term data, such as intraperitoneal chemotherapy after extensive peritoneum resection of widespread peritoneal surface cancers. The authors present considerable preliminary survival data that supports their explanations of complex procedures (i. e., technology), but their success still needs to be related to the biology of the particular cancers. Some low-grade lesions may have extensive peritoneal spread and a large body of literature exists to document this. Substantial bibliographies accompany the articles and are important for justification. This literature supports the concept of resecting adjacent organs in selected patients with advanced local cancers to achieve a good outcome at an acceptable cost.

The authors emphasize the "en-bloc" concept, which is of course essential for a good outcome. While many of the apparent attachments to adjacent organs by primary cancers may actually be inflammatory connections, the surgeon should usually assume that they are cancerous. Such adherence should almost always be used as an indication for the resection of the adjacent possibly involved structure, since blundering into an assumed inflammatory plane with attachment may be disastrous for the patient—because of violated cancer—if the assumption is wrong.

I commend this book to the surgical community, particularly the surgical oncology community, as it represents the experience, skills, and attitudes needed to carry out these extensive, potentially morbid and even potentially lethal surgical resections. Such extensive resections provide the optimum chance for cure in a select group of patients that frequently have a biological behavior that lends itself to longer-term survival.

Blake Cady

Preface

Multiorgan resections for cancer represent a special category of abdominal surgery. These complex procedures tend to push the boundaries of operability (i. e., the true indication for surgery) and resectability (i. e., the feasibility of achieving a complete resection). To be justifiable they must offer the patient a reasonable and meaningful chance of cure with acceptable morbidity and mortality. Thus, even more than in any other field of surgery, patient selection is of paramount importance and these operations must never be considered or undertaken lightly. The operation must benefit the patient and not the surgeon's ego. Precise, careful preoperative evaluation is now more readily available with modern 16- or 32-slice CT scanners using a properly administered contrast medium, different imaging planes, and 3D reconstruction technology. These must be fully exploited to provide maximal benefit. The patient must be carefully staged to rule out distant disease using the best techniques available, such as MRI to rule out brain metastases and PET scans when appropriate. Laparoscopy can allow occult peritoneal spread to be determined prior to submitting the patient to a full laparotomy. Lastly, the initial part of the operation should be considered a fact-finding mission to determine surgically the precise stage, extent, and ultimately the true resectability of the tumor. Under no circumstances must any irreversible step be taken before this operative assessment is complete.

The patient must be fit for surgery. Co-morbidities must be carefully evaluated and the patient's general and nutritional condition should be optimized prior to surgery, otherwise morbidity and mortality rates will be prohibitive.

These operations often require close cooperation between several surgeons. When planning one of these procedures it is important to recognize one's strengths and limitations so that the appropriate expertise is available at the time of surgery. These are complex, stressful procedures and it is important to remain within one's technical comfort zone. This ensures smooth surgery and minimizes the risk of intraoperative complications as well as shortening the actual length of the procedure. Thus, the team must be planned in advance. Furthermore, a cohesive team approach is required before, during, and after surgery to obtain the best results. The patient should be under the direct care of the principal surgeon, who is the team leader and who is ultimately responsible for the tactical decision-making and for the patient. The anesthetist and intensive care specialist are also key members of the team throughout these same three phases. If special blood requirements are anticipated the blood bank needs to be advised. Finally, these can be very long operations and special provisions may be required for the operating room staff. This all means that these operations require very meticulous planning and cannot be improvised at the last minute. The postoperative care must be equally attentive and rigorous and these are not good operations to do on a Friday.

From a technical perspective these are very complex operations. There are three distinct areas within the abdomen from top to bottom. Above the mesocolon the organs are disposed in a very asymmetrical manner, so surgery on the right or the left is quite different. The structures that will be resected tend to be close to the retroperitoneum and the critical abdominal blood vessels. Below the mesocolon there is a much greater degree of symmetry within the peritoneal cavity and the retroperitoneum is also more symmetrical. Symmetry is restored in the pelvis and the retroperitoneum is much less of a problem in terms of determining resectability. Surgical technique and tactics are based on this and on the relative mobility of the more superficial organs, whereas the deeper seated organs tend to be completely immobile. The surgeon needs to exploit this mobility and free up the more superficial organs before tackling the deeper ones.

These operations follow a very logical stepwise progression. The basic operative strategy is based on the organ where the tumor originates and the classic steps of its resection for cancer. The operation will progress down this path until the secondary organ becomes an obstacle. The secondary organ is one which has become involved by direct extension of the tumor into it. At this point the resection of the primary organ stops and the secondary organ is resected. This resection is the minimal resection required to achieve complete tumor clearance and does not necessarily necessitate all the steps that would be required if this were the primary organ (e. g., if the secondary organ is the colon, wide resection of the mesentery to achieve lymph node clearance is not performed). Once the secondary organ has been completely mobilized the resection of the primary organ resumes until its completion. Then the reconstruction required by both resections can be undertaken. A further aspect of these multiorgan resections can be the requirement for vascular resection and reconstruction to achieve the twin goals of complete tumor clearance and safeguarding the blood supply to the remaining vital structures in the abdomen or beyond.

This foreword is meant to give the reader a grasp of the basic philosophy of both this type of surgery and of this book. We have endeavored to present a systematic approach to these challenging resections organ by organ and to describe the detailed and practical approach to these complex problems. We hope that we will have described many little or unknown aspects of this surgery to our readers and that we have been as all-inclusive as possible.

Marco P Merlini
Ronald F Martin

Contributors

Michael Dusmet, FRCS
Consultant in Thoracic Surgery
The Royal Brompton Hospital
London
UK

Andres E Castellanos, MD
Assistant Professor
Department of Surgery
Drexel University College of Medicine
Philadelphia, PA
USA

Constantine Karakousis, MD, PhD, FACS
Professor of Surgery
State University of New York at Buffalo
Kaleida Health
Millard Fillmore Hospital
Buffalo, NY
USA

Ronald F Martin, MD, FACS
Staff Surgeon
Department of Surgery
Marshfield Clinic
Marshfield, Wisconsin
Clinical Associate Professor of Surgery
University of Vermont
Burlington, Vermont
USA

Marco P Merlini, MD, FACS, FRSM, FACA, FCCP
Professor of Surgery
Faculté de Biologie et Médecine
University of Lausanne
Head of the Department of Surgery
General Hospital
La Chaux-de-Fonds
Switzerland

William C Meyers, MD
Alma Dea Morani Professor
Chairman, Department of Surgery
Drexel University College of Medicine
Philadelphia PA
USA

Mustafa Oncel, MD, FASC, FASCRS
Research Fellow
Department of Colorectal Surgery
Cleveland Clinic Foundation
Cleveland, Ohio
USA

Ihor N Ponomarenko, MD
Griffin Hospital
Derby, Connecticut
USA

Roderick M Quiros, MD
Department of General Surgery
Rush University Medical Center
Chicago, Illinois
USA

Feza H Remzi, MD
Staff Surgeon
Department of Colorectal Surgery
Cleveland Clinic Foundation
Cleveland, Ohio
USA

Heather L Rossi, MD
Adjunct Instructor of Surgery
University of Minnesota
Minneapolis, Minnesota
USA

Theodore Saclarides, MD
Department of Surgery
Rush-Presbyterian-St.Luke's Medical Center
Chicago, IL
USA

Lee J Skandalakis, MD, FACS
Clinical Associate Professor of Surgical Anatomy
and Technique
Centers for Surgical Anatomy and Technique
Emory University School of Medicine
Atlanta, GA
USA

John E Skandalakis, MD, PhD, FACS
Chris Carlos Distinguished Professor and Director
Centers for Surgical Anatomy and Technique
Emory University School of Medicine
Atlanta, GA
USA

Paul H Sugarbaker, MD, FACS, FRCS
Professor of Surgery
Washington Cancer Institute
Washington, DC
USA

Valery Usatoff, MBBS (Hon), FRACS
Consultant Hepatobiliary and Pancreatic Surgeon
Monash University Department of Surgery
Alfred Hospital
Prahran, Victoria
Australia

Harold J Wanebo, MD
Department of Surgery
Roger Williams Medical Center
Boston University School of Medicine
Providence, RI
USA

Robin CN Williamson, MA, MD, MChir, FRCS
Professor of Surgery
Department of Gastrointestinal Surgery
Imperial College School of Medicine
Hammersmith Hospital
London
UK

Odysseas Zoras, MD, PhD
Associate Professor
Department of General Surgery
University Hospital of Heraklion
University of Crete Medical School
Heraklion, Crete
Greece

Table of Contents

4 Pelvis 131

5 Peritoneum 161

6 Retroperitoneum 179

Basic Principles & Anatomy

1

1 Surgical Indications

Marco P. Merlini and Michael Dusmet

The indications for multiorgan resections are complex to define because there are many variations in histologic type, pattern of invasion, number of organs involved, and situation in the peritoneal cavity or retroperitoneum. The timing of surgery and chemo- and/or radiotherapy (neo-adjuvant versus adjuvant) will also vary from case to case. Finally, the experience of the surgical team will also play a role.

More than in any other case a multidisciplinary approach to these tumors is essential. Medical oncologists, radiation oncologists, surgeons, and radiologists all have important contributions to make and multimodality therapy is frequently indicated.[1,2]

This chapter provides an overview of the principles of this challenging and difficult field of surgery. The tumors we will be discussing are by nature locally advanced. The twin goals in every case must be to achieve a complete resection and a curative resection, which are not necessarily synonymous, as shall be discussed throughout. Incomplete resections are of little or no benefit to the patient for they submit the patient to all the potential morbidity and mortality of the procedure without any of the benefit (i. e., the chance to be cured). The patient must be fit for the planned treatment for it is axiomatic that the patient can only be cured if he/she survives it. There is no place for expression of the surgical ego in this field of surgery and the desire to perform a "fantastectomy" must be banned. The only rationale must be a cold calculation of the true risks and benefits of the procedure. The patients that truly benefit from these complex procedures are an extremely highly selected group and improper patient selection will invariably lead to unacceptable outcomes, both in terms of morbidity/mortality and survival.

☐ Rationale

It has been shown that often the prognosis following the complete resection of a tumor that invades an adjacent organ is similar to that of a tumor which simply breaches the serosa. In gastric cancer, Bozzetti et al. examined the outcome of 143 tumors with invasion of an adjacent structure. The 5-year survival following complete resection of a pT4 N0 tumor was 29%, whereas this was 21% for pT3 N0 tumors.[3] A possible explanation might be that extension into a neighboring structure prevents shedding of cancer cells from the serosal surface and peritoneal carcinomatosis. Local invasion is certainly less ominous than loco-regional or distant spread. In the series of Bozzetti et al. lymph node involvement had a quite substantial negative impact on survival—the 5-year survival for pT3 N1 and pT4 N1 tumors were respectively only 2 and 5%. This is analogous to what has been shown in nonsmall cell lung cancer where much larger series are available. The 5-year survival following complete resection of a pT3 N0 tumor with chest wall invasion is 40–50%, which is similar to that of a pT1/2 N1 lesion and considerably better than the only 25–40% 5-year survival of patients with true minimal N2 disease. The 5-year survival of patients with completely resectable (as opposed to true minimal) N2 disease is only 9%.

☐ Indications

☐ Intraoperative Discovery

Despite careful preoperative evaluation the intraoperative staging, which is the mandatory first step in any cancer resection, will show invasion into an adjacent structure in a certain number of cases. There are areas where the normal close approximation of structures can make it impossible to accurately assess juxtaposition and invasion by CT or MRI. Again this situation is much more codified in thoracic surgery than in general surgery. In thoracic oncology (nonsmall cell lung cancer) it is commonly thought that in an ideal world the surgeon should have a 5% "open and shut" rate, i. e., cases where the intraoperative staging has shown a more advanced stage than predicted leading to the decision not to proceed with the planned resection. This prevents some patients being denied curative surgery due to over-interpretation of the preoperative imaging. A higher rate denotes an excessively cavalier attitude on the surgeon's behalf. In the abdomen these areas of juxtaposition vs. invasion, which can be delicate to assess on imaging, are the bile duct and the portal vein, the gastric antrum and the head of the pancreas, and the unciform process of the pancreas and the confluence of the mesenteric and portal veins. If this situation is anticipated or encountered it is essential that the patient should be cared for by a surgeon who feels comfortable performing these complex operations. Otherwise the patient should be referred to a tertiary referral center for the resection. What is essential is that the resection should be complete and that during the dissection the areas of tumor adhesion must not be meddled with surgically but encompassed by adequate resection margins.

Surgery after Induction Therapy

The term primary (chemo-, radio-, or chemo-radio) therapy implies that the object is to downstage the tumor so as to render an irresectable tumor resectable. Neo-adjuvant therapy is intended to improve the 5-year survival of a technically operable tumor which has an inherently poor prognosis. Induction therapy comprises both primary and neo-adjuvant therapy. However, the terms are often used interchangeably.

When primary tumors of the esophagus,[4–6] the stomach,[7–11] the ovary,[12–14] the rectum,[15,16] or the pancreas are irresectable at the time of presentation induction, therapy is often considered to try to downstage the tumor.[17–19] If there is a complete or partial response resection can be considered. Again it is worthwhile to remember that the definition of a partial response in many protocols is a reduction in size of >50% for the sum of the two greatest diameters. In some cases a high (five-fold, for example) reduction of the SUV on the PET scan can be used as a surrogate marker for tumor response to induction therapy. If the dissection planes between the organ of origin of the tumor and the involved second organ are not clear cut and clearly tumor free then a multiorgan resection should be performed.

In every case these operations require careful planning so that an appropriate team and instrumentation are available at the time of surgery. If a vascular substitute may be required (greater saphenous vein, internal jugular vein for example) the patient is positioned, prepped, and draped in preparation for this after ensuring that the anesthesiologist has not attempted to put lines into the vessel. Likewise at times ureteral catheters will need to be placed by cystoscopy prior to starting the operation itself.

Induction therapy followed by surgery is a potentially morbid combination that requires fit patients. The upper age in most trials is usually 70 years and this is worth remembering even outside of a trial setting. Even more than for multiorgan resections alone, patient selection is of paramount importance to obtain acceptable results.

Tumors which are Poorly Responsive to Chemo- and Radiotherapy

Some tumors, such as bile duct adenocarcinomas and retroperitoneal sarcomas do not respond to induction therapy in a satisfactory or reliable manner. This exposes the patient to a significant risk of tumor progression during induction therapy, which could mean progression to a completely irresectable stage. These are always very difficult situations to deal with both in terms of treatment decisions and the technical aspect of the resection itself. These are the operations which are liable to present the greatest technical challenges and therefore require the highest amount of preoperative planning and preparation. It is also essential that during the consent process the patient (and his/her family) is made aware not only of the risks of surgery, but also of the not insignificant risk of finding an irresectable tumor at the time of surgery which mandates retreat without resection (the so-called "open and shut" case).

Conditions

Below is the check-list of conditions which must be fulfilled for a patient to be a candidate for a multiorgan resection.

The Patient's General Condition

These are long, complex, occasionally hemorrhagic, sometimes staged procedures which put considerable physiologic stress on the patients. A careful and complete history is the mandatory first step in the evaluation of the patient and it is essential to quantify or rule out major organ dysfunction. Obviously routine blood work will be obtained to assess liver and kidney function. The threshold to obtain specialized investigations such as full pulmonary function tests, echocardiograms, thallium scans, or even coronary angiograms should be low. The overall performance score should be assessed. We use the Eastern Cooperative Oncology Group (ECOG) score which goes from 0 (no limitations whatsoever) to 4 (fully bed-bound).[20] Candidates for these complex operations will ideally all be in categories 0–2.

Distant Metastases

Appropriate investigations must be performed to rule out distant metastases. These will include CT of the chest, abdomen and pelvis, MRI of the brain (or at least CT if MRI is not readily available), PET scan if appropriate. If a PET scan is performed a bone scan is not necessary (PET has both higher sensitivity and specificity than the bone scan for bone metastases if the primary tumor is FDG avid). As a general rule the presence of distant metastases is an absolute contraindication to multiorgan resection. However, there is at least one report of thermoablation of limited liver metastases with radiofrequency in association with the resection of abdominal tumors.[21] This this is still controversial though and should only be considered in the setting of a prospective trial.

Peritoneal Carcinomatosis

There are at least two scoring systems for peritoneal carcinomatosis. Sugarbaker has described the Peritoneal Cancer Index.[22] The abdomen is divided up into 13 regions and a score from 0–3 is attributed to each one (0 = no tumor; 1 = tumor 0.5 cm; 2 = tumor 5 cm; 3 = tumor >5 cm or confluent tumor nodules). The total score can thus be between 0 and 39. This score can be used to predict the probability of complete tumor cytoreduction.

The Japanese Research Society for Gastric Cancer has divided peritoneal carcinomatosis into three stages[23]: stage P1 is limited to peritoneal metastases on the adjacent peritoneum, stage P2 denotes a few scattered distant peritoneal implants, and stage P3 means there are multiple distant peritoneal tumor nodules. They have reported the expected prognostic implications of increasing P stage following gastrectomy with wide systematic nodal dissection—with P1 carcinomatosis the median survival was 21.7 months. This figure was respectively 10.4 and 12.8 months for stage P2 and P3 disease.[24]

Diffuse peritoneal carcinomatosis precludes multiorgan resection. In favorable cases surgery might still be considered if there is very limited and completely resectable stage P1 disease in a very fit patient.

Peritonectomy and its different aspects are an important topic. That is why Chapter 13 is devoted to this subject, even if these techniques are not in the strict sense part of the topic of multiorgan resections. The evolution (reduction or disappearance) of peritoneal carcinomatosis following induction therapy can influence the decision regarding multiorgan resection. The findings at diagnostic laparoscopy before and after induction therapy will allow the peritoneum to be assessed and the final decision to be made.[25]

Predicted Survival

Multiorgan resection must always be done with curative intent. However, as shown by Martin et al. it is more the T and N stage that are the predominant predictors of survival rather than the number of resected structures.[26] In their series of 1133 gastrectomies for cancer, 286 patients underwent the resection of an adjacent organ. The median survival following gastrectomy alone was 63 months, whereas it was 32 months for gastrectomy in association with the resection of an adjacent organ. However, the authors reported that this was due more to the higher N stage of this second category of tumors than the multiorgan resection per se.

Peritoneal carcinomatosis has an impact on the survival following multiorgan resections: 5-year survival can be achieved for ovarian cancer but does not extend beyond 2 years for gastric cancer.

Requirement for a Stoma

Quality of life issues must also be taken into account in determining the indication for these resections. Especially in the lower abdomen these operations can require one or, at times, even two stomas to be constructed. These will influence the life style of patients in 80% of cases and their sexual activity will be curtailed in 40% of cases.[27] An ileostomy can allow better quality of life than a colostomy and this should be taken into account in deciding the best operative strategy.[28] Most centers that will be performing this type of surgery will have specialized stoma nurses who can have a considerable impact on lessening the negative impact of urinary or digestive stomas on the patient's quality of life.[29]

Paralyzing Sequelae

Pelvic and sacral resections have the risk of causing paresis or paralysis of the lower limbs as well as anorectal and/or urinary dysfunction, not to forget sexual dysfunction.

The resection of a sarcoma from the iliac fossa puts the femoral nerve at risk of temporary or permanent injury. This will limit flexion of the thigh. Usually the patient can get used to this limitation and with time the impact becomes fairly limited.

Resection of sacral nerves disturbs urinary, anorectal, and sexual function. If these are below the level of S3 the functional consequences are usually quite limited. Unilateral resections of the S1–S3 roots cause minor urinary dysfunction. Bilateral S1–S2 resections will often submit the patient to the requirement for occasional self-catheterization.

Chronic Lower Limb Edema

Preoperative lower limb edema is usually the harbinger of extensive retroperitoneal involvement and thus implies a poor prognosis. The indication for surgery must be evaluated very carefully and every effort must be made to image the retroperitoneal extension of the tumor. MRI can at times be helpful in this context. If extensive retroperitoneal involvement is found, palliative therapy in association with appropriate physiotherapy should be offered.[30]

Retroperitoneal Tethering

Extensive retroperitoneal tethering usually represents a contraindication to surgery because it often means that the celiac axis or the root of the mesentery is infiltrated. Tumors of the body of the pancreas are the most common example of this condition. That is why these tumors are only resectable in one quarter of all cases.[31] These tumors often invade the celiac axis, the retroperitoneal lymphatics, and the celiac plexus early in their course.

Diagnostic Laparoscopy

Laparoscopy is one of the most powerful staging tools available today. It can allow the extent of the tumor to be ascertained as well as tethering, loco-regional lymph nodes can be sampled for histologic verification, the peritoneum can be inspected for distant spread, and parts of the liver can be assessed for metastases. It can assist in the determination of the indication for surgery and/or induction therapy.

Esophagus

Transesophageal ultrasound with ultrasound guided fine needle aspiration biopsies (FNAB) has made the preoperative staging of the esophagus much more precise and in many cases offers the required information to make the appropriate management decisions (however transesophageal ultrasound alone without FNAB is an insufficiently precise tool to make a decision on suitability for resection). There are, however, cases where it will not resolve all the staging issues in a satisfactory manner. In these cases minimally invasive staging can be performed with laparoscopy and/or thoracoscopy. The sensitivity of thoracoscopy for mediastinal nodal staging could be as high as 93%. The same sensitivity (>93%) is seen for celiac axis nodes sampled by laparoscopy.[32] Thus, minimally invasive surgical staging can be precious in determining the indication for trimodal therapy.[33,34]

Stomach

Laparoscopy is better than CT and ultrasound in determining the precise stage of gastric carcinomas.[35] Diagnostic laparoscopy is performed in a reverse TNM sequence. Firstly, distant metastases (peritoneal) are ruled out, the loco-regional nodes are sampled and finally the tumor itself is assessed.[36] When combined with laparoscopic ultrasonography the sensitivity of the method is greater than 95%.[37,38] On the other hand the technical resectability cannot be determined with the same level of accuracy.[39]

Pancreas

Laparoscopy will allow liver and/or peritoneal metastases which were not detected to be seen, avoiding an unnecessary laparotomy. On the other hand the true resectability was accurately assessed in only 35% of cases. This is why staging laparoscopy cannot be considered to be a routine staging procedure for carcinoma of the pancreas at this time.[40,41]

References

1. Fukuchi SG, Offutt LA, Sacks J, Mann BD. Teaching a multidisciplinary approach to cancer treatment during surgical clerkship via an interactive board game. *Am J Surg.* 2000; 179:337–340.
2. Gross GE. The role of the tumor board in a community hospital. *CA Cancer J Clin.* 1987;37:88–92.
3. Bozzetti F, Regalia E, Bonfanti G, Doci R, Ballarini D, Gennari L. Early and late results of extended surgery for cancer of the stomach. *Br J Surg.* 1990;77:53–56.
4. Kato H, Fukuchi M, Manda R et al. The effectiveness of planned esophagectomy after noeadjuvant chemoradiotherapy for advanced esophageal carcinomas. *Anticancer Res.* 2004;24:4091–4096.
5. Yano M, Yasuda T, Miyata H, Fujiwara Y, Takiguchi S, Monden M. Correlation between histological effects of the main tumors and nodal status after chemoradiotherapy for squamous cell carcinoma of the esophagus. *J Surg Oncol.* 2005;89:244–250.
6. Greer SE, Goodney PP, Sutton JE, Birkmeyer JD. Neoadjuvant chemoradiotherapy for esophageal carcinoma: a meta-analysis. *Surgery.* 2005;137:172–177.
7. Persiani R, D'Ugo D, Rausei S et al. Prognostic indicators in locally advanced gastric cancer (LAGC) treated with preoperative chemotherapy and D2-gastrectomy. *J Surg Oncol.* 2005;89:227–238.
8. Barone C, Cassano A, Pozzo C et al. Long-term follow-up of a pilot phase II study with neoadjuvant epidoxorubicin, etoposide and cisplatin in gastric cancer. *Oncology.* 2004; 67:48–53.
9. Lindsey H. Preoperative chemoradiotherapy shows promise in gastric cancer. *Lancet Oncol.* 2004;5:519.
10. McDonald JS. Clinical overview: adjuvant therapy of gastrointestinal cancer. *Cancer Chemother Pharmacol.* 2004; 54(1):4–11.
11. Hartgrink HH, van de Velde CJ, Putter H et al. Neoadjuvant chemotherapy for operable gastric cancer: long term results of the Dutch randomized FAMTX trial. *Eur J Surg Oncol.* 2004;30:643–649.
12. Tate S, Hirai Y, Takeshima N, Hasumi K. CA 125 regression during neoadjuvant chemotherapy as an independent

prognostic factor for survival in patients with advanced ovarian serous adenocarcinoma. *Gynecol Oncol.* 2005;96: 143–149.

13. Markman M, Belinson J. A rationale for neoadjuvant systemic treatment followed by surgical assessment and intraperitoneal chemotherapy in patients presenting with non-surgically resectable ovarian or primary peritoneal cancers. *J Cancer Res Clin Oncol.* 2005;131:26–30.
14. Park TW, Kuhn WC. Neoadjuvant chemotherapy in ovarian cancer. *Expert Rev Anticancer Ther.* 2004;4:639–647.
15. Yang G, Wagner TD, Thomas CR. Multimodality approaches for rectal cancer. *Curr Probl Cancer.* 2004;28:316-342.
16. Zmora O, Dasilva GM, Gurland B. Does rectal wall tumor eradication with preoperative chemoradiation permit a change in the operative strategy? *Dis Colon Rectum.* 2004; 47:1607–1612.
17. Zimmermann FB, Schumacher C, Lersch C et al. Sequential and/or concurrent hypofractionated radiotherapy and concurrent chemotherapy in neoadjuvant treatment of advanced adenocarcinoma of the pancreas. Outcome and patterns of failure. *Hepato-Gastroenterology.* 2004;51: 1842–1846.
18. Sasson AR, Wetherington RW, Hoffmann JP et al. Neoadjuvant chemotherapy for adenocarcinoma of the pancreas: analysis of histopathology and outcome. *Int J Gastrointest Cancer.* 2003;34:121–128.
19. Fogelman DR, Chen J, Chabot JA et al. The evolution of adjuvant and neoadjuvant chemotherapy and radiation for advanced pancreatic cancer: from 5-fluorouracil to GTX. *Surg Oncol Clin N Am.* 2004;13:711–735.
20. Oken MM, Creech RH, Tormey DC et al. Toxicity and response criteria of the Eastern Cooperative Oncology Group. *Am J Clin Oncol.* 1982;5:649–655.
21. Berber E, Senagore A, Remzi F et al. Laparoscopic radiofrequency ablation of liver tumors combined with colorectal procedures. *Surg Laparosc Endosc Percutan Tech.* 2004;14:186–190.
22. Sugarbaker PH. *Management of Peritoneal Surface Malignancy using Intraperitoneal Chemotherapy and Cytoreductive Surgery.* Grand Rapids, Michigan: The Lundann Company; 1998.
23. Japanese Research Society for Gastric Cancer. *The General Rules for Gastric Cancer Study.* Tokyo: Kanahara Shuppan Co. Ltd; 1995.
24. Kikuchi S, Arai Y, Kobayashi N et al. Is extended lymphadenectomy valuable in palliatively gastrectomized patients with gastric cancer and simultaneous peritoneal metastasis? *Hepato-Gastroenterology.* 2000;47:563–566.
25. Gretschel S, Moesta KT, Hunerbein M et al. New concepts of staging in gastrointestinal tumors as a basis of diagnosis and multinodal therapy. *Onkologie.* 2004;27:23–30.
26. Martin RCG, Jaques DP, Brennan MF, Karpeh M. Extended local resection for advanced gastric cancer. Increased survival versus increased morbidity. *Ann Surg.* 2002;236: 159–165.
27. Nugent KP, Daniels P, Stewart B, Patankar R, Johnson CD. Quality of life in stoma patients. *Dis Colon Rectum.* 1999; 42:1569–1574.
28. Silva MA, Ratnayake G, Deen KI. Quality of life of stoma patients: temporary ileostomy versus colostomy. *World J Surg.* 2003;27:421–424.
29. Marquis P, Marrel A, Jambon B. Quality of life in patients with stomas: the Montreux Study. *Ostomy Wound Manage.* 2003;49:48–55.
30. Liao SF, Huang MS, Li SH et al. Complex decongestive physiotherapy for patients with chronic cancer-associated lymphedema. *J Formos Med Assoc.* 2004;103:344–8.
31. Tenchini P, Serio G, Nicoli N, Danieli D, Iacono C, Nifosi F. Primary malignant neoplasia of the exocrine pancreas: epidemiological findings, risk factors, early diagnosis. Personal case reports, 1970-1981. *Chir Ital.* 1983;35:147–156.
32. Krasna MJ, Mao YS, Sonett J, Gamliel Z. The role of thoracoscopic staging in esophageal cancer patients. *Eur J Cardiothorac Surg.* 1999;16:31–33.
33. Jiao X, Sonett J, Gamliel Z et al. Trimodality treatment versus surgery alone for esophageal cancer. A stratified analysis with minimally invasive pre-treatment staging. *J Cardiovasc Surg.* 2002;43:531--537.
34. Krasna MJ, Jiao X, Mao YS et al. Thoracoscopy/laparoscopy in the staging of esophageal cancer: Maryland experience. *Surg Laparosc Endosc Percutan Tech.* 2002;12:213–218.
35. Wakelin SJ, Deans C, Crofts TJ, Allan PL, Plevris JN, Paterson-Brown S. A comparison of computerized tomography, laparoscopic ultrasound and endoscopic ultrasound in the preoperative staging of esophago-gastric carcinoma. *Eur J Radiol.* 2002;41:161–167.
36. D'Ugo DM, Pende V, Persiani R, Rausei S, Picciocchi A. Laparoscopic staging of gastric cancer: an overview. *J Am Coll Surg.* 2003;196:965–974.
37. Stell DA, Carter CR, Stewart I et al. Prospective comparison of laparoscopy, ultrasonography and computed tomography in the staging of gastric cancer. *Br J Surg.* 1996;86: 1260–1262.
38. Burke EC, Karpeh MS, Conlon KC et al. Laparoscopy in the management of gastric adenocarcinoma. *Ann Surg.* 1997; 225:262–267.
39. Giger U, Schäfer M, Krahenbühl L. Technique and value of staging laparoscopy. *Dig Surg.* 2002;19:473–478.
40. Zhao ZW, He JY, Tan G, Wang HJ, Li KJ. Laparoscopy and laparoscopic ultrasonography in judging the resectability of pancreatic head cancer. *Hepatobiliary Pancreat Dis Int.* 2003;2:609–611.
41. Nieveen van Dijkum EJM, Romijn MG, Terwee CB et al. Laparoscopic staging and subsequent palliation in patients with peripancreatic carcinoma. *Ann Surg.* 2003;237:66–73.

2 Surgical Principles

Marco P. Merlini and Michael Dusmet

General Principles

Multiorgan resections follow the general principles of all oncological surgery. The patient must be operable, which means that all co-morbidities (cardiopulmonary, renal, etc) must be carefully assessed to determine the true operative risk. Distant metastases must be carefully ruled out by appropriate investigations. Complete local control of the tumor must be achieved. To obtain clear margins a rim of healthy tissue has to be resected with the tumor. Other prerequisites include systematic lymph node dissection, salvaging the blood supply to adjacent structures, the preservation of important nerves, the maintenance of adequate function of vital structures as well the preservation of their pathway of drainage (such as the ureter, for example). As for all major resectional surgery with curative intent, the projected postoperative quality of life is of paramount importance in determining the indication for surgery.[1–6] The impact of the surgery must be carefully and very openly discussed with the patient and it is essential to take into account the patient's perception of adequate quality of life and not to impose on the patient our own views on the subject.

It is not always easy to reconcile these ideals with multivisceral resections. The local control, the respect of the blood supply to adjacent structures, and the maintenance of the patient's quality of life are essential.[7,8] So to justify surgery the prognosis must be substantially better than what palliative surgery or chemotherapy and radiotherapy (either as isolated modalities or in combination) can offer. It is also important to recognize when palliative care (as a sole treatment modality) is the best option for the patient. Finally, the benefits of the surgery have to well outweigh the risks—a patient who dies following surgery cannot be cured.

There is no place for palliative multiorgan resections. To be effective palliation requires low morbidity and quick, uneventful recovery so that the patient can either undergo further therapy or have the best quality of life back as quickly as possible. The risks and recovery times of this type of extensive surgery are only justifiable in the context of curative intent.[9]

The philosophy of the resection itself follows on logically from these principles. The first and most important step of the operation is the determination of resectability before committing to it. The entire body cavity (chest or abdomen) is carefully inspected for signs of unexpected distant spread. Any areas of concern are biopsied and frozen section is performed. Nothing irreversible is done until these results are available. Any lymph node stations that would determine resectability are dissected out and again any areas of concern are sent for frozen section. Finally, the key areas of concern regarding technical resectability are dissected until the surgeon is sure that a complete resection will be achieved. This is when and only when the point of no return should be reached, which means that irreversible steps will be taken. Beyond this point the surgeon is committed to proceed with resection. Up to this point it is possible to choose to perform a much lesser, purely palliative procedure, or indeed to back out completely. The decision to proceed or to withdraw must always be a cold, clinical decision based on the probability for cure and on the expected quality of life, taking into account the patient's wishes as ascertained preoperatively. Implicit in the old-fashioned "it's his/her only chance" heroic attempt to resect the tumor at any cost is the very real ethical issue: is it licit to submit say 97 patients to a totally useless and dangerous operation (which is the case for all patients who are not cured) so that three can benefit (i. e., be cured)? The reader will please note that we have not introduced the difficult "cost per quality of life year gained" issue to this debate.

So, in reality, there are only a very few, very highly selected patients who actually truly qualify for this type of resection and it is of paramount importance to select patients rigorously and scrupulously and to be prepared to perform a lesser operation or to back out when adverse prognostic indicators are found during the initial evaluation phase of the operation. These issues must be fairly and openly discussed with the patient and his/her family prior to surgery as part of the consent process.

The "En Bloc" Resection

Any thoracic or abdominal tumor involving more than one organ must be resected en bloc with the surrounding involved structures.[10] This concept of en bloc resection is a constant theme throughout this book and a tenet common to all of its authors. Implicit in the term is the fact that there is only one operative specimen for

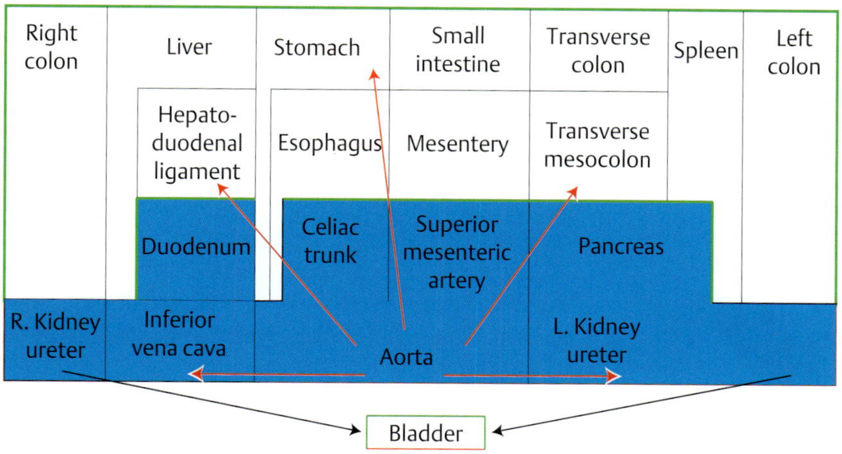

Fig. 2.**1** The abdominal organs are schematically represented. The anterior organs are mobile (small intestine, transverse colon) or can be mobilized if they have a contact with the retroperitoneum (ascending colon, liver, esophagus, stomach, spleen, descending colon). The retroperitoneal organs (duodenum, pancreas, major vessels are less easily mobilized). *Green line*: peritoneum. *Blue rectangles*: retroperitoneal organs.

the pathologist that contains all of the resected structures together. It is important to clearly identify all important structures and resection margins as well as any area of concern regarding tumor proximity so that the pathologist can take appropriate specimens. It is often very useful to go down to pathology immediately after surgery and to go over these complex specimens with the pathologist to help orientate the specimen for him/her and clarify areas of concern. During the operation itself it is important that frozen sections be clearly identified and if there are concerns about margins these areas should be marked with metal clips to help the radiotherapist to target these areas if postoperative radiotherapy would be an option.

These are very challenging operations from a purely technical point of view and require perfect knowledge of the surgical anatomy of the region of interest, including the usual and variant anatomy of neighboring blood vessels and nerves. Adhesions to surrounding structures represent a particular challenge. Obviously it is desirable to take down purely inflammatory adhesions at a distance from the tumor so as to avoid unnecessarily wide excisions, but it is equally of paramount importance not to breach the tumor during the dissection with the attendant risk of intracavitary seeding of the tumor and wound tumor implants.[11,12] This risk is not negligible with carcinomas and is considerable with sarcomas. If an inadvertent tumor breach does occur careful consideration should be given to washing out the body cavity with cytotoxic agents or even to proceed with formal intracavitary chemotherapy. As to tumor margins many surgeons prefer to rely entirely on respecting a clear macroscopic margin of healthy tissue around the tumor and deliberately avoid extensive frozen section examination of margins. If there are areas of adhesion these should be dealt with at a distance rather than risking breaching the tumor to obtain histologic confirmation by frozen section. Frozen sections are only justified at key "make or break" points during the explorative phase of the operation to decide if the tumor is technically resectable. If positive they imply retreat.

From Front to Back

The preoperative CT and MRI can be very useful to determine if the tumor is in contact with or invades the abdominal wall, especially in the area of the planned incision. If there has been no prior surgery the incision must avoid areas of tumor invasion. If there has been a previous operation it is customary to widely excise the full thickness of the previous incision.

Upon entering the abdomen, once the general inspection and any other distant dissection have been performed the tumor is usually approached from front to back. It is useful to consider the abdominal organs as being disposed in layers (Fig. 2.**1**). The most anterior layer, made up of the liver, stomach, small bowel, transverse colon, and spleen are mobile or readily mobilizable. The viscera are much more fixed and less readily mobilized as one gets further back in the abdomen. Moreover, towards the posterior peritoneum the organs are much closer to the main blood supply to the abdominal contents such as the celiac axis and the superior mesenteric artery as well as to the great veins and the central lymphatics. Thus, during a multivisceral resection the anterior organs are freed and prepared first, leaving them attached to the deeper organs. The surgeon can then progressively work around them, moving them side to side or up and down so as to free up the more posterior elements last.

The "Secondary" Organ

Multivisceral resections have two distinct components, even if an en bloc resection is always performed. The first is the resection of the organ in which the tumor originates. This will be done according to the usual

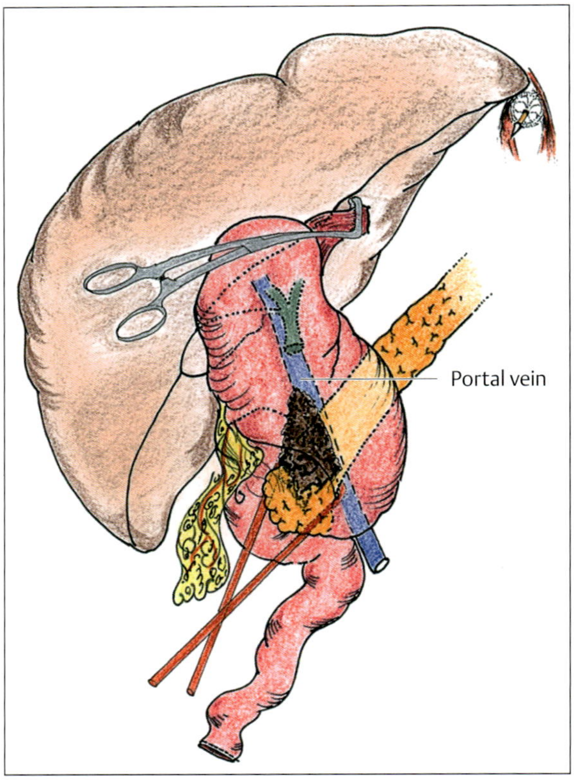

Fig. 2.**2** The first steps of the duodenopancreatectomy are completed: the hepatoduodenal ligament is dissected, the duodenum is Kocherized, the venous axis is prepared, the choledochus and first jejunal loop are divided. The greater curvature is now reflected on the right and the esophagus is divided. The further steps of the duodenopancreatectomy are then processed with the section of the isthmus of the pancreas.

principles guiding the resection of this organ for malignancy. The resection will deviate from this normal course in the area of involvement of the "secondary" organ. At the point where this interferes with the classic resection of the primary organ the dissection of the primary organ will stop to allow the secondary organ to be prepared. This will be done in the customary manner. Then the resection of the primary organ will resume. The operative strategy will of course need to include the reconstruction of all interrupted elements. An example is a tumor of the pancreas infiltrating the posterior wall of the stomach. The operation starts as a classic Whipple's procedure. After removing the gallbladder and performing a cholangiography, the hepatoduodenal ligament is dissected out separating the common bile duct, the hepatic artery, and taking up the gastroduodenal artery on a vessel loop. The portal vein is found and dissected free of the posterior aspect of the pancreas along with the terminal portion of the mesenteric vein. The duodenum is then freed up widely from the retroperitoneum then the right part of the gastrocolic ligament is picked up allowing the superior mesenteric vein to be dissected out from below the pancreas until the previous dissection from above is met. The first loop of jejunum is divided with a stapler and the ligament of Treitz is taken down allowing the proximal small bowel to pass under the mesentery. The gastroduodenal artery is divided as is the distal common bile duct. Normally the next step would be to divide the proximal duodenum with a stapler. However, now it is time to resect the "secondary" organ—namely the stomach. The gastrocolic ligament is taken down, the left gastric vessels are dissected at their origin and divided. The short gastric vessels are also divided and if a total gastrectomy is to be performed the distal esophagus is dissected circumferentially and will be progressively divided as a Prolene purse-string suture is placed allowing the anvil of an EEA stapler to be placed into the distal esophagus. If a subtotal gastrectomy is planned then the short gastric vessels are spared and the proximal stomach is divided with a stapler. The stomach is now completely free, but remains attached to the pancreas in the area of tumor invasion which has not been touched so as to in no way compromise the completeness of the resection (Fig. 2.**2**). At this point the pancreatectomy can proceed with the division of the pancreas through the isthmus. Then the dissection of the posterior aspect of the pancreas from the portal vein can be completed and the uncinate process can be dissected out taking down the retroportal lamina in the retroperitoneum. The operative specimen is now free and can be handed off. The reconstruction can now proceed, reestablishing intestinal continuity with either the distal esophagus or the stomach remnant.

□ The Point of No Return

In all complex operations there is a point beyond which the resection must proceed. It is important to ensure that no irreversible steps are taken until the surgeon is sure that it will be technically possible to resect the tumor. Mobilization of the omentum, the duodenum, or even dividing the intestine with a stapler are all examples of reversible steps in the evaluation of the tumor. However, once the blood supply to an organ is interrupted or that a solid organ itself is divided the point of no return has been breached.

Once the point of no return has passed it is essential to always bear in mind what must stay behind and to ensure that the blood vessels to these structures remain intact. For example, when proceeding with a combined gastrectomy-splenopancreatectomy the hepatic artery must be preserved with its origin at the celiac trunk. However, the left gastric and splenic arteries will be divided.

Centripetal Resection

Centripetal resection is a variant of the concept of front to back surgery. It is most commonly used in the superior part of the abdomen. It encompasses not only the resection of the organs which are involved by the tumor but also the systematic nodal dissection of the appropriate lymphatics which remain in continuity with the operative specimen. Thus, the primary organ and the secondary organ are first freed up anteriorly, then from above, below, and on both sides. The posterior aspect with the lymphatics is dissected last. The dissection becomes a sort of funnel. If we take the example of a combined gastrectomy-distal pancreatectomy-splenectomy for a stomach tumor invading the pancreas and/or spleen, the stomach is first prepared together with the omentum. The proximal duodenum is divided with a stapler. The spleen is freed from the diaphragm and retroperitoneum and mobilized to the right. This delivers the tail of the pancreas which is divided. The abdominal esophagus is dissected circumferentially and divided. The work at the mouth of the funnel is now done. Further dissection will follow the funnel down to the depths of the abdomen encompassing the nodal dissection. This usually starts at the hepatoduodenal ligament taking all the nodes off of the hepatic artery then along the top of the pancreas to the celiac trunk. The same dissection is then performed from left to right from the hilum of the spleen back to the celiac trunk. Only then will the left gastric and splenic vessels be divided. When this has been done the operative specimen will be free to be handed off. It will include in one specimen the stomach, distal pancreas, spleen, and the nodes draining all of these organs.

Lymphatic Drainage

The role of nodal dissection in the staging of abdominal cancer is well established.[13–16] This has direct prognostic implications and can influence subsequent management decisions. It is obviously of the same importance in multiorgan resections. The principle nodal dissection will be that of the primary organ.

Esophagus

The lymphatic drainage of the esophagus is complex, segmental, and interconnected. It includes the lower cervical, paratracheal, hilar, subcarinal, paraesophageal, paraaortic, paracardial, and celiac nodes (Fig. 2.**3**).[17,18]

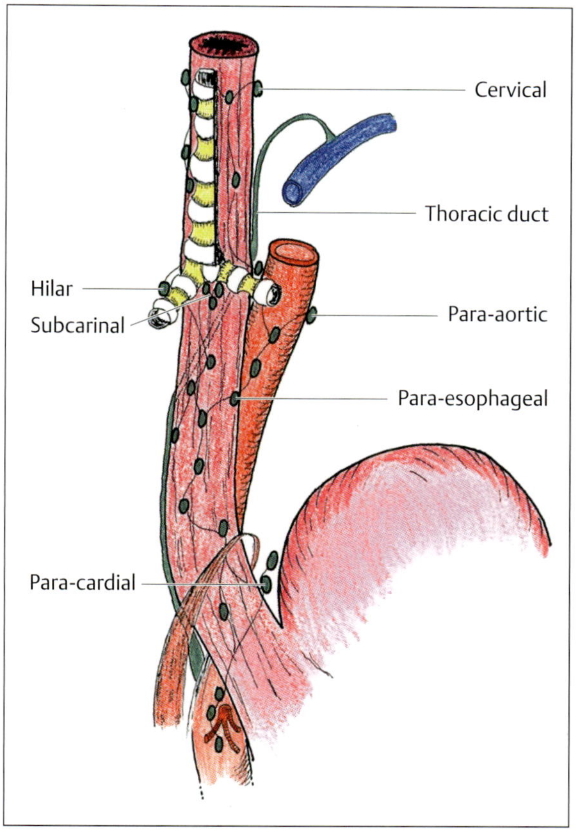

Fig. 2.**3** Diagram of the lymph nodes draining the esophagus.

Stomach

The Japanese Society for Research of Gastric Cancer has defined the different nodal territories for the stomach.[19] There are four concentric areas of nodal drainage.[20] The N1 nodes are closest to the stomach. They are labeled as follows: stations **1**-right paracardial; **2**-left paracardial; **3**-lesser curvature; **4**-greater curvature; **5**-suprapyloric; **6**-infrapyloric (Fig. 2.**4a**). A D1 resection will remove all of these nodes.

The N2 nodes are the second ring of nodes. They are around the celiac trunk and the splenic vessels. They are defined as: stations **7**-left gastric artery; **8a**-above the common hepatic artery, **9**-celiac trunk; **10**-hilum of the spleen; **11**-splenic artery (Fig. 2.**4b**). The resection of these nodes constitutes a D2 resection. This is the subject of some controversy.[21,22] It is recommended by most Japanese and German surgeons.[23–26]

The N3 nodes are deeper or further from the stomach. They are respectively: stations **8p**-behind the common hepatic artery; **12**-hilum of the liver; **13**-retropancreatic; **14**-root of the mesentery (Fig. 2.**4c**). The Japanese surgeons are the main proponents of the resection of N3 nodes.[27–29]

The N4 nodes make up the outside ring. They are respectively: stations **15**-middle colic artery; **16** (**a**,**b**,**c**,**d**)-pre- and paraaortic (Fig. 2.**4d**). They are the

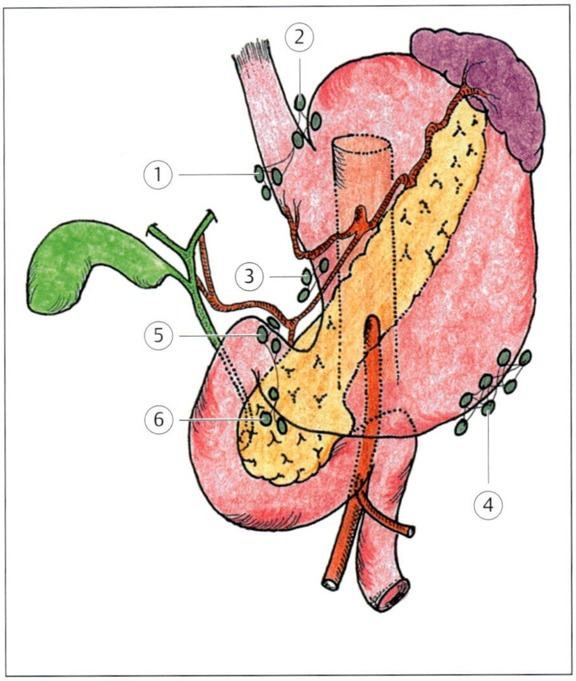

Fig. 2.**4a** Diagram of the N1 lymph nodes draining the stomach.

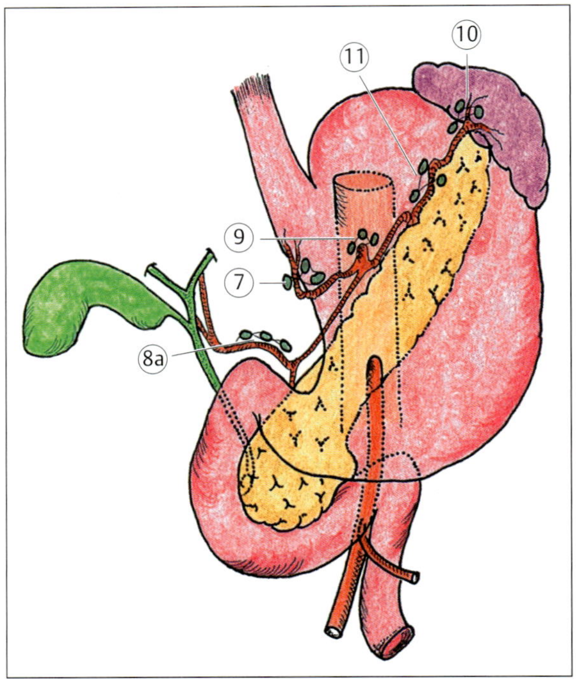

Fig. 2.**4b** Diagram of the N2 lymph nodes.

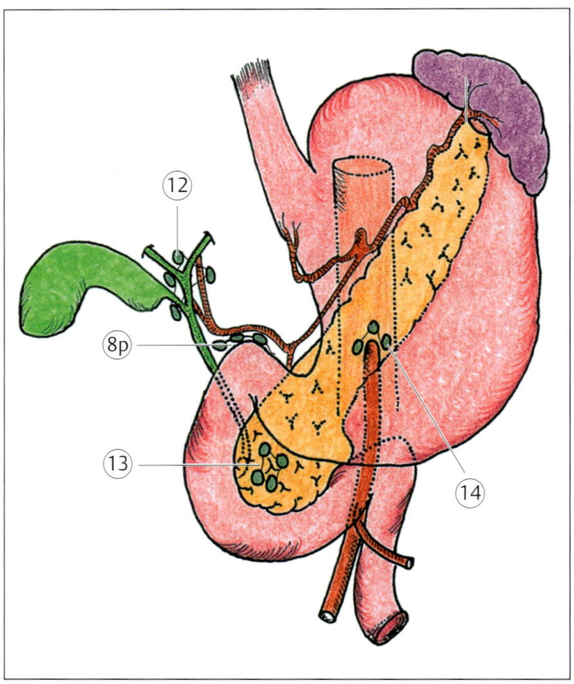

Fig. 2.**4c** Diagram of the N3 lymph nodes.

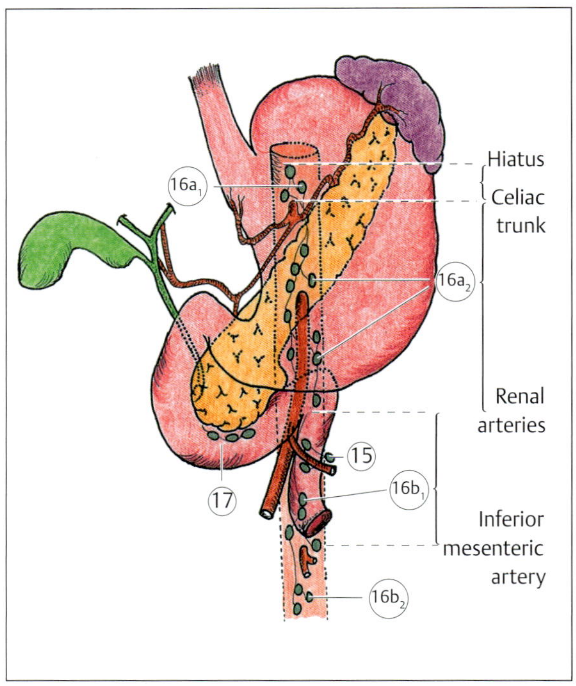

Fig. 2.**4d** Diagram of the N4 lymph nodes.

last nodes prior to drainage into the major lymphatics. The Japanese surgeons are practically the only ones who resect these nodes.[30–32]

Pancreas

The lymphatic drainage from the head and body of the pancreas is towards the celiac trunk nodes. The head of the pancreas drains to stations **7**, **8**, **9**, **11**, **12**, **13**, **14**, **15**, and **17** (anterior pancreaticoduodenal nodes) (Fig. 2.**5**).[33–35] The lymphatic drainage seems to follow

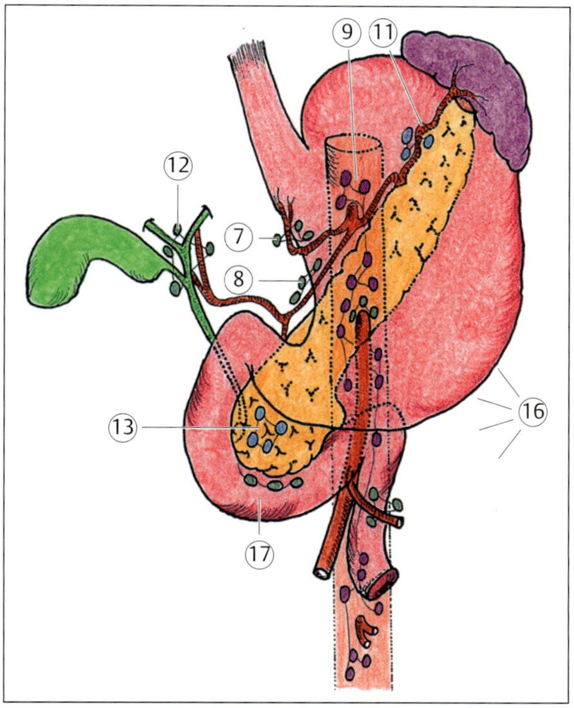

Fig. 2.5 Diagram of the lymph nodes draining the pancreas.

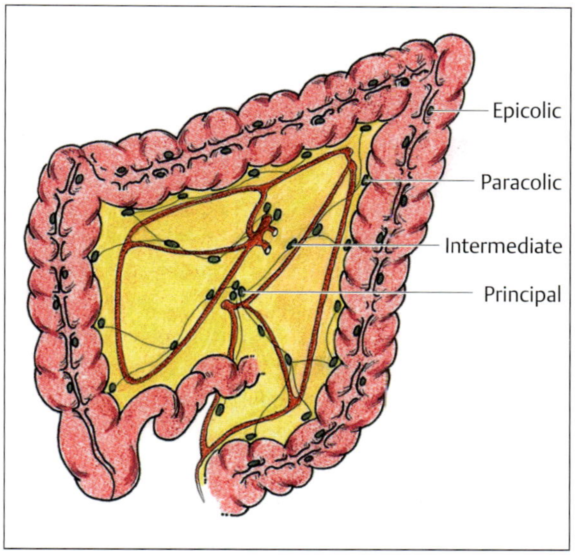

Fig. 2.6 Diagram of the lymph nodes draining the colon.

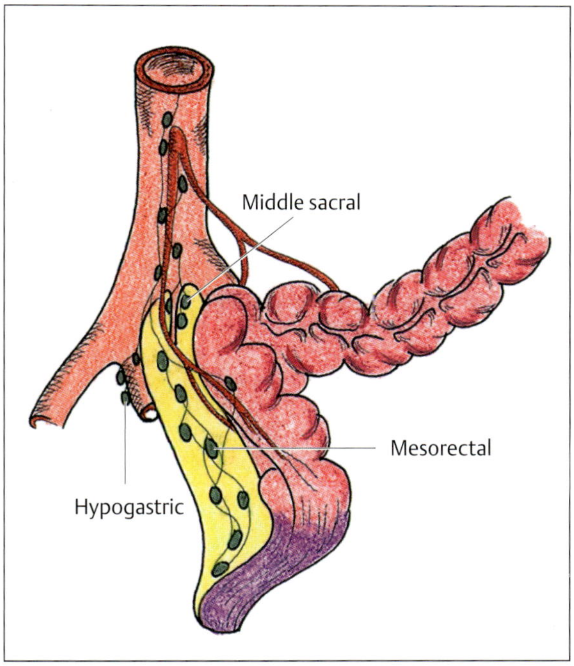

Fig. 2.7 Diagram of the lymph nodes draining the rectum.

the embryological development of the organ[36]: the ventral bud gives rise to the unciform process as well as to the retromesenteric and retroportal parts of the gland. The dorsal bud develops into the head and body of the organ. These two parts fuse at day 37 in utero. The drainage from the two parts seems separated by the axis of the superior mesenteric artery. The right part of the pancreas is drained by station **13** whereas the left part drains towards station **11**.[37] These two stations are next to last, draining into station **16**.

Colon and Rectum

There are several levels of nodal drainage. The colon has **epicolic nodes** along the taenias, then the **paracolic nodes** in the mesentery near the bowel. The drainage for the intestines is then towards the **intermediate nodes** which follow the blood vessels. The lymph then drains towards the **central nodes**. The small bowel and right colon then drain towards the **superior mesenteric nodes** whereas the left colon drains to the **inferior mesenteric nodes**. The last nodes are the **pre-** and **paraaortic nodes** (Fig. 2.**6**).[36]

The lymph drainage of the rectum is to the **nodes in the mesorectum** then the **paraaortic nodes**.[39] A second, deeper, set of nodes are the **midsacral nodes**, the **internal iliac nodes**, and the **obturator nodes**. These last two groups also drain the wall of the lesser pelvis (Fig. 2.**7**).[40]

□ Lavage

There are two roles for lavage. These are technically challenging operations and a clean operative field is a prerequisite for successful surgery. Regular washing will maintain clear visualization of structures. The second, more controversial role is to lyse any spilled tumor cells.[41] This can be accomplished by using sterile water, a 2% solution of hydrogen peroxide, or a solution of dilute Betadine.

Vascular Grafts

Multiorgan resections can at times require the resection of segments of vital vascular structures if they are involved by the tumor, such as the celiac trunk by a tumor of the body of the pancreas, the portal vein by a tumor of the head of the pancreas, the hepatic artery by a bile duct tumor, or the superior mesenteric artery by a sarcoma of the mesentery. In appropriately selected patients resecting affected vessels will allow a complete resection to be performed. When complete resection is achieved the vascular invasion in itself does not have a prohibitively negative prognostic implication. However, if vascular resection is considered it is important to have access to appropriate replacement vessels. Autologous tissue should often be preferred to synthetic grafts both for graft permeability and for their inherently better resistance to infection. There are three preferred options. Whenever it is thought that a graft may be required it is important to guarantee access to the vessel when positioning and draping the patient.

Saphenous Vein

The saphenous vein is a very good substitute for medium-sized arteries such as the superior mesenteric or hepatic artery. We always ensure access to it when performing multivisceral resections.

Internal Jugular Vein

This is a very good substitute for the portal vein or the external iliac vein.

Internal Iliac Artery

This makes a very good substitute for bifurcating arteries or when the saphenous vein is not available. The internal iliac artery can be used to replace the bifurcation of the hepatic artery.

Teamwork or "Tour de Force" by the Maestro?

Presently, many surgeons will not have the expertise to carry out all these long, complex, and stressful procedures, especially if specialized vascular, orthopedic, urological, or thoracic expertise is required. It is essential to remain within one's comfort zone of technical expertise and to recognize when help will or may be required so that appropriate colleagues will be available at the time of surgery. As in all fields of surgery expertise leads to shorter, smoother operations, and better outcomes. This is a field of surgery that does not tolerate the overambitious gladly at all.

As in all team endeavors it is important to have a designated leader. However, a cohesive team approach is necessary from the outset to ensure that the appropriate preoperative examinations are performed. Mutual respect will ensure technical excellence and a smooth operation. This starts with the positioning and draping of the patient in a way satisfactory to all. Likewise the incision(s) must be tailored to the needs of all.

Plenty of time should be set aside for these operations and if they will cover more than one shift adequate provisions need to be made by the nursing staff. It is virtually mandatory to have an ICU bed available for the immediate postoperative period. Careful consideration should be given to the use of transfusion sparing techniques. The use of cell-savers is considered inappropriate by some, controversial by others, and is acceptable to yet others. The blood bank should be warned if major vessels could be involved or if platelet transfusions are thought to possibly be necessary.

In the postoperative period the team must remain cohesive to obtain the best results and also to deal appropriately with possible complications. Each member must assume complete responsibility for his/her part of the operation, as for any other patient. This autonomy must be respected by all, especially the team leader. The patient should be officially referred to the surgeon who will be performing the bulk of the operation and follow-up. There is no scope for financial chicanery in this field of surgery. The old adage "proper planning and preparation prevent piss-poor performance" holds particularly true for this field of surgery.

Finally, it is essential that the anesthesiologist be actively involved in every aspect of the patient's care. This needs to be a named individual who will assume personal responsibility for every aspect of the patient's journey including the preoperative assessment, the intraoperative management and, ideally, the postoperative care.

The Patient

These operations are a major undertaking, both for the surgeon and for the patient. They can have significant morbidity and influence on quality of life so careful consideration must be given to the perceived prognosis before proposing this type of resection to a patient. If there is a perception that the risks outweigh the benefits the patient should be referred to the oncologist for palliative therapy. Good patient selection is of paramount importance to maintain acceptable morbidity and mortality as well as good results.

These are not operations for frail patients or the faint-hearted. The patient's active cooperation is essential in obtaining good results, as for all major surgery. The risks/benefits/uncertainties should be discussed very openly with the patient (and ideally with his/her family) and true informed consent is essential.

It is absolutely essential to have a complete preoperative work-up on these patients. Active coronary artery disease must be ruled out—there is scope for considerable blood loss and perioperative coronary events can have catastrophic consequences. If necessary, preoperative angiography and stent placement should be considered. This will mandate a 4-week delay in surgery so that the patient can receive adequate antiplatelet therapy while the endothelium covers the stent. Ideally the patient should be maintained on low-dose aspirin throughout the perioperative period to reduce the risk of stent occlusion. Similarly the patient needs to have adequate lung function. The patient's general and/or respiratory condition may require 2–3 weeks of optimization prior to surgery. This can have a considerable beneficial influence on outcome. Similarly the patient's nutritional status is of prime importance. If the patient has lost more than 10% of his/her body mass then surgery should be deferred for at least 2 weeks while the patient's nutritional status is corrected. Small bore feeding tubes with continuous or intermittent tube feeds in addition to a healthy diet can be of considerable benefit. This optimization of nutritional status can be an on-going process along with other measures to improve the patient's general condition, integrated with smoking cessation, bronchial toilet, and a graded exercise program. All necessary specialists should be called in (cardiology, respiratory medicine, nutritionists, and physiotherapists). The principle surgeon should keep a close eye on the patient—the logistics of these procedures can be quite complex and any change in plan will involve many people. Keeping them informed of progress focuses the team on these rather special patients. This also helps to motivate the patient.

☐ Specific Principles

☐ Above the Mesocolon

This part of the abdomen is quite asymmetrical and the surgery is quite different on each side. The retroperitoneal structures, especially the pancreas, will play a key role. Multiorgan resections are highly dependant on the vascular anatomy and lymphatic drainage which have considerable influence both on the operation itself and its prognosis.

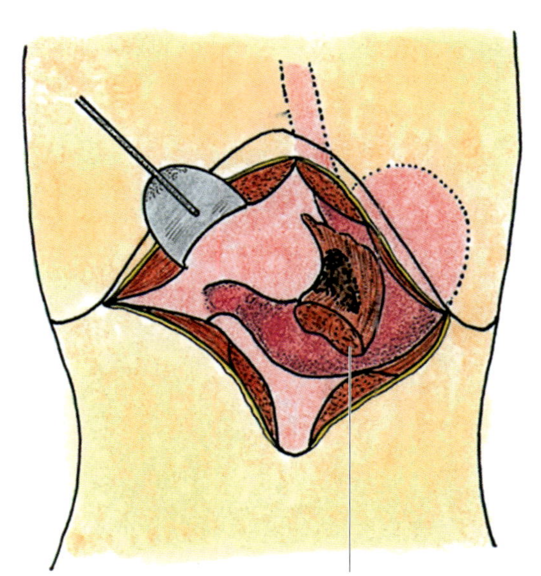

Fig. 2.**8** Gastric cancer invading the left rectus muscle. A bilateral subcostal incision allows the approach to the aponeurosis of this muscle. The left rectus is then divided at a distance above and below the tumoral invasion and remains attached to the stomach.

Stomach

Gastric tumors can invade a variety of adjacent structures.

Anterior Abdominal Wall

If the muscles of the abdominal wall are involved (laparoscopy can help to determine this) the incision must be planned to be at a distance from this area. This can be either a vertical or an oblique incision. The full thickness of the involved muscle is then resected (Fig. 2.**8**). Then the gastrectomy can proceed in the usual manner. The abdominal wall defect should be reconstructed with a nonresorbable material. Some materials, such as PTFE, can be allowed to be in direct contact with the abdominal contents.

Hiatus and Posterior Diaphragm

It is not uncommon for the hiatus or the left crus of the diaphragm to be involved by tumors of the distal esophagus or cardia. First of all the surgeon needs to ascertain if the celiac trunk is also involved. If so this must be dealt with first and the hepatic artery reconstructed. The celiac trunk can then be divided at its base. If the celiac trunk is not involved then the stomach is mobilized in the customary manner, the duodenum is divided. The lymph node dissection is performed and the gastric vessels are divided. The diaphragm is then incised above the hiatus through nor-

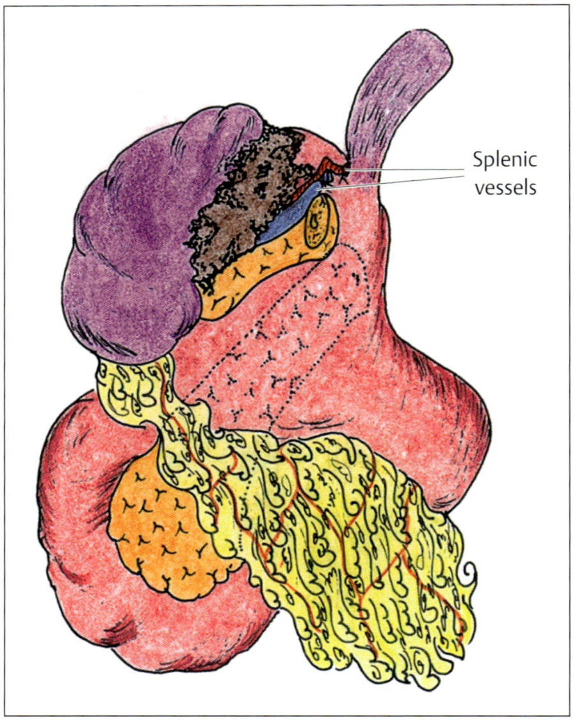

Fig. 2.**9** Proximal gastric cancer invading the spleen and tail of the pancreas. The stomach is reflected on the right en bloc with the spleen. The tail of the pancreas is divided. The splenic vessels are ligated.

mal tissues. As much of the diaphragm and its crura are resected as necessary to achieve a complete resection. Posteriorly the plane of dissection will be the along the wall of the aorta. The esophagus can then be encircled above the tumor and divided. The anvil of the EEA stapler is then placed in the esophagus in the usual manner to allow the gut to be reconstructed.

Spleen, Tail of Pancreas, Splenic Flexure of Colon

Whenever a gastric tumor involves the spleen, the tail of the pancreas, or the splenic flexure of the colon the operation always starts by gaining access to the lesser omental cavity by lifting the omentum up from right to left.[42] The proximal duodenum is divided and the left gastric vessels are divided. The distal esophagus is divided. If the spleen and tail of the pancreas are involved they become the secondary organ. The gastrectomy is now halted and the spleen is mobilized off of the posterior abdominal wall and is retracted forward with the stomach, pulling the tail of the pancreas up with it. The posterior aspect of the pancreas is mobilized, the splenic vessels are divided proximal to the tumor invasion, and the pancreas itself is divided at this level (Fig. 2.**9**). The gastrectomy can then proceed with the lymph node dissection and division of the remaining gastric vessels.

If the splenic flexure of the colon is also involved then during the preparation of the secondary organs the adjacent transverse and descending colon need to be mobilized. Then the mesentery can be divided, the colon divided proximal and distal to the tumor infiltration with the GIA stapler and the continuity will subsequently be re-established.

Transverse Colon

The transverse colon and its mesentery are the most frequently involved secondary structures.[42] This is usually fairly straightforward to deal with. The colon is stapled off on either side of the tumor and the adjacent mesentery is resected as required (Fig. 2.**10**). However, it is not uncommon for the middle colic artery to be involved. Depending on the quality of the arterial arcade this can require an extensive colon resection to be

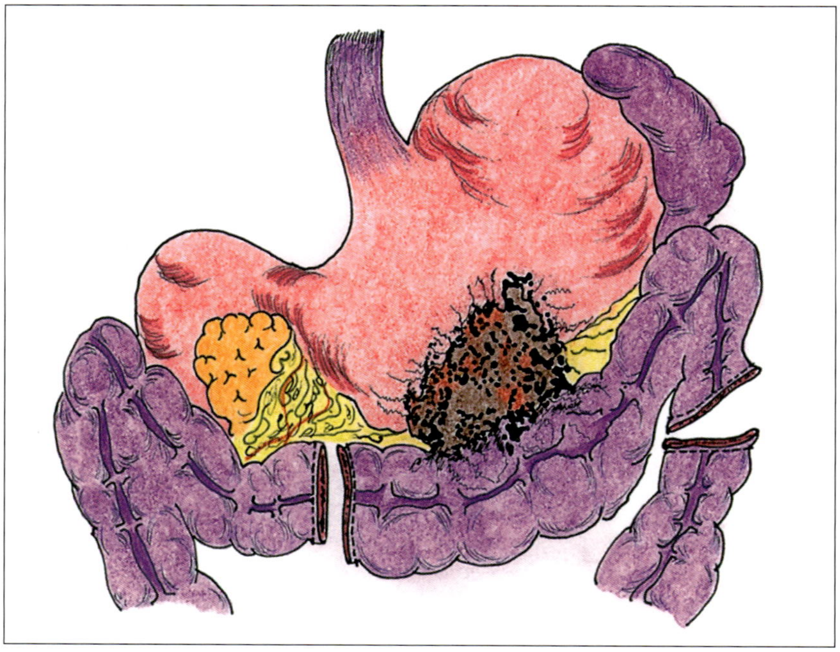

Fig. 2.**10** Gastric cancer invading the transverse mesocolon, the middle colic vessels, and the transverse colon. The colon is stapled and removed with the stomach.

performed based on the adequacy of blood supply to the remaining colon.

Head of the Pancreas

When an antral tumor involves the head of the pancreas,[42] this will require that a duodenopancreatectomy be performed in addition to the subtotal gastrectomy. First, the omentum is picked up and the lesser cavity is accessed then the stomach is divided obliquely with a stapler. Then instead of dividing the proximal duodenum the duodenopancreatectomy is performed dissecting the hepatoduodenal ligament, preparing the hepatic artery, dividing the bile duct, mobilizing the duodenum, dividing the proximal jejunum which is mobilized, freeing up the posterior aspect of the head of the pancreas from the portal and mesenteric veins. The unciform process is dissected and the isthmus of the pancreas is transected (Fig. 2.**11**). Then the gastrectomy can resume with the nodal dissection and the division of the left gastric vessels.

Body of the Pancreas

This is a technically challenging situation. Both operations (primary and secondary organs) get more or less mixed up. After opening up the lesser cavity the invasion of the pancreas can be ascertained. Then the superior mesenteric vein is found and followed up, dissecting it off of the back of the pancreas. The stomach is then mobilized along the greater curvature along with the spleen which is also freed up from the abdominal wall and diaphragm. Then the esophagus is dissected out and transected, placing the anvil of the stapler into it. The hepatic artery and portal vein are now followed down behind the pancreas. The gastric nodal dissection and division of the gastric vessels is now performed. The proximal duodenum is divided following which the isthmus of the pancreas can now be divided after ligating the splenic vessels at this level (Fig. 2.**12**). The stomach is reflected on the left and the isthmus of the pancreas can be worked out from the right. The isthmus is divided and the specimen (stomach, spleen, body of the pancreas) is removed.

In summary, this complex technique implies steps from front to back and of the secondary organ:

- Opening the lesser cavity (gastrectomy);
- dissection of the superior mesenteric vein (secondary organ);
- mobilization of the greater curvature and spleen (gastrectomy and secondary organ);
- transection of the esophagus (gastrectomy);
- dissection of the hepatoduodenal ligament (hepatic artery, portal vein) (secondary organ);
- nodal dissection (gastrectomy);
- stapling of the duodenum (gastrectomy);
- transection of the pancreas isthmus (secondary organ).

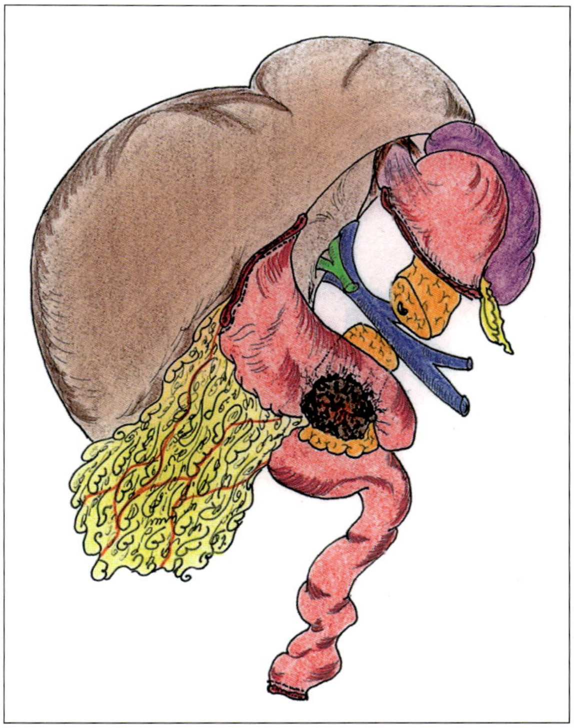

Fig. 2.**11** Gastric tumor invading the head of the pancreas. The proximal stomach is stapled and reflected to the right with the omentum. The hepatoduodenal ligament is dissected and the choledochus is divided. The isthmus of the pancreas is sectioned and the venous mesentericoportal axis is exposed.

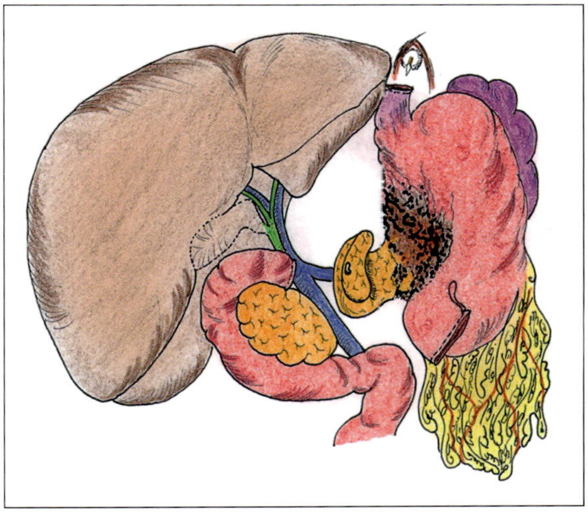

Fig. 2.**12** Gastric tumor invading the body of the pancreas. The stomach is completely mobilized with the omentum and spleen. The esophagus is divided. Posteriorly, the hepatoduodenal ligament is prepared, the pancreas isthmus is transected and the venous axis is visible.

The pancreatic resection margin can now be dealt with. First, the pancreatic duct needs to be carefully oversewn with 5–0 Prolene sutures. Then the margin itself can be closed with interrupted 3–0 or 4–0 resorbable sutures (some surgeons staple the pancreatic resection margin).

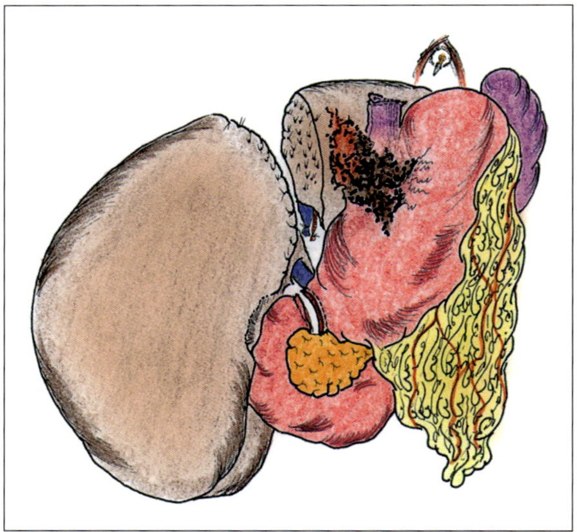

Fig. 2.**13** Gastric tumor invading the left liver lobe. The omentum is elevated, the gastric fundus is separated from the spleen, the cardia is divided and the anvil is placed in the abdominal esophagus. The proximal duodenum is stapled. The hepatoduodenal ligament is dissected and the left hepatic vessels are divided. The left liver lobe is separated and is removed en bloc with the stomach.

Liver

A tumor of the lesser curvature can infiltrate the left lobe of the liver. The operation starts by lifting the omentum and taking down the short gastric vessels. The distal esophagus and the proximal duodenum are then divided. The attention is then directed to the liver. If the liver involvement is minimal an atypical resection of segment III can be performed. Otherwise segments II and III will need to be formally resected (liver = secondary organ). First, the hilum is dissected and the left hepatic artery is identified and divided. The left branch of the portal vein is divided. The left bile duct is identified and taken up on a loop. Cholangiography will confirm the correct anatomy—the bile duct from segment VI can drain into the left bile duct (Hjortsjo's anomaly).[43,44] Any division of the bile duct must be to the left of such an anomaly. The left hepatic vein is identified and divided then the liver is cut to the left of the round ligament (Fig. 2.**13**). Thereafter, the gastrectomy can continue as described above.

Pancreas

Head and Uncinate Process

Invasion of the portal vein is not a contraindication to surgery.[45–50] If this is suspected access to the saphenous vein is planned. During the dissection the invasion of the portal vein is confirmed. The operation is started as usual. The bile duct is divided; the duodenum is mobilized and divided as is the proximal jejunum. Then, when the isthmus is to be cut the portal, splenic, and superior mesenteric veins are clamped. If the invasion is limited and superficial a tangential resection of the portal vein can be performed. Otherwise it is resected with the operative specimen. Then the vein is sutured if only a minimal amount was resected. A patch of saphenous vein can be used to repair a tangential resection. If a segment of portal vein is resected, it can generally be reconstructed by an end-to-end superior mesentericoportal vein suture, mobilizing the mesentery if necessary.

Invasion of the superior mesenteric artery is usually considered to be a contraindication to surgery because of its ominous prognostic implications.

Body

Tumors of the body of the pancreas are often irresectable because they have often invaded the root of the mesentery,[51–54] the retroperitoneum, or the celiac trunk. Their retroperitoneal lymphatic spread also contributes to their poor prognosis. There can be circumstances where local invasion does not preclude meaningful resection and should be carefully explored. If the tumor seems to be infiltrating the lesser curvature of the stomach and the left gastric artery in front and above and the portal and splenic veins posteriorly, then the first thing to do is to ensure that the hepatic artery is not involved, which would constitute an indication to abandon the resection. The next step is to ensure that any invasion of the mesentery is only superficial and does not include invasion of the superior mesenteric artery, which would again be an indication of nonresectability. If the stomach is involved as described above then the pancreatectomy will need to be associated with a total gastrectomy, which means an exenteration of the left upper quadrant. If the head of the pancreas is involved then a total pancreatectomy will have to be considered.

Technically the combined resection of the body of the pancreas and total gastrectomy starts with the vascular exploration described above. Then the hepatoduodenal ligament is opened and the bile duct and portal vein are dissected out. The duodenum is mobilized, then the lesser cavity is entered. The spleen is mobilized from the abdominal wall and the diaphragm. The distal esophagus is transected, as are the lesser omentum and the proximal duodenum. The mesentery is dissected off of the pancreas and the proximal jejunum is transected and freed so as to pass below the mesentery. The spleen and pancreas are then retracted to the front and right together with the splenic vessels, taking them off of the left adrenal and the left renal vein. The superior mesenteric vein and portal veins are clamped and divided, the pancreas is transected and the operative specimen is handed off (Fig. 2.**14**). The portal vein is reconstructed and the intestinal continuity is re-established.

The Bile Duct

The Distal Bile Duct

When an adenocarcinoma of the distal bile duct is in contact with the pancreas a Whipple procedure will be required. However, the bile duct will need to be resected much higher, up to the main bile duct or the confluence. If there is posterior invasion the portal vein will need to be resected. The operation itself is pretty much like a standard duodenopancreatectomy except that the portal vein and the common bile duct will be transected at the same time. Second, the reconstruction of the portal vein is much more difficult without a graft as the vein must be divided near to its bifurcation. If the portal vein has to be resected, it is best to use autologous tissue. Our preferred graft is the internal jugular vein.

The bile duct and portal vein are prepared as high as possible above the tumor. The hepatoduodenal ligament is dissected free and the hepatic and gastroduodenal arteries are looped. Then the lesser cavity is opened and the superior mesenteric vein is prepared. The duodenum is Kocherized, the first loop of jejunum is stapled, and the duodenum is divided. The anterior step is now completed (from front to back).

The posterior step starts with the transection of the pancreas isthmus. The splenic vein is next dissected. The superior mesenteric, portal, and splenic veins are clamped and divided. The pancreas is then dissected from below up freeing the specimen from the retroperitoneum (Fig. 2.**15**). The veins are reconstructed in the usual manner, except that yet again the bile duct anastomosis will be much higher than usual which can be a bit challenging technically.

The Proximal Bile Duct

Tumors of the proximal bile duct can involve the hepatic artery to the left of the hepatic pedicle as well as the portal vein behind. In this case the bile duct is prepared above the tumor and below, at the level of the pancreas. The hepatic artery is also dissected out above and below the tumor. The artery will be reconstructed with a saphenous vein graft with an end-to-end anastomosis at either end (using 7–0 Prolene). The portal vein is reconstructed with an internal jugular vein graft. The bile duct is reconstructed using a retrocolic loop of jejunum which is anastomosed to the bile duct remnant (Fig. 2.**16**).

□ Below the Mesocolon

This area is less asymmetrical than the upper abdomen. Within the peritoneal cavity the lateral limits are the ascending and descending colon. Above there is the transverse colon. The small bowel fills the space in the middle. In the retroperitoneum the two great vessels (inferior vena cava and aorta) lie on either side of

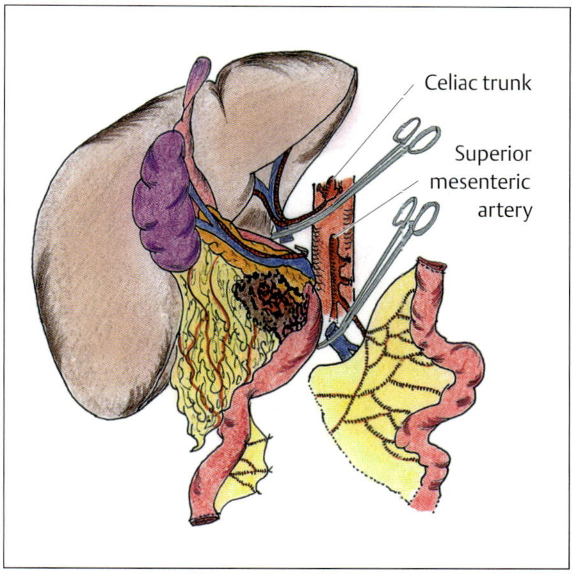

Fig. 2.**14** Tumor of the head and body of the pancreas invading the stomach, the splenic and portal veins, preserving the hepatic and superior mesenteric arteries. The hepatoduodenal ligament is dissected. The first jejunal loop is stapled and reflected to the right. The stomach, spleen, and the pancreas are retracted on the right. The last maneuver before removing the surgical specimen en bloc is the resection of the portal vein after the application of two vascular clamps.

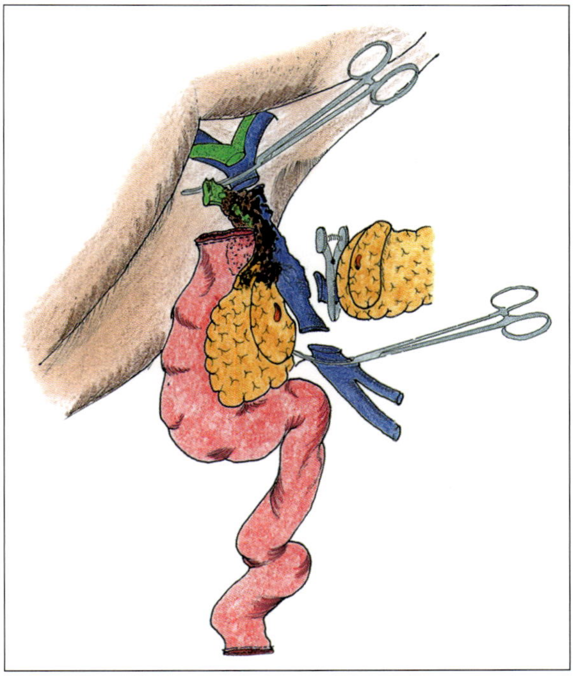

Fig. 2.**15** Tumor of the choledochus invading the portal vein. The hepatic duct is divided as high as possible. The proximal duodenum and the first jejunal loop are stapled. The neck of the pancreas is divided. The portal, splenic, and superior mesenteric veins are clamped and divided. The hepatic duct and choledochus are removed with the head of the pancreas and duodenum.

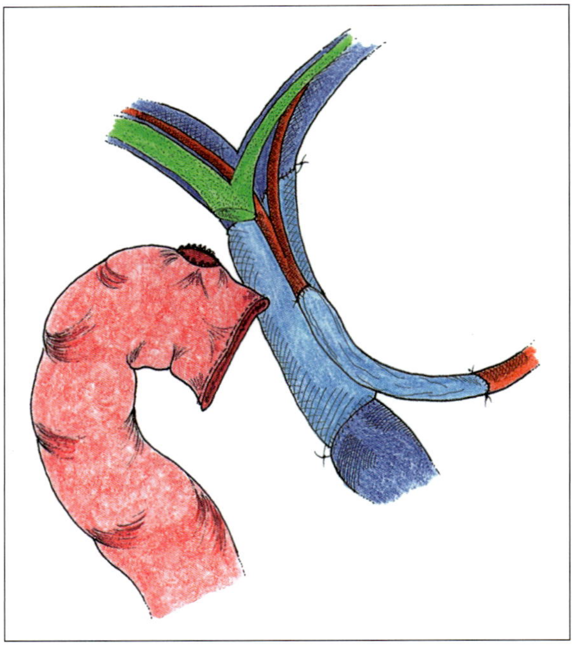

Fig. 2.**16** Removal of the hepatoduodenal ligament for a proximal biliary tract tumor. An internal jugular vein graft is used to bypass the portal vein and a saphenous vein for the hepatic artery. The hepatoenteric anastomosis is then performed.

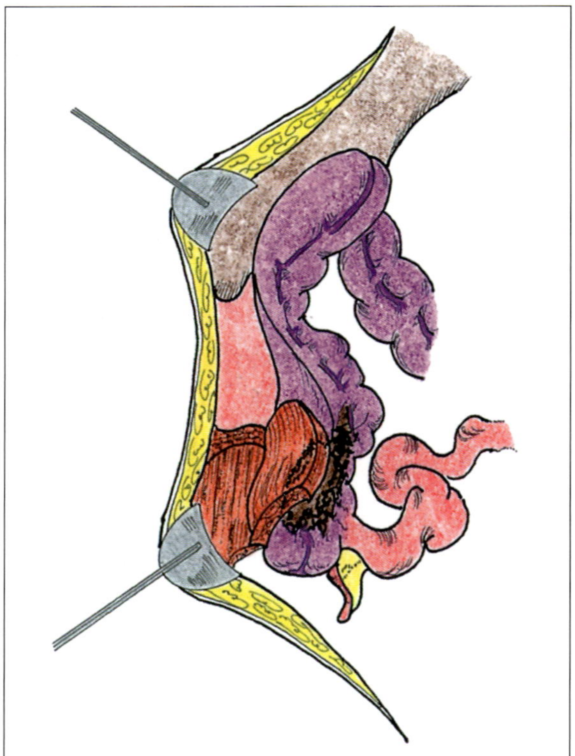

Fig. 2.**17** Tumor of the caecum invading the abdominal wall. The muscular abdominal wall is removed with the ascending colon.

the spine and the adrenals, kidneys, and ureters are more or less symmetrical in position.

The Right Side (Tumors of the Ascending Colon)

Lateral and Anterior Abdominal Wall

When a tumor of the ascending colon invades the abdominal wall the right hemicolectomy starts in the usual way with the preparation and section of the distal ileum and transverse colon. The dissection and resection of the mesentery are performed in the usual way. The colon is freed from the abdominal wall and retroperitoneum in the usual way at a distance from the tumor, but when the dissection gets near to the area of invasion the incision is deepened into the abdominal wall taking the full thickness of one or more of the abdominal muscles so as to have completely clear resection margins. The retroperitoneal dissection can then proceed as normal (Fig. 2.**17**). The bowel anastomosis is performed. If a full thickness muscle resection is performed we tend to reconstruct this area with a resorbable mesh. If there is a weakness of the abdominal wall this can be dealt with at a later stage using nonresorbable material. There are concerns about using nonresorbable material when there is a nearby large bowel anastomosis.

Kidney and Ureter

If the ureter is involved a segmental resection can be necessary. The ureter can also be re-implanted into the bladder. If this is not feasible then a loop of small bowel can be used to drain the ureter. Chapter 8 describes these techniques in detail. If the kidney is involved a nephrectomy will be required.

Duodenum and Pancreas

A tumor of the right colon which is invading the pancreas will require an en bloc resection of the colon, the duodenum, and the head of the pancreas. Now that effective chemotherapy is available for carcinoma of the colon careful consideration should be given to induction therapy before embarking on such a considerable resection.

The first step is to assure resectability of the duodenopancreatic bloc and that the superior mesenteric artery is not infiltrated, which would indicate that resection should be abandoned. It is also important to ensure that the portal and superior mesenteric veins are free. The right hemicolectomy starts in the usual way, dividing the distal ileum and the transverse colon and taking down the mesentery with its lymph nodes. The right colon is taken off of the lateral abdominal wall and the retroperitoneum up to near the area of duodenopancreatic involvement. The duodenum and pancreas become now the secondary organs. The hepatoduodenal ligament is dissected out followed by the steps of the duodenopancreatectomy already described. When the pancreas is transected at the isthmus, the specimen is reflected on the right. The last retroperitoneal attachments are separated and the operative specimen is delivered (Fig. 2.**18**).

Right Lower Quadrant

A large tumor of the caecum with deep invasion of the right lower quadrant may require a wide ilioinguinal approach as described in detail in Chapter 11.

The Left Side (Tumors of the Descending Colon)

Small Bowel

Whenever a loop of small bowel is involved it will be resected along with the primary tumor by dividing the small bowel at a short distance from the area of tumor involvement and resecting a triangle of mesentery (down to its root). The colon resection can then proceed in the customary manner. Both small and large bowel continuity will then be restored in the usual manner.

Spleen, Tail of the Pancreas, Left Kidney

Tumors of the splenic flexure can invade posteriorly into the spleen, the tail of the pancreas, or the left kidney. If there is infiltration of the spleen alone, a simple splenectomy will suffice. This will be integrated into the colectomy at the appropriate time.

If the tail of the pancreas is involved then, after ensuring that the tumor appears to be technically resectable, the colectomy will proceed as far as possible until the posterior involvement hinders progress. The posterior step begins with the separation of the spleen from the posterior abdominal wall. The spleen and tail of the pancreas are retracted downwards and to the right. The splenic vessels are ligated. Then the splenopancreatectomy will be performed as describe above. Finally, the colon resection will resume and the bowel continuity will be restored.

If the left kidney is involved, the posterior dissection takes the left kidney in conjunction with invasion of the tail of the pancreas. At that time the renal vein is dissected out and divided, then the renal artery is divided. The ureter is interrupted and the distal end tied off and abandoned (Fig. 2.**19**). When the secondary organ(s) is (are) completely free the colectomy will resume and finally bowel continuity is restored.

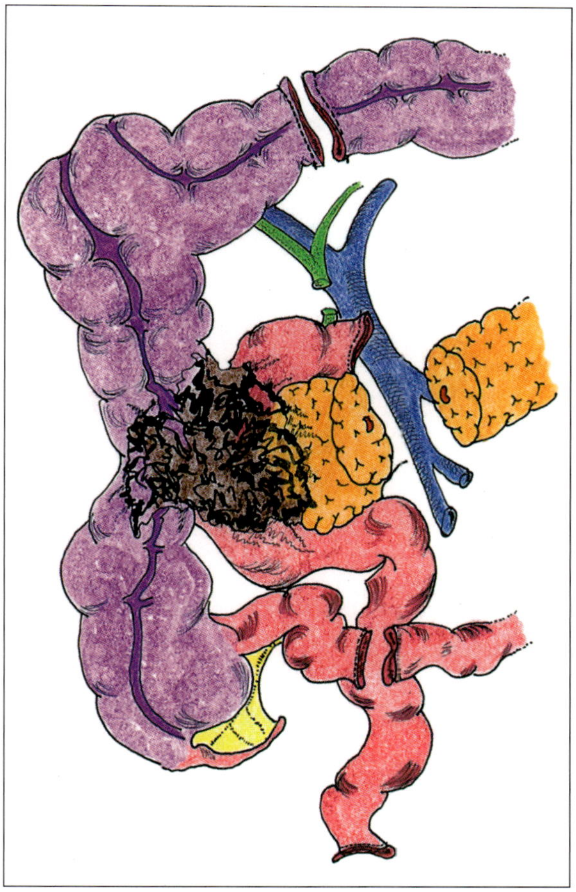

Fig. 2.**18** Ascending colon tumor invading the duodenum and head of the pancreas. The venous mesentericoportal axis is first explored. The choledochus and proximal duodenum are divided. The proximal jejunum is then stapled and the isthmus of the pancreas is transected. The further steps of the right hemicolectomy (stapling of the distal ileum and proximal transverse colon) are now carried out.

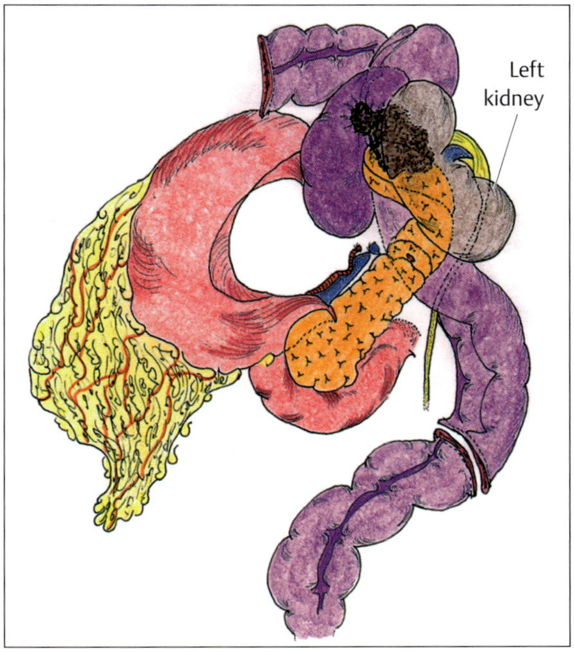

Fig. 2.**19** Splenic flexure tumor invading the spleen, tail of the pancreas, and left kidney. The stomach is reflected on the right. The splenic flexure, spleen, tail of the pancreas, and left kidney are dissected en bloc. The transverse and descending colon are stapled. The splenic vessels are ligated. The tail of the pancreas is divided.

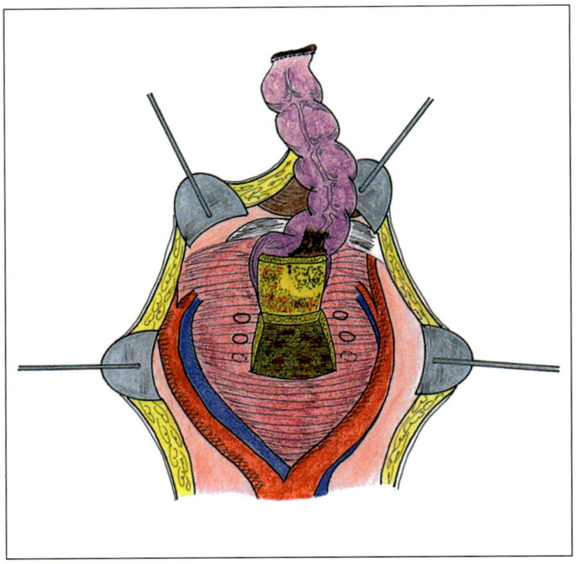

Fig. 2.**20** Rectal tumor invading the sacrum. The lower anterior resection removes the tabula interna of the sacrum.

Central Compartment (Tumors of the Mesentery)

These tumors will usually mandate a more or less extensive bowel resection. The more central the tumor, the greater the resection will be. It is obviously essential to determine whether this represents a prohibitive bowel resection before any irreversible steps are taken. The origin of the superior mesenteric artery, above the tumor is an essential first step. In some cases a reconstruction with a saphenous vein graft will permit the resection to proceed. The special aspects of the management of the superior mesenteric artery are discussed in Chapter 14.

☐ Lesser Pelvis

The lesser pelvis is fairly symmetrical and has both an intra- and a retroperitoneal component. This last compartment contains the lower rectum, the rectal mesentery (with its lymph nodes), blood vessels, lymphatics, nerves, and the ureters.

Median Anterior Tumors

Gynecologic tumors can infiltrate the bladder or bladder tumors can infiltrate the uterus. This requires an anterior pelvic exenteration, which is a classic, standard operation.[55] Uterine and ovarian tumors can also involve the adjacent bowel. If a loop of small bowel is involved, it is resected as described above and bowel continuity will be restored at the end of the operation. If the adjacent rectum is involved the hysterectomy will proceed as usual until the uterus is freed and gives posterior access to the rectum. Then the secondary organ operation starts. This will be either a standard sigmoid resection if the tumor is at the dome of the uterus, or a low anterior resection if the rectum is involved. The large bowel or rectum resection is then performed in the customary manner, then the specimen (uterus and sigmoid/rectum) is delivered and the bowel continuity is restored.

Median Posterior Tumors

When a rectal tumor infiltrates the bladder or prostate a pelvic exenteration will be required. Again the usual sequence of events takes place. The bowel resection (with its mesentery and lymph nodes) proceeds as far as possible then the secondary organ resection is performed, then the bowel resection is completed. If a low anterior resection is being performed the bowel anastomosis is performed before the urinary tract reconstruction. If a definitive colostomy is planned then the pelvic floor is reconstructed, the anal wound is dealt with (preferentially synchronously by a separate surgical team), the urinary tract reconstruction is done, the colostomy is fashioned, the abdominal wall is closed, and the colostomy is opened.

The combined resection of the sacrum and the rectum is described in Chapter 12. However, when the tumor infiltration into the bone is minimal the en bloc resection of the tabula interna of the sacrum in continuity with the rectum is a worthwhile and less invasive technique (Fig. 2.**20**).

Lateral Tumors

Invasion of the Ureter or the Iliac Vessels

With paramedian tumors the CT and MRI can show the relationship of the posterior aspect of the tumor to the ureter and the iliac vessels. Preoperatively it can be helpful to place catheters in the ureters. If these cannot be passed that might indicate that they are involved. If invasion of the iliac vein is suspected access to the jugular vein should be planned for. After making a low midline incision, this can be extended into an ilioinguinal one if further access to the retroperitoneal structures as well as to the iliac fossa and the crural area is required.

The dissection starts with the mobilization of the tumor by incising the peritoneum and mobilizing the tumor medially as far as possible, if necessary through the psoas muscle. At this point it is important to gain control of the iliac vessels. The iliofemoral vessels are taken up on vessel tapes above and below the tumor at whatever level is required. An effort is made to gain control of the internal iliac vessels from below and medially, but this is often impossible. The ureter is also taken up on a vessel loop above the tumor. Now it is possible to clamp the iliofemoral vessels above and below the tumor. The internal iliac vessels are also clamped if possible. If not the division of the iliofe-

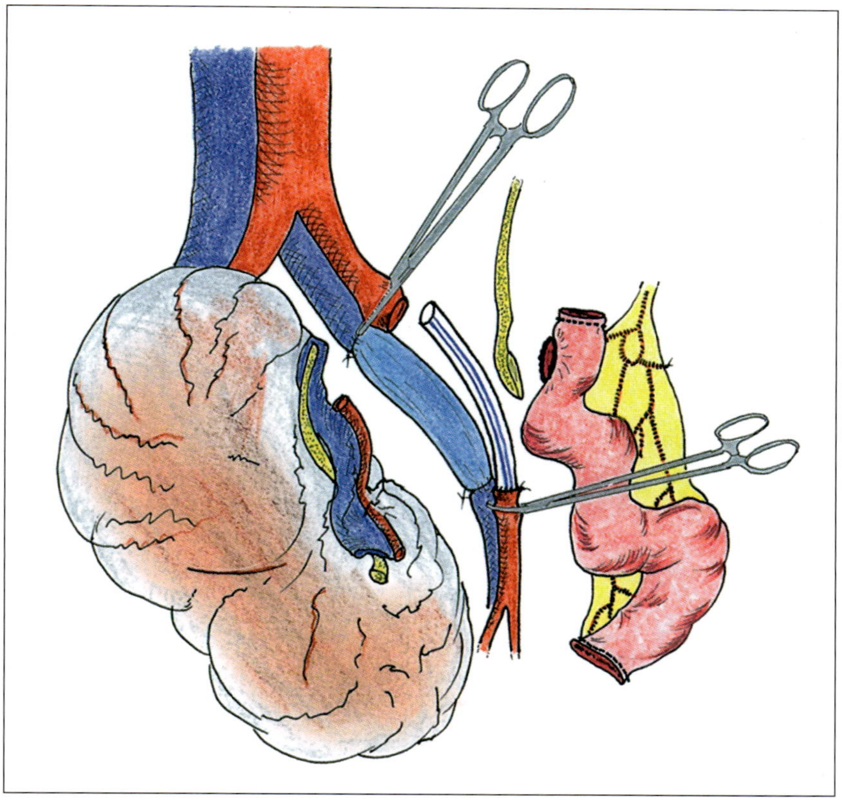

Fig. 2.**21** Tumor (sarcoma) of the pelvis invading the left ureter and iliac vessels. The tumor is retracted to the right and is removed with the invading structures. A jugular vein and prosthetic arterial bypass is performed. An ileal conduit joins the ureter to the bladder.

moral vessels should be put off as long as possible and bleeding from the internal iliac vessels will be contained by compression. The ureter will be divided as necessary (Fig. 2.**21**). The specimen will finally be removed with the iliac vessels and the ureter in one piece. The internal iliac vessels can now be sutured closed with 4–0 and/or 5–0 Prolene sutures with large needles.

The iliofemoral vessels can now be reconstructed. The vein is done first, using the internal jugular vein as a graft. A 7–8-mm synthetic graft is used for the artery. The ureter can be reconstructed using a loop of small bowel which is anastomosed to the bladder (see Chapter 14).

Invasion of the Lumbo-Sacral Plexus

This is discussed in detail in Chapters 12 and 14.

□ Conclusion

The keystone of multivisceral resections is the en bloc technique. The basic principle is to work from front to back around the tumor. The primary organ determines the overlying operative strategy and this includes the systematic nodal dissection of the primary organ. In the pelvis the peritoneum is often also resected. When the involvement of the secondary organ inhibits progress the steps leading to the resection of the secondary organ are carried out. This will free up the tumor to allow the resection of the primary organ to proceed. Finally, all necessary reconstructions are performed.

Throughout the operation it is essential to preserve the blood supply to the remaining viscera. To this end in many of these operations the first key stage is to determine the status of the superior mesenteric artery.

The upper abdomen is quite asymmetrical. So most of the decision making and strategy hinge on the pancreas as well as the celiac trunk and its principal branches. Below the mesocolon the structures are much more symmetrical both in the peritoneal cavity and in the retroperitoneal space. The key element here tends to be whether or not the superior mesenteric artery is involved. In the pelvis there is again a large degree of symmetry and the key tends to be the control and management of the ureters and the iliac vessels.

These operations are complex and require meticulous planning both in terms of investigation and strategy but also in terms of time, resources, and manpower. It is essential to have a cohesive team to look after these patients and this cannot be improvised at the last minute.

Finally, these are huge operations. Patient selection and preparation are key elements in the success of the undertaking. If all of these caveats are carefully respected good results can be achieved both in terms of morbidity/mortality and survival.

References

1. Kumar D, Kubota H, Tachibana M et al. Prognosis of T4 gastric carcinoma patients: an appraisal of aggressive surgical treatment. *J Surg Oncol.* 2001;76:278–282.
2. Koregana D, Okamura T, Baba H, Saito A, Sugimachi K. Results of resection of gastric cancer extending to adjacent organs. *Br J Surg.* 1988;75:12–15.
3. Kodama I, Takamiya H, Mizutani K et al. Gastrectomy with combined resection of other organs for carcinoma of the stomach with invasion of adjacent organs: clinical efficacy in a retrospective study. *J Am Coll Surg.* 1997;184:16–22.
4. Bozzetti F, Regaglia E, Bonfanti G, Doci R, Ballarini D, Gennari L. Early and late results of extended surgery for cancer of the stomach. *Br J Surg.* 1990;77:53–56.
5. Isozaki H, Tanaka N, Tanigawa N, Okajima K. Prognostic factors in patients with advanced gastric cancer with macroscopic invasion to adjacent organs treated with radical surgery. *Gastric Cancer.* 2000;3:202–210.
6. Kitamura K, Tani N, Koike H et al. Combined resection of the involved organs in T4 gastric cancer. *Hepato-Gastroenterology.* 2000;47:1769–1772.
7. Koregana D, Orita H, Okuyama T, Moriguchi S, Maehara Y, Sugimachi K. Quality of life after gastrectomy in patients with carcinoma of the stomach. *Br J Surg.* 1992;79: 248–250.
8. Thybusch-Bernhardt A, Schmidt C, Küchler T, Schmid A, Henne-Bruns D, Kremer B. Quality of life following radical surgical treatment of gastric carcinoma. *World J Surg.* 1999; 23:503–508.
9. Bloeschle C, Izbicki JR, Limmer J et al. Multivisceral resection for locally advanced gastric cancer. *Acta Chir Belg.* 1995;95:72–75.
10. Hulscher JBF, Van Sandick JW, Offerhaus GJA, Tilanus HW, Obertop H, Van Landschot JJB. Prospective analysis of the diagnosis yield of extended en bloc resection for adenocarcinoma of the oesophagus or gastric cardia. *Br J Surg.* 2001;88:715–719.
11. Shchepotin B, Chorny VA, Nauta RJ, Shabahang M, Buras RR, Evans SRT. Extended surgical resection in T4 gastric cancer. *Am J Surg.* 1998;175:123–126.
12. Sugarbaker PH, Yonemura Y. Palliation with a glimmer of hope: management of respectable gastric cancer with peritoneal carcinomatosis. *Hepato-Gastroenterology.* 2001;48: 1238–1247.
13. Guadagni S, de Manzoni G, Catarci M et al. Evaluation of the Maruyama computer program accuracy for preoperative estimation of lymph node metastases for gastric cancer. *World J Surg.* 2000;24:1550–1558.
14. Noguchi M, Miyazaki I. Extended lymph node dissection in gastrointestinal cancer. *J Surg Oncol.* 1997;65:57–65.
15. Bozzetti F. Rationale for extended lymphadenectomy in gastrectomy for carcinoma. *J Am Coll Surg.* 1995; 180: 505–508.
16. Gervasoni JE, Taneja C, Chung MA, Cady B. Biologic and clinical significance of lymphadenectomy. *Surg Clin N Am.* 2000;80:1631–1673.
17. Akiyama H, Tsurumaru M, Udagawa H et al. Radical lymph node dissection for cancer of the thoracic esophagus. *Ann Surg.* 1994;364.
18. Skandalakis JE, Gray SW, Skandalakis LJ. Surgical Anatomy of the Esophagus. In: Jamieson GG, ed. *Surgery of the Esophagus.* Edinburgh: Churchill Livingstone; 1988: 19–35.
19. Japanese Research Society for Gastric Cancer. The general rules for gastric cancer study in surgery and pathology. *Jpn J Surg.* 1981;11:127–145.
20. Wu CW, Hsieh MC, Lo SS et al. Morbidity and mortality after radical gastrectomy for patients with carcinoma of the stomach. *J Am Coll Surg.* 1995;181:26–32.
21. Bonenkamp JJ, Hermans J, Sasako M, van de Velde CJH. Extended lymph node dissection for gastric cancer. *N Engl J Med.* 1999;340:908–914.
22. Cuschieri A, Weeden S, Fielding J et al. Patient survival after D1 and D2 resections for gastric cancer: long-term results of the MRC randomized surgical trial. *Br J Cancer.* 1999;79:1522–1530.
23. Siewert JR, Böttcher K, Stein HJ, Roder JD. Relevant prognostic factors in gastric cancer. Ten-year results of the German Gastric Cancer Study. *Ann Surg.* 1998;228:449–461.
24. Kasakura Y, Mochizuki F, Wakabayashi K, Kochi M, Fujii M, Takayama T. An evaluation of the effectiveness of extended lymph node dissection in patients with gastric cancer: a retrospective study of 1403 cases at a single institution. *J Surg Research.* 2002;103:252–259.
25. Sendler A, Etter M, Böttcher K, Siewert JR. Resektionsausmass in der Chirurgie des Magenkarzinoms. *Chirurg.* 2002;73:316–324.
26. Liu KJM, Atten MJ, Donahue PE, Attar BM. Extended lymphadenectomy for gastric cancer: results in a teaching hospital. *Am Surg.* 2002;68:365–372.
27. Results of resection of gastric cancer with distant metastases. *Hepato-Gastroenterology.* 1998;45:592–596.
28. Ramacciato G, Aurello P, D'Angelo F, Cicchini C, Sternberg CN. Does extended lymphadenectomy influence prognosis of gastric carcinoma after curative resection? *Hepato-Gastroenterology.* 2000;47:1470–1474.
29. Adachi Y, Mimori K, Mori M, Maehara Y, Sugimachi K. Morbidity after D2 and D3 gastrectomy for node-positive gastric carcinoma. *J Am Coll Surg.* 1997;184:240–244.
30. Maeta M, Saito H, Kondo A et al. Effects of super-extended paraaortic lymphadenectomy (PAL) on biological responses in totally gastrectomized patients with T3 or T4 gastric cancer. *Gastric Cancer.* 1998;1:57–63.
31. Maeta M, Yamashiro H, Saito H et al. A prospective pilot study of extended (D3) and superextended paraaortic lymphadenectomy (D4) in patients with T3 or F4 gastric cancer managed by total gastrectomy. *Surgery.* 1999; 125:325–331.
32. Baba M, Hokita S, Natsugoe S et al. Paraaortic lymphadenectomy in patients with advanced carcinoma of the upper-third of the stomach. *Hepato-Gastroenterology.* 2000;47:893–896.
33. Nakao A, Harada A, Nonami T et al. Lymph node metastases in carcinoma of the head of the pancreas region. *Br J Surg.* 1995;82:399–402.
34. Kayahara M, Nagakawa T, Futagami F, Kitagawa H, Ohta T, Miyasaki I. Lymphatic flow and neural plexus invasion associated with carcinoma of the body and tail of the pancreas. *Cancer.* 1996;78:2485–2491.
35. Yoshida T, Matsumoto T, Sasaki A, Shibata K, Aramaki M, Kitano S. Outcome of paraaortic node-positive pancreatic head and bile duct adenocarcinoma. *Am J Surg.* 2004; 187:736–740.
36. O'Morchoe CCC. Lymphatic system of the pancreas. *Microscopy Research and Technique.* 1997;37:456–477.
37. Pissas A. Anatomoclinical and anatomosurgical essay on the lymphatic circulation of the pancreas. *Anat Clin.* 1984;6:225–280.

38. Barnes G Jr. Colon and Appendix. In: *Anatomic Basis of Tumor Surgery.* Wood WC, Skandalakis JE, eds. St Louis: Quality Medical Publishing Inc; 1999: 390–423.
39. Heald RJ, Smedh RK, Kald A, Sexton R, Moran BJ. Abdominoperineal excision of the rectum—an endangered operation. *Dis Colon Rectum.* 1997;40:747–751.
40. Canessa CE, Miegge LM, Bado J, Silveri C, Labandera D. Anatomic study of lateral pelvic lymph nodes: implications in the treatment of rectal cancer. *Dis Colon Rectum.* 2004;47:297–303.
41. Averbach AM, Jacquet P. Strategies to decrease the incidence of intra-abdominal recurrence in resectable gastric cancer. *Br J Surg.* 1996;83:726–733.
42. Martin RCG, Jaques DP, Brennan MF, Karpeh M. Extended local resection for advanced gastric cancer. Increased survival versus increased morbidity. *Ann Surg.* 2002;236:159-165.
43. Launois B, Jamieson GG. Left Hepatectomy and Extended Left Hepatectomy. In: Launois B, Jamieson GG, eds. *Modern Operative Techniques in Liver Surgery.* Edinburgh: Churchill Livingstone; 1993: 37–41.
44. Hjortsjo CH. The topography of the intrahepatic duct systems. *Acta Anat.* 1951;11:599–615.
45. Imaizumi T, Hanyu F, Harada N, Hatori T, Fukuda A. Extended radical Whipple resection for cancer of the pancreatic head: operative procedure and results. *Dig Surg.* 1998;15:299–307.
46. Taschieri AM, Elli M, Rovati M et al. Surgical treatment of tumors invading the spleno-mesenteric-portal vessels. An Italian multicenter surgery. *Hepato-Gastroenterology.* 1999;46:492–497.
47. Nakao A, Kaneko T, Takeda S et al. The role of extended radical operation for pancreatic cancer. *Hepato-Gastroenterology.* 2001;48:949–952.
48. Takahashi S, Ogata Y, Tsuzuki T. Combined resection of the pancreas and portal vein for pancreatic cancer. *Br J Surg.* 1994;81:1190–1193.
49. Fuhrman GM, Leach SD, Staley CA et al. Rationale for en bloc vein resection in the treatment of pancreatic adenocarcinoma adherent to the superior mesenteric-portal vein confluence. *Ann Surg.* 1996;223:154–162.
50. Leach SD, Lee JE, Charnsangavej C et al. Survival following pancreaticoduodenectomy with resection of the superior mesenteric-portal vein confluence for adenocarcinoma of the pancreatic head. *Br J Surg.* 1998;85:611–617.
51. Mayumi T, Nimura Y, Kamiya J et al. Distal pancreatectomy with en bloc resection of the celiac artery for carcinoma of the body and tail of the pancreas. *Int J Pancreatology.* 1997;22:15–21.
52. Kimura W, Han I, Furukawa Y et al. Appleby operation for carcinoma of the body and tail of the pancreas. *Hepato-Gastroenterology.* 1997;44:387–393.
53. Furukawa H, Hiratsuka M, Iwanaga T et al. Extended surgery-left upper abdominal exenteration plus Appleby's method—for type 4 gastric carcinoma. *Ann Surg Oncol.* 1997;4:209–214.
54. Isozaki H, Tanaka N, Fujü K, Tanigawa N, Okajima K. Improvement of the prognosis of gastric cancer with extensive serosal invasion using left upper abdominal evisceration. *Hepato-Gastroenterology.* 2001;48:1179–1182.
55. Brunshwig A. Complete excision of pelvic viscera for advanced carcinoma. *Cancer.* 1948;1:177–183.

3 Posterior Aspect of the Abdominal Viscera and Retroperitoneum

John E. Skandalakis, Lee J. Skandalakis, and Odysseas Zoras

"Many a clinical reputation lies buried behind the peritoneum. In this hinterland of straggling mesenchyme with its vascular and nervous plexuses, its weird embryonic rests, its shadowy fascial boundaries, the clinician is often left with only his flair and his diagnostic first principles to guide him."[1]

☐ Definition

The retroperitoneal space, or area, or just "retroperitoneum" is the region or space behind the peritoneal cavity. To be more anatomically correct, the retroperitoneum is the area of the posterior abdominal wall which is located between the posterior parietal peritoneum and the deep lamina of the transversalis fascia. This space is a vast territory lacking an accurate knowledge and accepted map. We, anatomists, need more work to uncover and understand this vast hidden area, this uncharted sea.

Embryologically and anatomically, the retroperitoneal space is related to the thorax above and the lower extremities below. This anatomic highway is responsible for the dissemination of any pathologic entity originating in the retroperitoneal space. The retroperitoneal space is also closely related to the intraperitoneal anatomical entities. Therefore, traumatic, benign and malignant, and local or diffuse inflammatory processes may spread upward or downward in the peritoneal cavity with connective tissue the pathway of these pathologic entities. An excellent example is the fluid of pancreatitis which can travel practically everywhere: up in the thorax or as low as the triangle of Scarpa.

The peculiar and poorly understood lymphatic pathways and blood vessels are also responsible for the metastatic process of malignant disease of the retroperitoneal space. For all practical purposes, the pericardial space and tunica vaginalis are the only two spaces isolated from the overall continuity of the space-at-large formed by the peritoneal and pleural spaces.

☐ Embryogenesis

The formation of the primitive coelom takes place at the end of the third week or the beginning of the fourth week of embryonic life. Around the third week, the intraembryonic mesoderm is responsible for the differentiation which causes the formation of the lateral plate, the intermediate mesoderm, and the paraxial mesoderm. Further differentiation of the somatic and splanchnic mesoderm divides the lateral plate into layers. Between the somatic and splanchnic mesoderm, on either side of the midline, is the intraembryonic coelom. The right and left intraembryonic coelom unite, forming a single large cavity, which later subdivides to form the pleural, pericardial, and peritoneal cavities and the tunica vaginalis.

At the time of somite formation early in the fourth week, clefts appear in the embryonic mesoderm, occupying a horseshoe-shaped area lateral to the neural plate. They pass across the midline, anterior to the developing head fold of the embryo, and coalesce to form a continuous cavity extending backward beside the head to communicate with the coelomic spaces of the rapidly forming myotomes. The bend in the horseshoe represents the future pericardial cavity. The lateral arms represent the pleural canals, and later, the pleural cavities. These lateral prolongations become dorsal by the rotation of the pericardium under the pharynx. They extend above the septum transversum and lie on either side of the foregut. Ventrally, the ventral parietal recesses (two corresponding prolongations) end blindly.

The pericardial cavity is very large, while the future pleural cavities are narrow, leading into a small peritoneal cavity. As the lungs develop, the pleural cavities enlarge faster than the pericardial cavity. The pleural cavities expand cranially into the somatic mesoderm beyond the cranial limits on the pericardium. The portion of the pericardial wall formed by the pleuropericardial membrane enlarges to form the whole of the lateral walls of the adult pericardium with the rest of the pericardium forming from the portions attached to the anterior and posterior mediastinum, the superior mediastinum, and the diaphragm.

The mesodermal cells lining the intraembryonic cavity change to mesothelial cells by further differentiation. The parietal and visceral layers of the serous membranes are produced from these cells. The somatic mesoderm forms the parietal layer of the serous membrane, eventually lining the pleural and peritoneal cavities. The splanchnic mesoderm forms the visceral layer of the serous membrane covering the abdominal and thoracic viscera. The space subjacent to the serous membrane defines the single subserous space. This is the subperitoneal space of the abdomen and pelvis and the subpleural space of the thorax in the adult. Thus, the formation of the omenta, mesenteries, and ligaments is the result of several embryogenetic steps. The gastrointestinal tract is closed, associated, and fixed with the dorsal and ventral mesentery.

Surgical Anatomy

Topography and Relations

Within the retroperitoneal space are embryologically related organs which are referred to as the retroperitoneal viscera. These include the adrenals, kidneys, and ureters. There are also numerous vascular and neural structures, including the aorta and its branches, the inferior vena cava and its tributaries, the lymphatics and the lymph nodes, the lumbar plexus with its branches, and the sympathetic trunks.

In addition to the organs and tissues that develop in the retroperitoneum, several other organs attain a secondarily retroperitoneal position in later embryologic development. These include most of the duodenum, the pancreas, and major portions of the ascending and descending colon.

Within the greater retroperitoneal space, there are also several small spaces or subcompartments. Loose connective tissue and fat surround the anatomic entities, and, to a variable degree, occupy the smaller spaces. The parietal peritoneum is in continuity with the visceral peritoneum and vice versa.

To be more specific, the visceral organs within the retroperitoneal space are: right and left adrenal, right and left kidney, urinary bladder, ascending colon, descending colon, upper 2/3 of the rectum (approximately), proximal vagina, vas deferens (partially), abdominal aorta, iliac arteries, abdominal inferior vena cava and iliac veins.

The following anatomic entities have a partial relation to the retroperitoneal space: distal esophagus (abdominal esophagus), proximal stomach, liver, and spleen.

Retroperitoneal (Extraperitoneal) Connective Tissue

Hinman subdivided the retroperitoneal connective tissue into three layers (strata)[2]: outer stratum, intermediate stratum, and inner stratum. The outer stratum forms the abdominopelvic fascia which is the transversalis fascia. The intermediate stratum forms the renal fascia (the fascia of Gerota). The inner stratum is merely the peritoneum and the so-called fusion-fascia (Fig. 3.**1**) present at the junction of "*an intraperitoneal organ (the pancreas, the duodenum, or the ascending or descending colon) with the undersurface of the primitive celomic epithelium.*"

Hinman further stated that the inner stratum covers the gastrointestinal viscera and its blood supply.[2] The

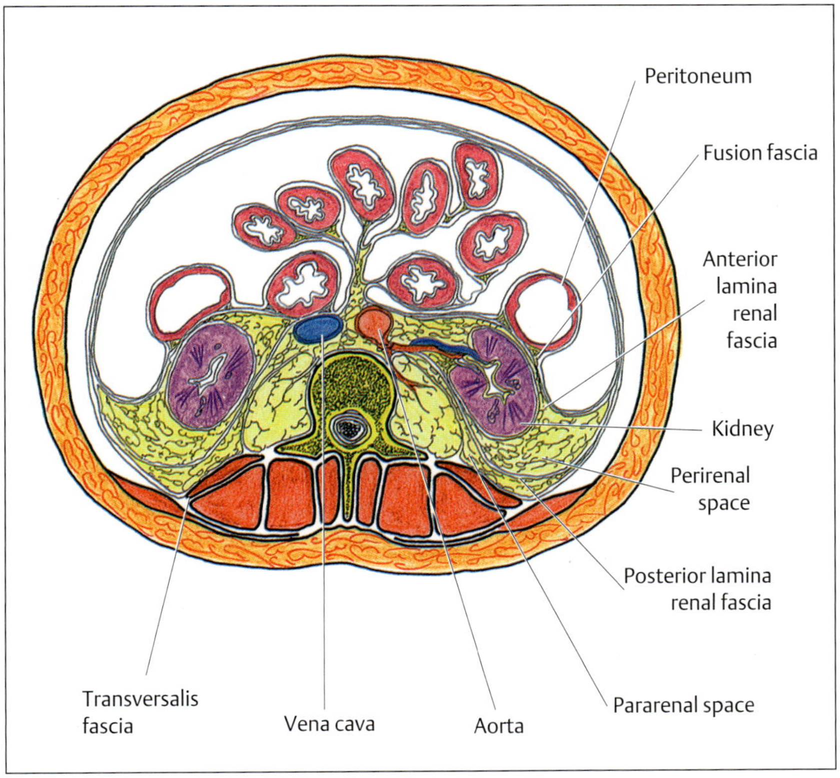

Fig. 3.**1** Distribution of retroperitoneal fasciae (reproduced from Skandalakis JE, Colborn GL, Weidman TA, Foster RS Jr, Kingsnorth AN, Skandalakis LJ. *Surgical Anatomy: The Embryologic and Anatomic Basis of Modern Surgery*. Athens, GR: Paschalidis Medical Publication; 2004)[3] (view from below).

intermediate stratum envelops the adrenals, kidneys, ureters, and the vessels and nerves. The outer stratum forms the internal fascia lining the body wall. We would add the thought that the intermediate stratum represents the extraperitoneal connective tissues that are associated with the anterior, lateral, and posterior walls of the abdominopelvic cavity. These tissues are locally condensed, or otherwise specialized in form, in association with distinct organs such as the kidneys.

Boundaries of the Retroperitoneal Region (Space)

The possible boundaries of the retroperitoneal region are as follows.

Above: T12 and 12th rib.

Below: Base of the sacrum, the iliac crest, the upper rami of the pubic bones, and the pelvic diaphragm.

Lateral: The vertical line between the erector spinae muscle (sacrospinalis) and the three flat abdominal muscles or to the lateral border of the quadratus lumborum muscle. Pack and Tabah extended the space as follows[4]: "*In a practical sense, we would extend this space more laterally to the tip of the twelfth rib at a line dropped perpendicularly downward to a point on the iliac crest situated approximately at the junction of the anterior half with the posterior half of the iliac crest. This line corresponds with the point at which the transversus abdominis muscle becomes aponeurotic, by which aponeurosis it arises from the tips and borders of the transverse processes of the lumbar vertebrae.*"

Medial: Lumbar and sacral vertebrae with the abdominal aorta and inferior vena cava and their branches; the sympathetic chains and nerve plexuses; the lymphatic elements.

Anterior: The anatomic entities related to the anterior wall and parietal peritoneum of the retroperitoneal space are: part of the liver and its bare area, part of the duodenum, part of the ascending colon, part of the descending colon, and much of the pancreas within the lesser sac. The colon, duodenum, and pancreas are intraperitoneal organs during much of their embryologic development but become fixed in their definitive retroperitoneal positions by fusion of their peritoneal investment with the posterior parietal peritoneum.

Posterior: The posterior wall of the space is related to several muscles. From lateral to medial, they are: the aponeurosis of the transversalis abdominis; the quadratus lumborum muscle; most medial, the psoas muscle. These three muscles are covered by a relatively tough layer of fascia which is common for the iliopsoas muscles. However, the anterior layer of the thoracodorsal fascia covers the quadratus lumborum. These boundaries form the lumbar area of the retroperitoneal space, which is the home of the right adrenal gland, the right kidney, the ascending colon, the duodenum, the left adrenal gland, the left kidney, and the descending colon.

There are several subdivisions or zones of the retroperitoneal space, such as: (1) Two fossae: lumbar and iliac; (2) Three zones: Zone 1 (centromedial), Zone II (lateral right and left), Zone III (Pelvic).

Nunn et al.[5] proposed a realistic anatomic division of the retroperitoneal space into three zones for description and decision-making in the treatment of retroperitoneal injury. These zones, their boundaries, and their contents are as follows:

Zone I (centromedial):
- Upper: Diaphragmatic, esophageal, and aortic openings.
- Lower: Sacral promontories.
- Lateral: Psoas muscles.
- *Contents*:
  Abdominal aorta, inferior vena cava, pancreas, duodenum (partial).

Zone II (lateral):
- Upper: Diaphragm.
- Lower: Iliac crests.
- Lateral: Psoas muscles.
- *Contents*:
  Kidneys and their vessels, ureters and their abdominal parts, ascending and descending colon, hepatic and splenic flexures.

Zone III (pelvic):
- Anterior: Space of Retzius.
- Posterior: Sacrum.
- Lateral: Bony pelvis.
- *Contents*:
  Pelvis in toto, pelvic wall, rectosigmoid colon, iliac vessels, urogenital organs (partial).

Falcone et al.[6] reported that a moderate to severe Zone I hematoma after blunt injury identified by computed tomography (CT) coupled with either multiple intraabdominal injuries or a solid viscus score (SVS) greater than 4 indicated a need for urgent exploration.

Trerotola et al.[7] reported the following locations of retroperitoneal hematomas secondary to femoral catheterization in 21 patients (seven patients had hematomas in two locations): retroperitoneum (12), peritoneum (3), groin and thigh (8), and abdominal wall (5).

Radiologic evaluation of the retroperitoneum was investigated by Chaffanjon et al.[8] They studied the anatomy of cadavers and healthy subjects using magnetic resonance imaging (MRI) and CT. They postulated that the orientation of the retroperitoneal viscera (the pancreas, the adrenal glands, and the kidneys) depends both on individual morphology and the size of the liver. There are two hepatic landmarks for radiologic imaging: the middle hepatic vein and the portal bifurcation.

They recommend oblique sectional planes be used for retroperitoneal studies.

We recommend the excellent book of MA Meyers, *Dynamic Radiology of the Abdomen*, a storehouse of embryologic, anatomic, and pathologic information.[9] The interested student should also be familiar with the multiple publications of Oliphant and colleagues.[10–14]

Iliac Fossa

The iliac fossa is lined with peritoneum which covers the extraperitoneal fat. It continues medially to the retroperitoneal space (lumbar area), then downward to the pelvic wall, as well as forward to the anterior abdominal wall. Just behind the fat is the multilaminar iliacus fascia.

The floor of the iliac fossa is the iliacus muscle. The iliohypogastric nerve usually crosses the iliacus fascia from medial to lateral behind the lower portion of the kidney. Other branches of the lumbar plexus pass through the psoas major and lie deep to the iliac fascia as they cross the iliac fossa. The femoral nerve descends in the lateral part of the interval between the psoas and iliacus muscles.

The common and external iliac arteries and veins, running inferiorly around the brim of the true pelvis on the medial surface of the psoas, are covered with a medial extension of the iliacus fascia. Inferiorly, the fascia iliaca contributes to the formation of the iliopubic tract together with the transversalis fascia and the transversus abdominis muscle.

Pelvic Sidewall

The pelvic sidewall may be presented from a surgicoanatomic standpoint as five surgicoanatomic layers associated with specific anatomic entities.

First layer	Peritoneum, which is associated with several organs of the digestive, urinary, and genital tracts.
Second layer	Abdominal aorta and abdominal inferior vena cava.
Third layer	Parietal fascia and visceral fascia.
Fourth layer	Nerves of the pelvis.
Fifth layer	Muscles: piriformis and obturator internus.

Psoas Muscle

For all practical purposes, the psoas muscle extends from the posterior mediastinum to the thigh. On its way downward, it is closely associated with the perirenal space and, perhaps, with the posterior pararenal space. One of the authors (JES) witnessed a tuberculous psoas abscess pointing at the medial upper thigh just below the inguinal ligament (Scarpa's femoral triangle).

Abscesses of pyogenic organisms may be formed by a retrocecal perforated appendix, colonic diverticulitis, or Crohn's disease. Santaella et al.[15] stated that an abscess involving the iliopsoas area should be drained surgically and not percutaneously.

The pathway of renal inflammatory processes is from the perirenal space directly to the psoas muscle. Hematomas in the psoas muscle have been reported. Other pathologic processes involving the muscle are malignant neoplasms of the retroperitoneal space. Such a case was presented by Nathanson and Sonnino.[16] They excised the tumor and the entire muscle via the retroperitoneal approach without violation of the peritoneal cavity.

□ Compartments of the Retroperitoneal Space

Three compartments of the retroperitoneal space are related to the kidney:

- Anterior pararenal compartment.
- Posterior pararenal compartment.
- Perirenal compartment.

The renal fascia, a collagenous connective tissue of mesodermal origin enveloping the kidney, is responsible for this compartmentalization.

The fascial layers and the spaces related to the kidney are as follows, from anterior to posterior:

- Peritoneum.
- Anterior pararenal space (with a variable quantity of loose connective tissue and fat).
- Anterior lamina of Gerota's fascia.
- Perirenal space (the kidney and the ureter; the adrenal in a separate subcompartment; fat).
- Posterior lamina of Gerota's fascia.
- Posterior pararenal space (usually with a large content of more compact fat).
- Thoracolumbar (lumbodorsal) fascia and the fascia of the psoas muscle.

To generalize, the muscle fascia lining the abdomen is referred to as the transversalis fascia (Fig. 3.**2**). More specifically, however, the transversalis fascia, which is the fascial lining of the transversus abdominis muscle, is continuous with the subdiaphragmatic fascia above. Medially, it is continuous with the psoas fascia and the thoracolumbar (or lumbodorsal) fascial investment (anterior lamina) of the quadratus lumborum muscle. Below, it is continuous with the fascia of the iliacus muscle and the parietal muscular fascia of the true pelvis.

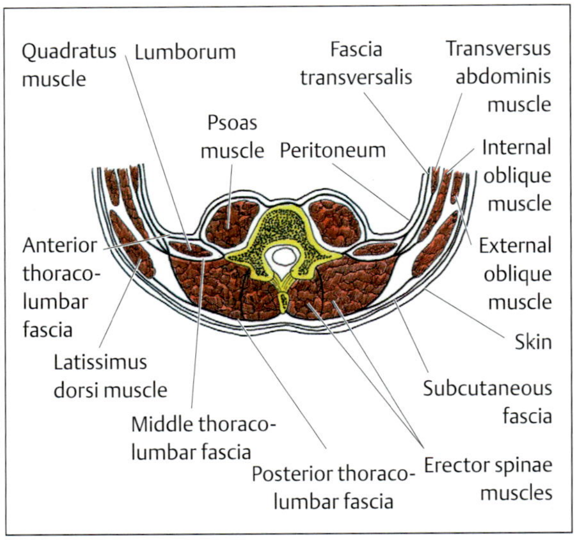

Fig. 3.**2** Diagrammatic cross section through posterior body wall in lumbar region.

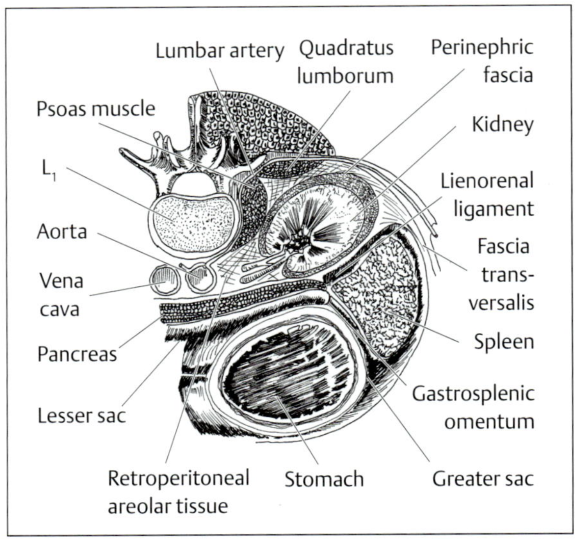

Fig. 3.**3** Horizontal section through left kidney, spleen, and stomach.

Perirenal Space

The perirenal space is the home of the kidneys. Therefore, each organ lies between the posterior lamina and the anterior lamina of the fascia of Gerota. Because of the compartmentalization of the retroperitoneal space by the various retroperitoneal connective tissues and fasciae, the kidney is enveloped by the anterior and posterior laminae of the renal fascia (fascia of Gerota or perinephric or perirenal fascia) and by the fatty tissue inside and outside the fascia.

The anterior lamina is also known as the fascia of Toldt and the posterior fascia is known as the fascia of Zuckerkandl.

Last[17] called the renal fascia a "*vague condensation of the areolar tissue between the parietal peritoneum and the posterior abdominal wall.*" However, he added that "*certain of its attachments are worthy of note since they serve to restrain the extenuation of a perinephric abscess*" (Fig. 3.**3**).

The renal fascia has a peculiar pathway. It covers the fat of the anterior and posterior surface of the kidney. There is some medial fixation with the adventitial coverings of the renal vessels with extension to the aorta on the left and the inferior vena cava (IVC) on the right. Above and toward the adrenal gland and the diaphragm, the anterior and posterior laminae unite, or perhaps fuse and finally, join the subdiaphragmatic fascia. However, at the upper pole of the kidney, there is a fascial septum separating the adrenal gland from the kidney.

After an anatomic examination of 10 cadavers, Reich et al.[18] reported a vascularized, wide-based borderline lamella (corresponding to the anterior lamina of Gerota's fascia) remaining in the area of the 2nd and 3rd parts of the duodenum. It covered the inferior vena cava but was fixed with the abdominal aorta.

The lower extent of both the anterior and posterior laminae of the renal fascia is enigmatic. Some anatomists and surgeons believe that the two laminae fuse. However, others believe that they do not fuse, existing in a state of nonunion which thereby permits the kidney alone and not the adrenal gland to travel downward (ptotic kidney, nephroptosis, or floating kidney). Some investigators trying to explain nephroptosis refer to weight loss and, therefore, loss of the perinephric fat which they think keeps the kidney in its normal position. Others support the idea of a weak union which can be ruptured from above by the collection of fluid in the perirenal space downward to the pelvic wall.

Raptopoulos et al.[19] reported that perirenal disease does not extend into the pelvis because of the fusion of renal fasciae and the formation of a cone which acts as a barrier to disease extension. The supporters of nonunion theorize that the inferior extensions of the anterior and posterior laminae form the so-called periureteral sheath.

One of the authors (JES) remembers vividly the era of retroperitoneal air insufflation (presacral pneumography). Air was injected into the retroperitoneal space by insertion of a needle anterior to the sacrum and posterolateral to the rectum. This now-discarded procedure, done prior to CT, MRI, etc., precisely outlined the renal contents within the perirenal space. It also indicated pathologic anomalies (if any), especially those of the adrenal glands[20] (Fig. 3.**4**).

In many dissections, the ureter is seen descending from behind the anterior lamina of the sheath, bringing with it a mesentery-like membrane, presumably derived from the perirenal fascia. Downward extension of Gerota's fascia merges with the pararenal fatty tissue in the infrarenal space.

The posterior renal lamina unites with the anterior renal fascia close to the posterolateral surface of the ascending or descending colon to form the so-called lateroconal fascia. This fascia continues to blend with the parietal peritoneum somewhere at the right or left gutter area anterolaterally. However, it is often seen to be reduced to a thinner mantle of connective tissue intervening between the peritoneum and the transversalis fascia.

Kudos belongs to Meyers and his associates[9,10,21] and Parienty et al.[22] for their studies of the anatomic and radiologic anatomy of the renal fascia and the compartments it defines (Figs. 3.**5** and 3.**6**). These workers found that both laminae (anterior and posterior) of Gerota's fascia can be seen radiologically in 50% of patients. The same authors stated that the posterior lamina is thicker in comparison with the anterior lamina. The posterior lamina is also more frequently visualized. The anterior fascia is more prominent on the left side.

The causes of perirenal fluid collection are as follows:

- Bleeding due to blunt abdominal trauma, rupture of a vessel or aortic aneurysm, or spontaneous bleeding secondary to benign or malignant neoplasia.
- Urinoma secondary to obstructive uropathy, blunt abdominal trauma, or iatrogenic injury (secondary to surgery or diagnostic instrumentation).
- Abscess secondary to either pyelonephritis or an infected urinoma.

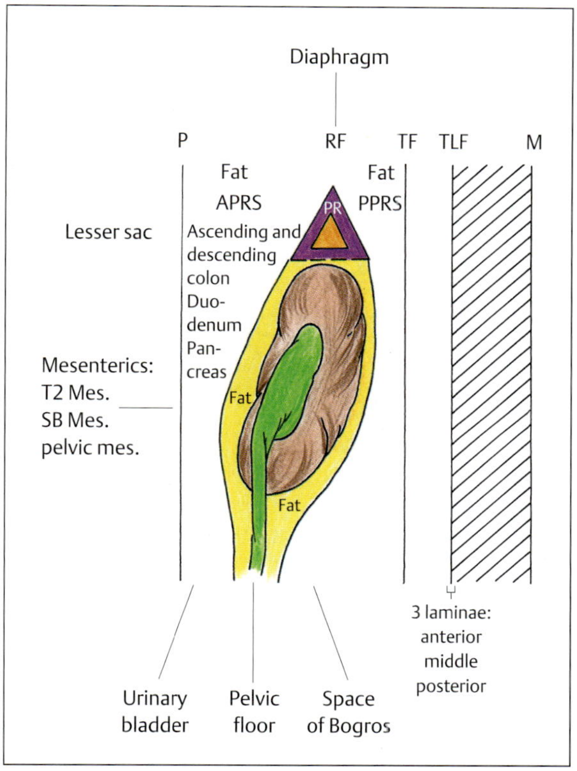

Fig. 3.**4** Retroperitoneal spaces (highly diagrammatic). Δ, adrenal gland; *PR*, perirenal space; *RF*, renal fascia (Gerota's); *P*, peritoneum; *APRS*, anterior pararenal space; *PPRS*, posterior pararenal space; *TLF*, thoracolumbar fascia; *TF*, transversalis fascia; *M*, muscles (reproduced from Skandalakis JE, Colborn GL, Weidman TA, Foster RS Jr, Kingsnorth AN, Skandalakis LJ. *Surgical Anatomy: The Embryologic and Anatomic Basis of Modern Surgery*. Athens, GR: Paschalidis Medical Publication; 2004).

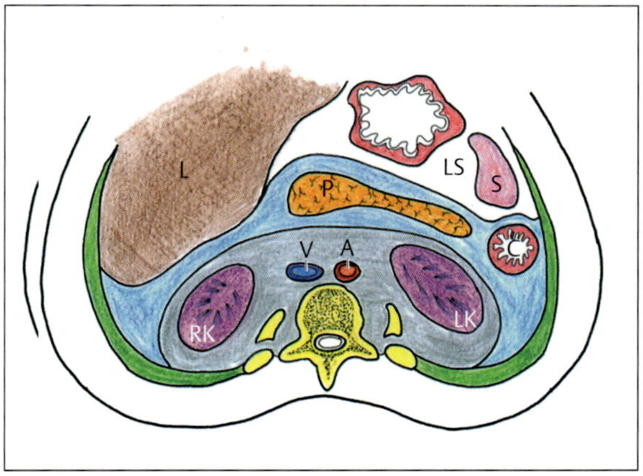

a

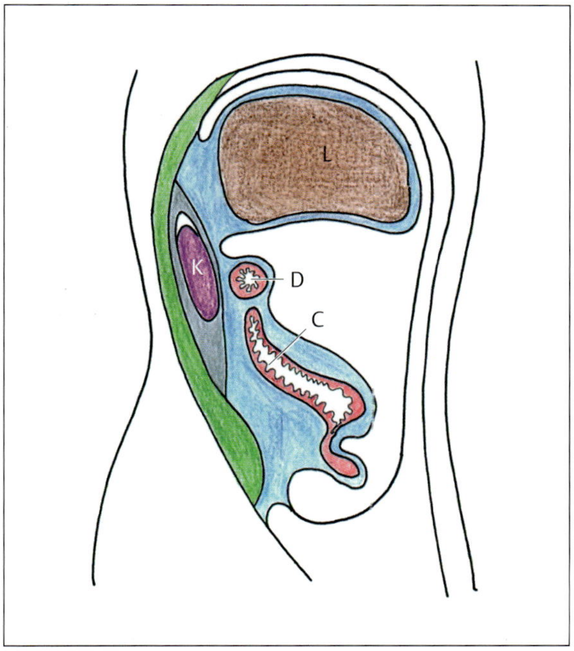

b

Fig. 3.**5a,b** **a** Axial diagram at level of kidneys. **b** Sagittal diagram in plane of right kidney. Three major retroperitoneal compartments shown: anterior pararenal space (*in blue*), perirenal space (*in grey*), posterior pararenal space (*in green*). *L*, liver; *P*, pancreas; *LS*, lesser sac; *S*, spleen; *V*, vena cava; *A*, aorta; *RK*, right kidney; *LK*, left kidney; *C*, colon; *D*, duodenum (reproduced from Korobkin M, Silverman PM, Quint LE, Francis IR. CT of the extraperitoneal space: normal anatomy and fluid collections. AJR 1992;159:933–941).[25]

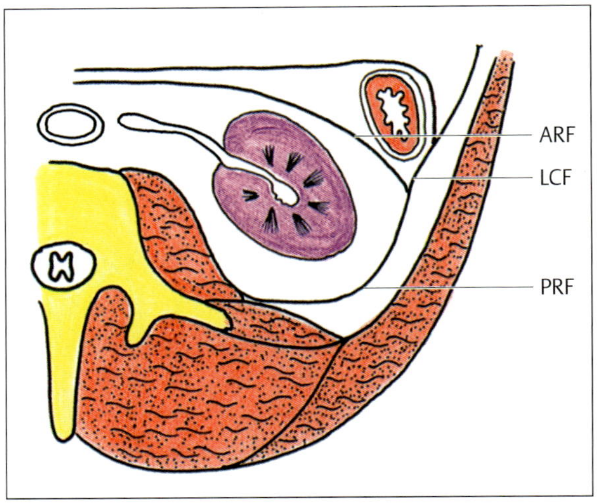

Fig. 3.**6** Diagram at the level of the left kidney. *ARF*, anterior renal fascia; *LCF*, lateroconal fascia; *PRF*, posterior renal fascia (reproduced from Korobkin M, Silverman PM, Quint LE, Francis IR. CT of the extraperitoneal space: normal anatomy and fluid collections. AJR 1992;159:933–941).[25]

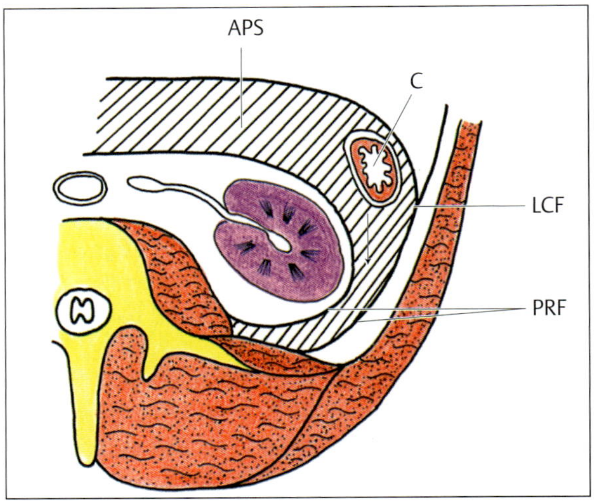

Fig. 3.**7** Retrorenal extension of pancreatitis fluid. Diagram shows fluid (*hatched area*) dissecting layers of posterior renal fascia. *APS*, anterior pararenal space; *C*, descending colon; *LCF*, lateroconal fascia; *PRF*, two layers of posterior renal fascia (reproduced from Korobkin M, Silverman PM, Quint LE, Francis IR. CT of the extraperitoneal space: normal anatomy and fluid collections. *AJR*. 1992;159:933–941).[25]

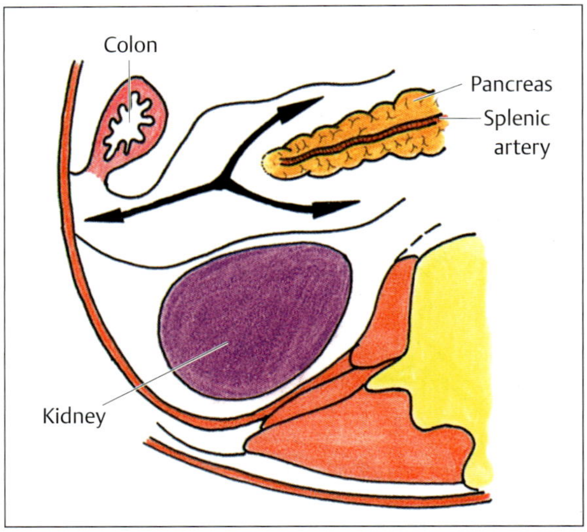

Fig. 3.**8** Pathway of extravasations from the tail of the pancreas. (reproduced from Meyers MA. *Dynamic Radiology of the Abdomen*. 5th ed. New York: Springer; 2000).[9]

Anterior Pararenal Compartment

We agree with Rubenstein et al.[23] that the anterior pararenal compartment (Fig. 3.**7**) is a distinct retroperitoneal space and not an intraperitoneal space as Dodds et al.[24] reported.

According to Korobkin et al.,[25] fluid collection is more common on the left side than on the right perhaps due to pancreatitis of the tail (Fig. 3.**8**). Fluid collection on the right is secondary to duodenal perforation or pancreatitis.

Posterior Pararenal Compartment

Fluid collection in this space is a rare phenomenon. According to Mindell et al.,[26] it can occur if sufficient fluid is present.

☐ Communication of the Retroperitoneal Spaces

The communications of the several retroperitoneal spaces are highly controversial. According to Korobkin et al.,[25] the anterior and posterior pararenal spaces merge caudal to the cone of the renal fascia (perhaps conveniently, this area is called the infrarenal retroperitoneal space) which communicates with the prevesical space and other compartments of the pelvic wall.

Raptopoulos et al.[27] and Feldberg et al.[28] studied the medial attachment of the posterior renal lamina. They reported that the attachment is not always the same, inserting near the anterior or the posterior surfaces of the psoas muscle. According to these authors, the attachment is most likely at the posterior aspect of the psoas muscle, or occasionally, at the quadratus lumborum muscle at the area of the lower renal pole.

The medial extension of the anterior lamina is highly controversial. To what extent does it continue across the midline? If such continuation exists, do right and left perirenal spaces communicate? It is our opinion, from an anatomic standpoint, that communication between the right and left perirenal spaces is somewhat questionable. However, Kneeland et al.[29] and Mindell et al.,[26] using radiologic and cadaveric studies, reported that the perirenal spaces may communicate across the midline anterior to the aorta and the inferior vena cava (IVC) and posterior to the anterior laminae of the renal fascia. If this is true, a midline vascular pathology, such as an aortic aneurysm, may travel to the left or even to the right perirenal space. Hopper et al.[30] disagreed, advising that the pathway of the blood from such a rupture is to the psoas muscle and then into the posterior pararenal space. Last[17] may have been correct that this "layer" is just areolar tissue. Raptopoulos et al.[27] agree with Last that the anterior lamina is thin.

Since the anterior lamina is thin, perhaps the lateroconal fascia is the product of the posterior lamina only. The water is muddy, the anatomy is confused; perhaps we cannot interpret the radiologic images of the anatomy 100% correctly. In the operating room, many times have surgeons been unsure about the formation of compartments, the pathway of fluids and, finally, the accurate localization of compartmental collection. Maybe Last[17] *was* right. Or, perhaps, the amount of blood (bleeding from injury to the retroperitoneal organs) or inflammatory potentialities (secondary, perhaps, to pancreatitis) play a greater or lesser role in the final picture.

According to Korobkin et al.,[25] an abscess or infected fluid can be found in any compartment. Pancreatic fluid secondary to pancreatitis is most likely to collect in the anterior pararenal space, or perhaps, in all retroperitoneal compartments. We agree. As a matter of fact, we (JES, LJS) have seen a case of intraperitoneal pancreatic extravasation presenting as hydrocele secondary to collection at the tunica vaginalis.

Hureau et al. reported the following[31,32]:

- The anterior pararenal space is almost virtual (*quasi virtuel*), demonstrating its existence through pathologic manifestations such as acute pancreatitis.
- The posterior pararenal space continues to the space of Bogros (Fig. 3.**9**) which is a lateral extension of the retropubic space of Retzius. The space of Bogros is formed laterally by the iliac fascia, anteriorly by the transversalis fascia, and medially by the parietal peritoneum.
- The perirenal spaces continue down to the bladder and the prevesical space.

We want to emphasize that we do not have all the answers about these spaces, which extend to the diaphragm and to the pelvis, assuming the guided migration of pathologic processes. However, we must always remember the upward and downward continuation of the retroperitoneal space: thorax and neck as well as pelvis and triangle of Scarpa (Figs. 3.**10**–3.**12**).

There are several other spaces and anatomic entities related to the retroperitoneal space, such as the subperitoneal pelvic space (extraperitoneal), the vesicoumbilical fascia and vesical spaces. It is not within the scope of this chapter to present all these spaces.

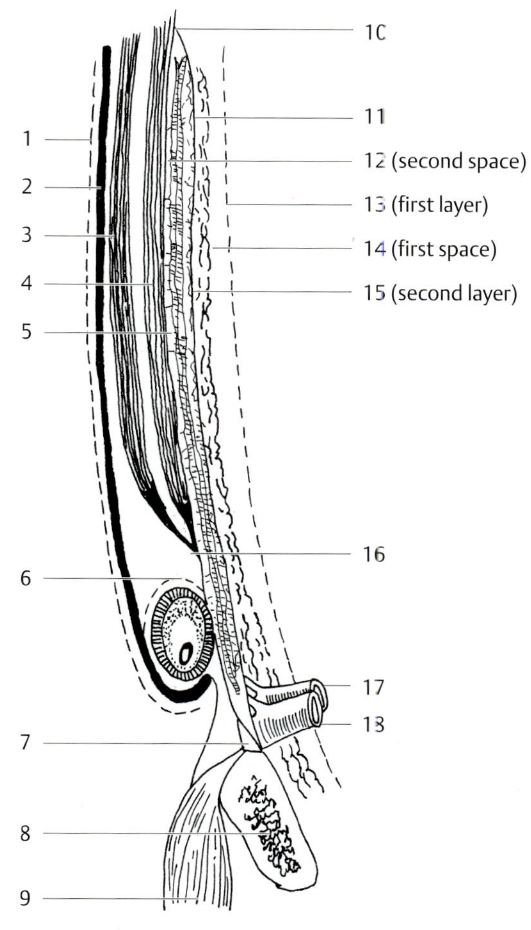

Fig. 3.**9** Highly diagrammatic representation of the layers of the abdominal wall and inguinal area. *1*, External oblique fascia (fascia of Gallaudet); *2*, external oblique aponeurosis; *3*, internal oblique muscle; *4*, transversus abdominis muscle and its aponeurosis; *5*, transversalis fascia anterior lamina (third layer); *6*, external spermatic fascia; *7*, Cooper's ligament; *8*, pubic bone; *9*, pectineus muscle; *10*, possible union of transversalis fascia laminae; *11*, transversalis fascia posterior lamina (second layer); *12*, vessels (second space); *13*, peritoneum (first layer); *14*, space of Bogros (first space); *15*, preperitoneal fat; *16*, transversus abdominis aponeurosis and anterior lamina of transversalis fascia; *17*, femoral artery; *18*, femoral vein (modified from Skandalakis JE, Colborn GL, Androulakis JA, Skandalakis LJ, Pemberton LB. Embryologic and anatomic basis of inguinal herniorrhaphy. *Surg Clin North Am*. 1993;73:799–836; with permission. Drawn with R.C. Read).

Visceral Blood Supply

The abdominal aorta and its branches, the abdominal IVC and its tributaries, all represent the visceral blood supply of the several anatomic entities within the retroperitoneal space or within the peritoneal cavity.

Therefore, the retroperitoneal space is the home of the great vessels of the abdomen: the abdominal aorta and abdominal IVC. Aortic branches and venous tribu-

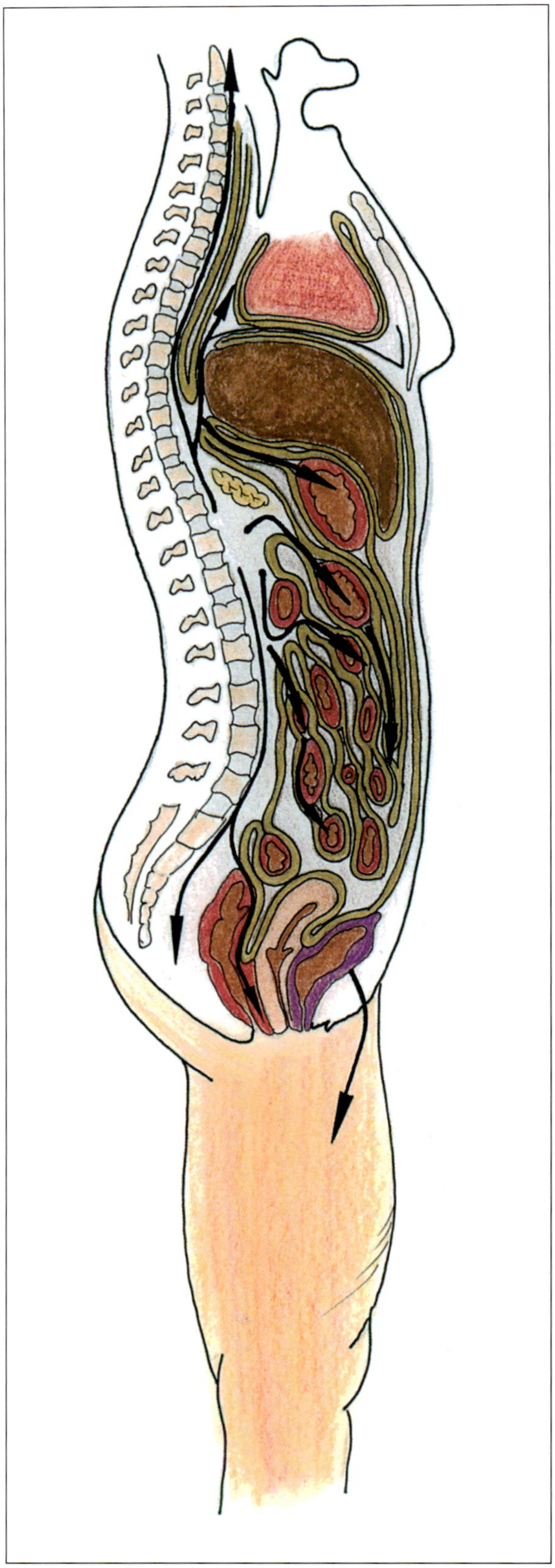

Fig. 3.10 Communication of the retroperitoneal spaces: midsagittal view (female).

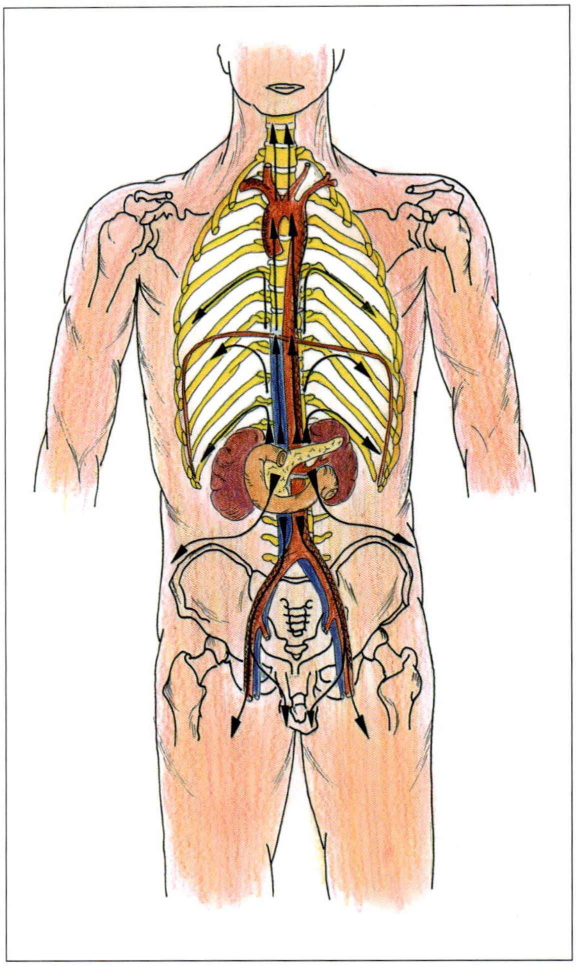

Fig. 3.11 Communication of the retroperitoneal spaces: anterior view (male).

taries are responsible for the blood supply of the gastrointestinal canal and the three unpaired glands as well as the three paired glands and the roof and walls of the abdomen (Fig. 3.**13**).[33]

Abdominal Aorta and its Collateral Branches

- Celiac artery.
- Superior mesenteric artery (SMA).
- Inferior mesenteric artery (IMA).
- Suprarenal arteries.
- Renal arteries.
- Gonadal arteries.
- Inferior phrenic arteries.
- Lumbar arteries.
- Median sacral artery.

The celiac artery or trunk is located at the level of the disc between the 12th thoracic and 1st lumbar vertebrae. It is very closely related to the median arcuate

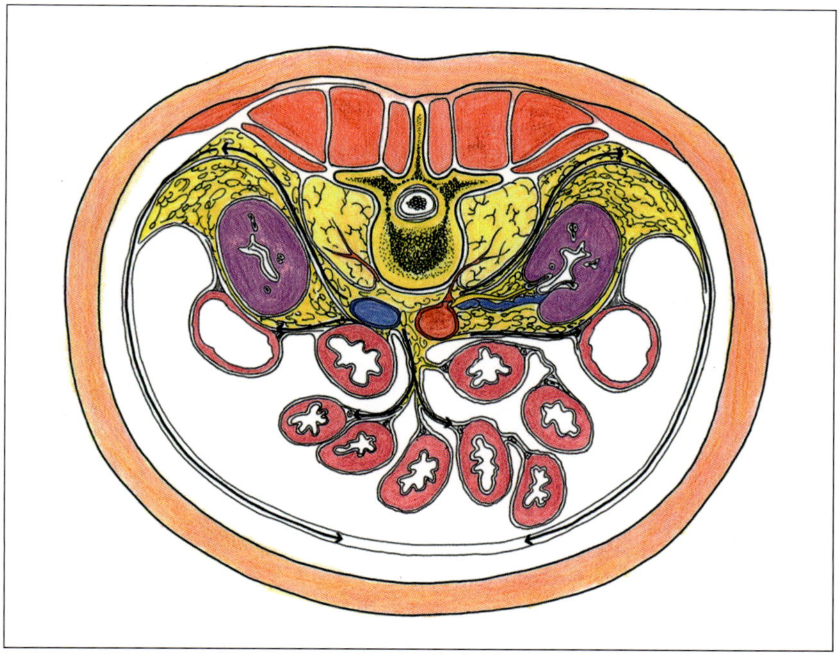

Fig. 3.**12** Communication of the retroperitoneal spaces: transaxial view at L2 (view from above).

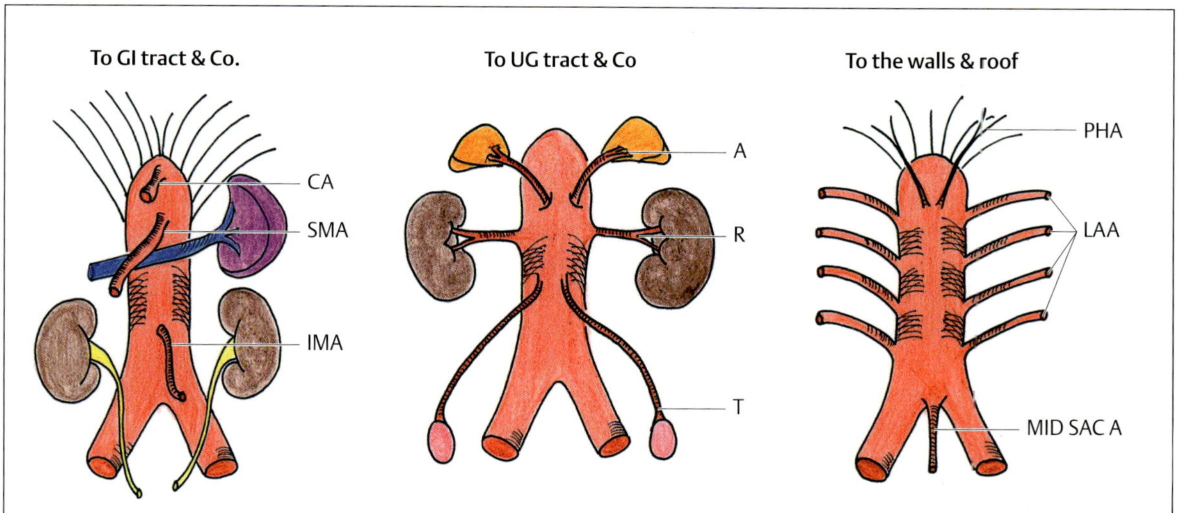

Fig. 3.**13** The branches of the abdominal aorta arranged according to the planes they occupy (see Fig. 3.**15**). *CA*, Celiac artery; *SMA*, superior mesenteric artery; *IMA*, inferior mesenteric artery; *GI*, gastrointestinal; *UG*, urogenital; *MID SAC A*, median sacral artery; *LAA*, lumbar arteries; *PHA*, phrenic artery; *A*, adrenal artery; *R*, renal artery; *T*, testicular artery.

ligament which bridges the two diaphragmatic crura and which is in front of the celiac artery.

The superior mesenteric artery originates from the aorta just below the origin of the celiac artery behind the neck of the pancreas and behind the splenic vein. On its pathway downward, a clamp mechanism is formed by the SMA and aorta. Within this angle formation there are three anatomic entities from above downward: the left renal vein, the uncinate process of the pancreas, and the third portion of the duodenum (Fig. 3.**14**).

The inferior mesenteric artery originates from the aorta approximately 1–2 inches above the aortic bifurcation, behind the third portion of the duodenum, and in front of the third lumbar vertebra.

The right and left renal arteries originate just inferior to the origin of the SMA and behind the right and left renal vein. The gonadal arteries (testicular or ovarian) arise just below the renal arteries. The right and left suprarenal arteries arise just above the renal arteries.

According to Greig et al.,[34] the right and left inferior phrenic arteries originate from the aorta (46.1%), from

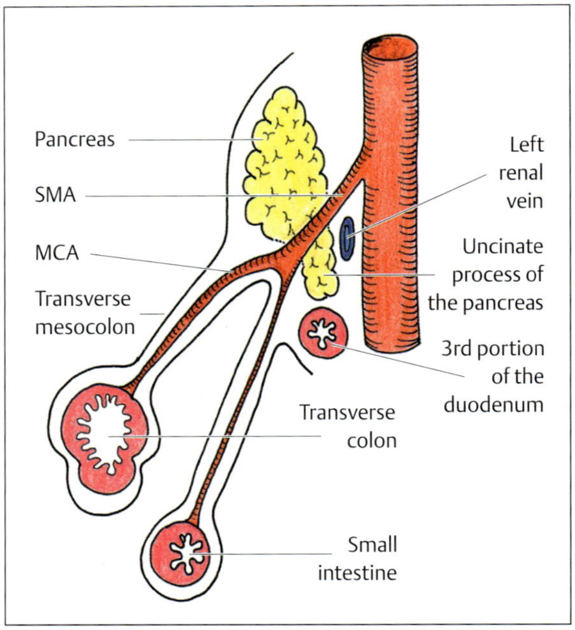

Fig. 3.**14** Diagrammatic sagittal section through the neck of the pancreas. The uncinate process and the third part of the duodenum lie posterior to the superior mesenteric artery (*SMA*). The midline colic artery (*MCA*) leaves the SMA at the inferior pancreatic margin to travel in the transverse mesocolon.

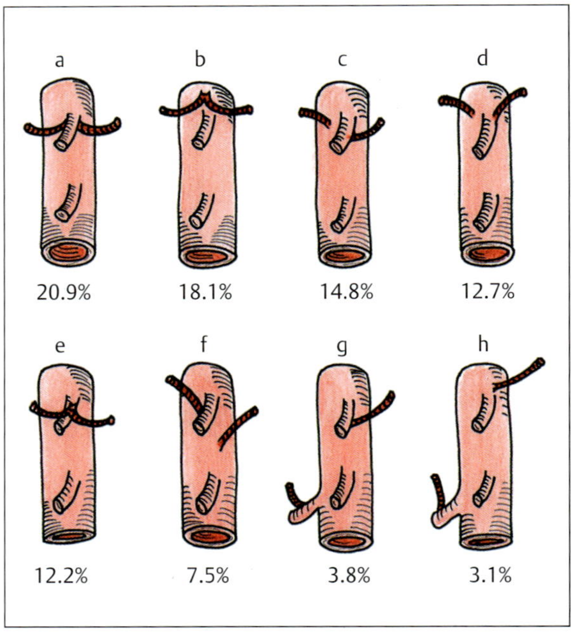

Fig. 3.**15** Origins of the inferior phrenic arteries in more than 90% of 850 body halves; *a* through *f* show origins from the celiac artery, the aorta, or both; *g* and *h* show origin of the right phrenic artery from the right renal artery.

the celiac artery (41.4%), or from other branches (renal, left gastric, hepatic, etc). Not only the diaphragm benefits from these arteries but also the adrenals, the lower esophagus, and the right lateral hepatic segment (Fig. 3.**15**).

The four pairs of the right and left lumbar arteries are located dorsal and medial of the psoas muscle and the sympathetic trunk and arise from the aorta. The fifth pair, the right and left iliolumbar arteries, originate from the internal iliacs. Remember: the right lumbar arteries pass behind the inferior vena cava. The right and left first lumbar arteries pass behind the diaphragmatic crura.

The median sacral artery is the downward continuation of the abdominal aorta. It is located anterior to the fifth lumbar vertebra and behind the left common iliac arteries.

Arterial Variations

Aberrant and accessory renal arteries are found in 20–25% of patients. These occasionally originate at the common iliac and gonadal arteries.[35]

Venous Drainage

Inferior Vena Cava and its Tributaries

The abdominal IVC is formed by the right and left common iliac veins approximately at the level of the fourth lumbar vertebra, just behind and to the right of the bifurcation of the aorta. Its upward path is behind the duodenum and the pancreas. Approaching the liver and diaphragm, it is located within the hepatoduodenal ligament between the right adrenal gland and portal vein.

Veins of the Three Paired Glands

The suprarenal, the renal, and the gonadal veins (the veins of the three paired glands) enter the inferior vena cava as follows. On the right side, each vein enters the IVC separately. On the left side, the veins unite to form the left renal vein which is located behind the pancreas and splenic artery and vein, anterior to the aorta, just below the origin of the SMA.

The senior author (JES) and colleagues studied the collateral flow and anomalies of the left renal vein.[36] The anatomy of this vein is extremely important to the modern surgeon since division of the left renal vein is common in many procedures. We found no evidence of additional tributaries off the left renal vein. Opening of the left gonadal and left suprarenal veins did not reveal any direct connections to the IVC. There was evidence of a systemic collateral flow system draining the left kidney once the left renal vein was divided.

Veins of the Body Wall

The right and left inferior phrenic veins drain diaphragmatic blood to the inferior vena cava. According to Grant and Basmajian,[37] the left vein in most of the cases empties into the left renal vein. The lumbar veins empty

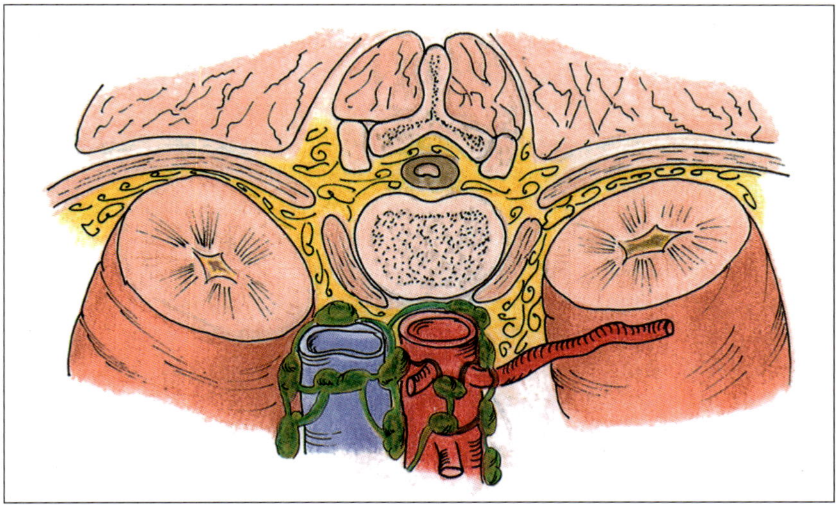

Fig. 3.**16** Retroperitoneal lymphatics: pre-, retro-, paraaortic and pre-, retro-, paracaval groups.

into the IVC, the right and left iliolumbar veins into the right and left common iliac veins. The left common iliac vein accepts the median sacral vein.

There is a link in the venous network of the retroperitoneal space. The right and left ascending lumbar veins together bridge the right and left lumbar veins. The ascending lumbar vein begins at the common iliac vein and ends in the azygos or hemiazygos.

The portal vein is the main vessel of the gastrointestinal trunk and the three unpaired glands. It is formed by the splenic vein and superior mesenteric vein. In rare cases, the inferior mesenteric vein also takes part, draining into the junction of the superior mesenteric vein and splenic vein. The venous blood passes the hepatic parenchyma through the branches of the portal vein and enters the thoracic inferior vena cava through the hepatic veins to reach the heart.

Venous Variations

Anomalies of the left renal venous drainage system included bifurcation of the gonadal vein, bifurcation of the suprarenal vein, an inferior phrenic vein draining into the left renal vein distal to the SMA, and the presence of a lumbar vein draining into the left renal vein. The lumbar veins may perhaps represent a normal variant. A supernumerary left renal vein was also reported.[36]

Multiple renal veins occur in 25% of patients. Duplication of the renal vein (1–3%), clamping behind the aorta (1.8%), and loop formation around the aorta (1.5%) may be found with anomalies of the IVC.[37]

☐ Retroperitoneal Lymphatics

The general surgeon should be familiar with the lymph nodes of the gastrointestinal tract and the three unpaired glands (liver, spleen, pancreas). The urologist must know the groups of lymph nodes pertaining to the kidney, ureter, bladder, prostate, penis, and testicles. The gynecologist deals with the lymph nodes of the uterus, fallopian tubes, ovaries, and vulva.

From an anatomic standpoint, the retroperitoneal lymph nodes can be rather difficult to classify. The retroperitoneal lymphatics form a very rich and extensive chain from the inguinal ligament and pelvis to the respiratory diaphragm and posterior mediastinal nodes. Usually, these lymph nodes are located close to the aorta and IVC. The right paraaortic lymph nodes are in very close relationship with the left paracaval lymph nodes. The number of abdominal and pelvic lymph nodes is approximately 230.[38]

The following classification is very simple, logical, and anatomic (Fig. 3.**16**):

Aortic Group:

- Preaortic nodes.
- Retroaortic nodes.
- Paraaortic nodes.

Caval Group:

- Precaval (prevenous) nodes.
- Retrocaval (retrovenous) nodes.
- Paracaval (laterovenous) nodes.

Pelvic Group:

- Common iliac nodes.
- External iliac nodes.
- Internal iliac (hypogastric) nodes.
- Obturator nodes.
- Sacral nodes.

Complete, total, and accurate mapping of lymph nodes of the retroperitoneum is necessary prior to radical retroperitoneal lymphadenectomy. Since the topography of the retroperitoneal lymph nodes is very closely related to the vasculature, perhaps the best approach is thoracoabdominal. This involves skeletonization of the abdominal aorta and its branches and the IVC and its branches.

Aortic Group

Preaortic Nodes

One to three celiac nodes are located around the base of the celiac artery. They are very closely related to the celiac ganglion and the lymph nodes of the superior mesenteric artery. These nodes receive lymph from the stomach, liver, pancreas, and superior mesenteric nodes. Efferents from the celiac nodes form the intestinal lymph trunk which enters the abdominal lymph complex called the cisterna chyli.

According to Rhee and Gloviczki, in about 50% of patients, the cisterna chyli is located anterior to the second lumbar vertebra between the abdominal inferior vena cava and abdominal aorta. The right and left lumbar trunks, the gastrointestinal trunks, and a pair of lower intercostal trunks all terminate in the cisterna chyli, which becomes the thoracic duct after passing through the aortic hiatus. With injury, closure should be attempted using 7–0 monofilament.[39]

Two or three superior mesenteric nodes receive lymph from the small bowel, right colon part of the transverse colon, and pancreas. They communicate with inferior mesenteric nodes and drain to the celiac nodes. The two nodes of the IMA receive lymph from the left colon.

Retroaortic Nodes

The retroaortic lymph nodes provide a station of communication between the pre- and paraaortic lymph nodes in front of the third and fourth lumbar vertebrae. Healey and Hodge stated that the retroaortic lymph nodes are variable in number and are not true regional lymph nodes.[40]

Paraaortic Nodes

The right lateral paraaortic nodes, together with the left paracaval nodes, form the right lumbar chain of nodes which can be found intimately related to the inferior vena cava. The left paraaortic (left lumbar) lymph nodes form a group of five to ten lymph nodes drained by the left lumbar trunk posterolateral to the abdominal aorta. The right and left lumbar lymph trunks communicate with the common iliac nodes distally and drain into the abdominal confluence (cisterna chyli) proximally. The paraortic nodes are primary sites of testicular neoplasms.[41]

Caval Group

Precaval Nodes

Precaval lymph nodes are located at the anterior wall of the inferior vena cava. Healey and Hodge[40] stated that two of these nodes, one at the aortic bifurcation and one at the termination of the left renal vein, are constant.

Retrocaval Nodes

Retrocaval lymph nodes are located on the psoas muscle and the right crus of the diaphragm.

Paracaval Nodes

Paracaval nodes are found at the right lateral side of the vena cava. One node at the entrance of the right renal vein to the inferior vena cava is the metastatic site for right testicular malignancy. The left paracaval nodes are in close association with the right aortic nodes.

Pelvic Group

Common Iliac Nodes

There are four to six common iliac lymph nodes which are located around the artery. The medial nodes of this group lie against the body of the fifth lumbar vertebra and are called the nodes of the promontory. Efferents pass to the lumbar nodes.

External Iliac Nodes

There are eight to ten external iliac lymph nodes. These are located lateral, medial and, occasionally, anterior to the external iliac artery. The medial group is, essentially, the internal continuation of the deep inguinal lymphatics, receiving lymph from the superficial and deep inguinal nodes. They receive lymph from the glans, clitoris, anterior abdominal wall, the region of the obturator vessels, the neck of the bladder, the prostate, and the internal iliac nodes. The posterior (intermediate) group, situated deep to the external iliac artery near the femoral ring, receives lymph from the bladder, prostate, cervix, and upper part of the vagina.

Internal Iliac Nodes

The internal iliac lymph nodes are located chiefly at the points of origin of the branches of the internal iliac artery. The nodes receive lymph from the tissues supplied by the respective arterial branches which pass to the perineum, gluteal region, posterior thigh, and pelvic organs.

Obturator Nodes

There are one or two obturator lymph nodes. They are located at the obturator foramen close to the obturator neurovascular structures.

Sacral Nodes

The sacral lymph nodes are located in or near the midline, close to the median and lateral sacral vessels. They receive afferents from the prostate and rectum and drain to the internal iliac and lumbar nodes.

Retroperitoneal Innervation

Six nerves (Fig. 3.**17**) and the lumbar sympathetic chains are present in the retroperitoneal space. The six nerves are branches of the lumbar plexus which is formed by a branch of T12 as well as by the anterior primary rami of the first four lumbar nerves. Most of the branches of the plexus are related to the psoas major muscle, passing through it or behind it or being formed within it.

The nerves formed by the plexus are:

- Iliohypogastric.
- Ilioinguinal.
- Genitofemoral.
- Lateral femoral cutaneous.
- Obturator.
- Femoral.

Iliohypogastric Nerve: T12–L1

Arising from T12–L1 or L1 only, the iliohypogastric nerve (Fig. 3.**17a**) is the first nerve of the lumbar plexus. It emerges from the lateral border of the psoas muscle. After passing between the lower pole of the kidney and the quadratus lumborum muscle, it pierces the transversus abdominis muscle above the iliac crest and travels downward between the internal oblique muscle and the transversus abdominis muscle, supplying these muscles. It divides into two branches: the lateral cutaneous branch for the anterolateral skin of the gluteal area and the anterior cutaneous branch. The anterior cutaneous branch pierces the internal oblique 2–3 cm medial to the anterior superior iliac spine and, thereafter, penetrates the aponeurosis of the external oblique above the superficial inguinal ring. The iliohypogastric nerve supplies the skin of the suprapubic region.

Ilioinguinal Nerve: L1

The ilioinguinal nerve (Fig. 3.**17b**) has the same general pathway as the iliohypogastric nerve, piercing the internal oblique just medial to the anterior superior iliac spine. The two nerves may be combined prior to their separation in the vicinity of the superficial inguinal ring. Usually, the ilioinguinal nerve traverses the inguinal canal together with the spermatic cord, emerging through the superficial inguinal ring to supply the skin of the upper inner thigh, the root of the penis and the scrotal skin or the mons pubis and the labium majus. When the combined ventral ramus divides very late, the ilioinguinal nerve may appear as a singular entity just above the external inguinal ring, crossing

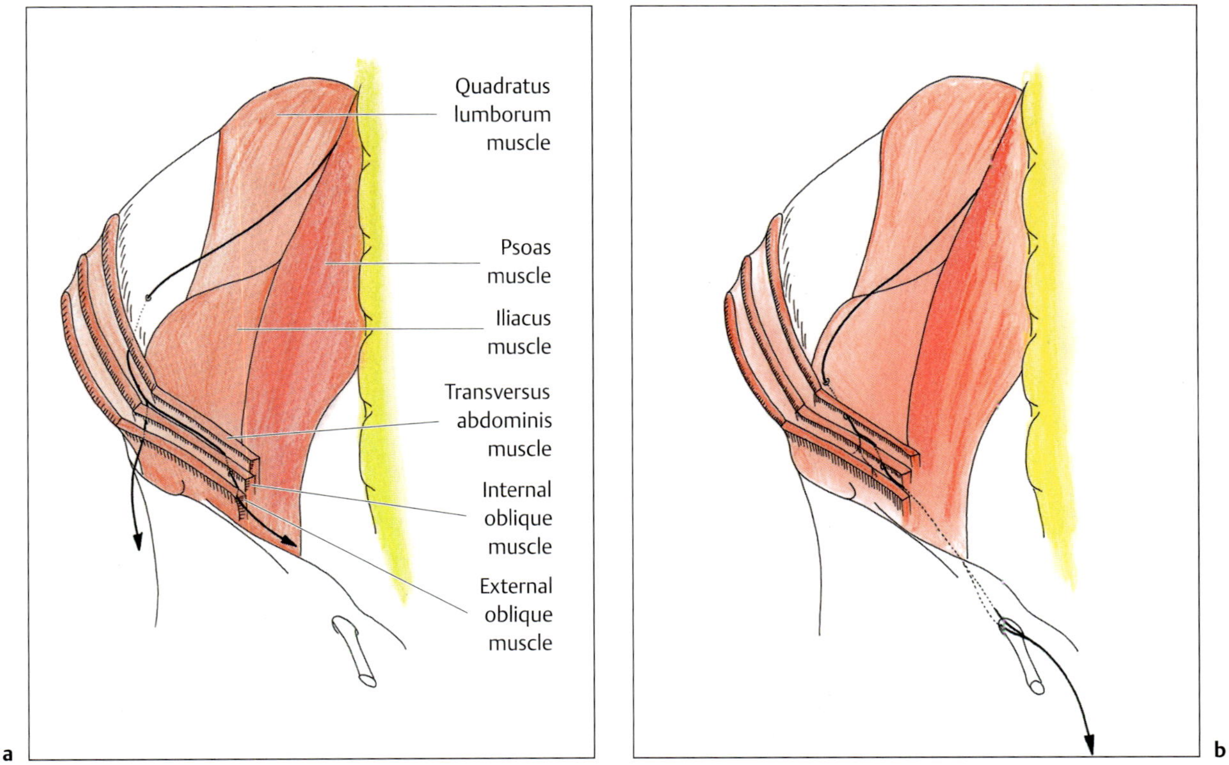

Fig. 3.**17a, b** Nerves of the retroperitoneum.

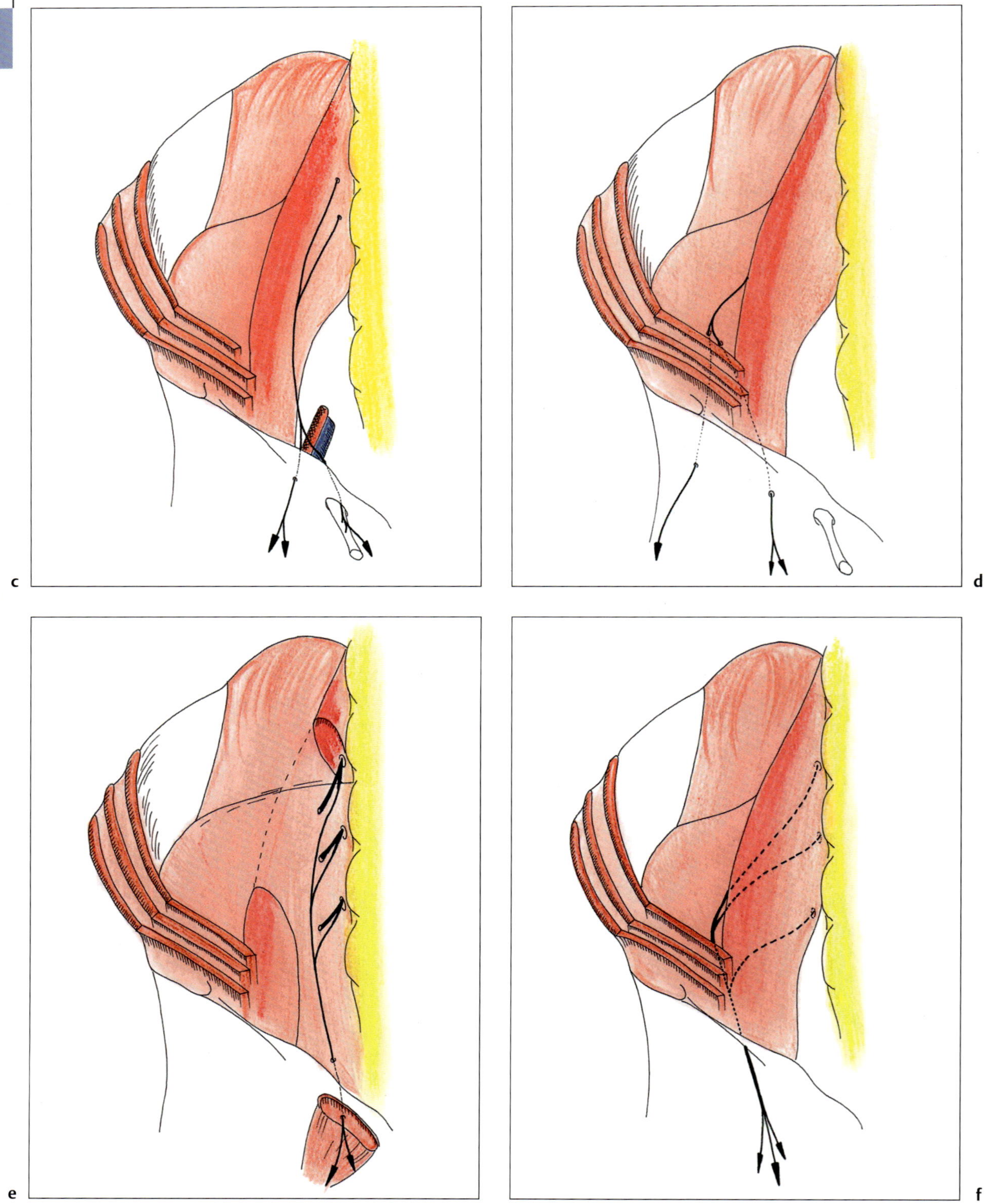

Fig. 3.**17c–f** Nerves of the retroperitoneum.

the spermatic cord obliquely to reach its lateral side and exit the lateral aspect of the ring. All or part of the ilioinguinal nerve may accompany the lateral femoral cutaneous nerve across the iliac fossa, thereafter penetrating the muscular wall to reach the inguinal canal.

Genitofemoral Nerve: L1 and L2

The genitofemoral nerve (Fig. 3.**17c**) pierces the psoas muscle anteriorly. In some cases, the two roots of the genitofemoral nerve may remain separate through their passage in the psoas muscle, joining as they emerge from the muscle. It gives origin to two branches: the genital branch and the femoral branch. The genital branch leaves the ventral surface of the psoas, passes ventral to the external iliac vessels and crosses ventral to the iliopubic tract to enter the inguinal canal just lateral to the inferior epigastric artery and the origin of the cremaster branch of the inferior epigastric artery. Passing through the inguinal canal, it supplies the cremaster muscle and part of the scrotal skin. The femoral branch passes below the inguinal ligament within the anterior layer of the femoral sheath and participates in the innervation of the skin of the triangle of Scarpa (femoral triangle).

Lateral Femoral Cutaneous Nerve: L2 and L3

The lateral femoral cutaneous nerve (Fig. 3.**17d**) emerges from the lateral border of the psoas muscle approximately at the level of L4. After perforating the inguinal ligament or passing deep to it close to the superior anterior iliac spine, it passes posterolaterally to supply the lateral aspect of the thigh.

Obturator Nerve: Anterior Divisions of L2, L3, L4

The obturator nerve (Fig. 3.**17e**) rises and courses beneath the medial border of the psoas muscle. Then, entering the true pelvis, it passes on its lateral wall to reach the obturator foramen. It traverses the obturator canal with the obturator vessels, continuing downward to innervate the adductor muscles and the skin of the medial part of the thigh.

Femoral Nerve: Posterior Divisions of L2, L3, L4

The femoral nerve (Fig. 3.**17f**) emerges from the lateral border of the psoas muscle. It is more or less concealed beneath the iliopsoas fascia between the lateral edge of the psoas and the iliacus as it passes inferiorly. It passes through the lacuna musculorum under the inguinal ligament and is closely associated with the iliopsoas muscle. It supplies the muscles of the anterior compartment of the thigh and provides sensory fibers to the anterior and medial thigh and the medial side of the leg.

Lumbar Sympathetic Chains

The right and left lumbar sympathetic chains lie right and left, respectively, along the medial border of the psoas muscle. Each chain is located anterior to the lumbar vertebrae, covered by the IVC at the right and the right paraaortic nodes at the left. Each is formed by four ganglia which vary in size and position. They communicate with each other, as well as with the thoracic trunk above and the pelvic trunk below.

Several lumbar splanchnic nerves arise from the right chain posterior to the IVC and emerge between the cava and the aorta to join the preaortic nerve plexus. The splanchnic branches of the left sympathetic chain pass laterally around the aorta to enter the nerve plexus. Lumbar splanchnic branches of the left chain pass around the lateral aspect of the aorta to enter this plexus. Communicating rami pass posterolaterally from the sympathetic chains between the lumbar vertebral discs and the tendinous origin of the psoas muscle to join the ventral primary rami of the lumbar nerve plexus.

☐ Retroperitoneal Pathology and Neoplasia

☐ Pathology

The literature on pathology of the retroperitoneal region is extensive. Chronic and acute inflammatory processes, benign and malignant neoplasms (primary or metastatic), and parasites such as filaria[42] may be found in this large, anatomically enigmatic space which extends for all practical purposes from the posterior mediastinum and neck to the pelvis and both lower extremities.

Retroperitoneal hematoma may be produced by blunt or penetrating injuries.[43] For all practical purposes, the retroperitoneum is an areolar space without geographic limitation. Therefore, hematoma may be localized or it may spread rapidly.

Khaw et al.[44] presented six cases of male patients with groin masses secondary to ruptured abdominal aortic aneurysms. They reported that the anatomic pathway from the perirenal space is the transversalis fascia leading to the inguinal area, then to the inguinal sac and finally to the scrotum. Thus, if the hematoma travels behind the transversalis fascia along the iliac vessels, it will reach the femoral ring and then the femoral triangle (Fig. 3.**18**).

Retroperitoneal hematoma may be divided into upper and lower. Most likely the lower is secondary to pelvic fractures and the upper to duodenal, pancreatic, or renal acute injury.

Remember:

- If the retroperitoneal hematoma is expanding, exploration is a must.
- If the retroperitoneal hematoma is located in the upper abdomen and related to the duodenum, pancreas or renal vessels, then exploration is also a must even if the hematoma is not expanding.

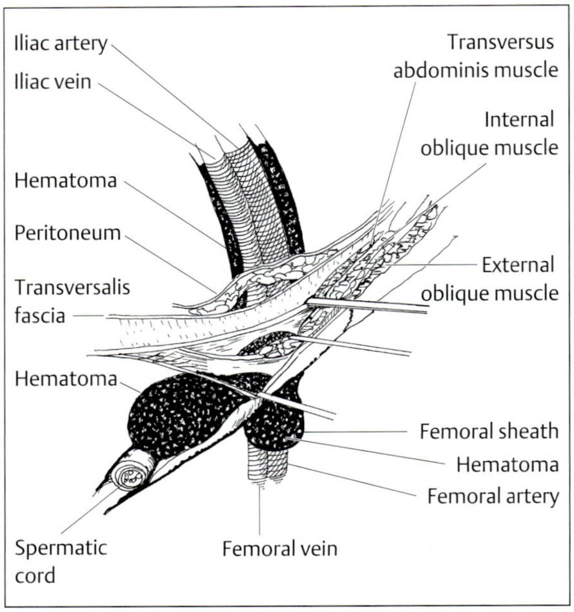

Fig. 3.**18** Hematoma from ruptured aortic aneurysm contained in retroperitoneal space by transversalis fascia. Note hematoma at superficial inguinal ring and femoral sheath.

Nobel et al. reported femoral nerve palsy secondary to iliacus hematoma.[45]
Any inflammatory process within the retroperitoneal space may involve the space in toto or just produce a localized abscess. According to Altemeier and Alexander,[46] a retroperitoneal abscess is palpable in approximately 50% of cases. This abscess may travel up to the thorax, down to the triangle of Scarpa, into the peritoneal cavity and, occasionally, may reach the anterior and posterior abdominal wall.

The genesis of a retroperitoneal abscess is due to a benign or malignant inflammatory process of parts of the digestive tract (appendix, cecum, duodenum, pancreas) or from the kidneys. Edwards and Eckhauser[47] discussed retroperitoneal perforation of the appendix presenting as subcutaneous emphysema. Paule et al.[48] described retroperitoneal lymphocele secondary to surgery of the abdominal aorta. Retroperitoneal polyarteritis nodosa[49] and necrotizing retroperitoneal fascitis[50,51] have been reported.

Remember that despite the modern armamentarium of the surgeon such as the CT scan, the etiologic factors, the pathogenesis, and the pathway of the abscess are occasionally difficult to deduce. Crepps et al.[52] stated that the most common causes of isolated retroperitoneal abscesses in their series were renal disease and postoperative infection. Limited drainage or wide exploration of the retroperitoneal space are the treatments of choice. Michel and Pagliano[53] reported a retroperitoneal abscess with rupture to the peritoneal cavity, comparing it to intraperitoneal rupture of a pyonephrosis.

Retroperitoneal collection of chyle is secondary to injury of the cisterna chyli. Chyle collection secondary to injury of a duct is possible but rare. The cisterna chyli or any affected duct may be ligated with impunity.

The pathway of retroperitoneal collection is very peculiar. It may travel upward (thoracic cavity: through the esophageal hiatus), downward (scrotum, femoral triangle: under the inguinal ligament), or laterally (right or left paracolic gutter). The pressure of gas (air) in the retroperitoneal space is most likely secondary to perforation of the gastrointestinal tract. Such perforations may be secondary to trauma, infection, and occasionally gas secondary to hidden retroperitoneal abscess.

Retroperitoneal fibrosis (RPF) is a rare idiopathic medical entity of the retroperitoneal layers and spaces. It involves retroperitoneal organs such as ureters, vessels, parts of the gastrointestinal tract, etc. Ureteric and colonic obstruction has been reported secondary to RPF.[54]

Dagradi et al.[55] reported the removal of a cystic mass from the "*upper retroperitoneal space*" of a 47-year-old patient. The mass had been present since birth and contained hairs and bony structures.

☐ Neoplasia

There is an abundance of embryonic connective tissue which is of mesodermal and neural crest ectodermal origin in the retroperitoneal space. This is the mesenchyme which becomes loose connective tissue as well as adipose tissue.

This agrees with the histologic picture of mesenchyme since loose areolar and adipose-reticular tissue perhaps compose most of the retroperitoneal connective tissue which for all practical purposes is a support network for the anatomic entities which are located in the retroperitoneal space.

According to Foster and Skandalakis,[56] retroperitoneal soft tissue sarcomas are not common tumors, since they comprise 10–20% of all soft tissue sarcomas in adults. If sarcomas originating in the adrenal glands or the kidneys are removed from the total, then retroperitoneal malignancies rise to 40–70%. Lymphomas account for 15–30% of the total with other less common tumors making up the remainder. Liposarcoma is the most frequent retroperitoneal sarcoma. Singer et al.[57] stated that retroperitoneal sarcoma is less than 1% of all malignant tumors and perhaps 10% of all sarcomas. Bautista et al.[58] reported that liposarcomas (61%) are the most common pathology, leiomyosarcomas (30%) and other tumors such as histiocytoma and hemangioendothelioma perhaps 8–9%.

Retroperitoneal sarcomas should be removed in toto with a healthy margin.[43] As we know, cancer does not respect spaces, subspaces, territories, or frontiers. In the retroperitoneal space, as everywhere else, the word is invasion. Cervical, uterine, prostate, bladder, and colon cancers can metastasize to the retroperitoneal lymph nodes.[41] Therefore, anatomic or surgicoanatomic territories will not stop the extension of cancer up and down, medially and laterally as well as deep.

Levine et al.[59] presented the occurrence of bilateral diffuse orbital retrobulbar masses and retroperitoneal fibrosis. Retroperitoneal fibrosis with scirrhous gastric cancer was reported by Dohmen et al.[60] Retroperitoneal fibrosis as a host response to papillary renal cell carcinoma was reported by Fromowitz and Miller.[61]

Gheysens et al.[62] reported a case of retroperitoneal Castelman's disease. Miyashita et al.[63] reviewed the literature on primary retroperitoneal synovial sarcoma.

Hida et al.[64] removed a retroperitoneal schwannoma, a lumbar paraspinal lesion. De Peralta et al.[65] stated that retroperitoneal cysts of muellerian type require excision, rather than less radical procedures, because of a possible malignant component. Retroperitoneal ganglioneuroma was reported by Lambruschi et al.[66] Posner et al.[67] reported diffuse retroperitoneal amyloidosis. Retroperitoneal sarcoidosis was reported by Bach and Vellet[68] and a retroperitoneal bronchogenic cyst was reported by Foerster et al.[69]

☐ Surgery

The retroperitoneum can be approached and explored by several routes including the transperitoneal route and the extraperitoneal route. Flummerfelt and Karakousis[70] advised a combination of extraperitoneal and transperitoneal dissection for the removal of retroperitoneal tumors. Incision is made with the patient in a lateral supine position.

Malerba et al.[71] reported the radical surgical treatment of 42 patients with primary retroperitoneal soft tissue sarcomas. The 5-year survival was 48.1% and 5-year disease-free rate was 38.8%. The authors recommended wide surgical excision as the best chance for long-term survival.

There are two accepted procedures used for diagnosis of retroperitoneal injuries and for exploration of the involved anatomic entities. The Cattell maneuver exposes right-sided structures. The Mattox maneuver exposes left-sided structures.

Cattell maneuver (Fig. 3.**19**):

- Step 1 Incise the lateral peritoneum along the cecum, ascending colon, and hepatic flexure.
- Step 2 Divide the white line of Toldt (peritoneal reflection at the area of the lateral wall of the cecum and ascending colon).
- Step 3 Perform duodenal mobilization (Kocherization).
- Step 4 Mobilize all right-sided anatomic entities anteromedially.

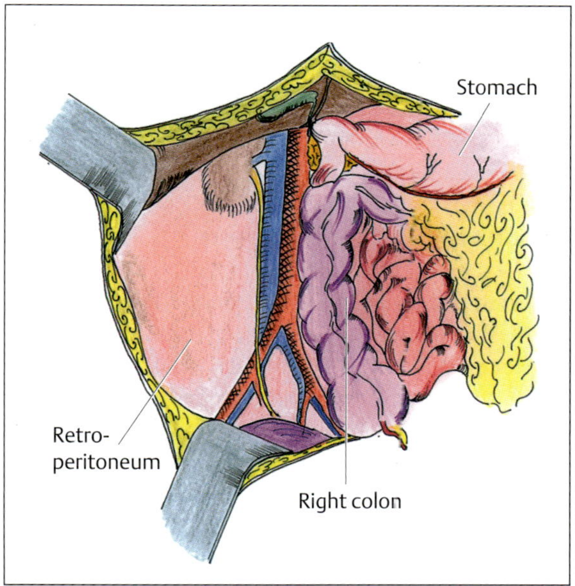

Fig. 3.**19** Right-sided approach to exposure of retroperitoneal structures using Cattell maneuver.

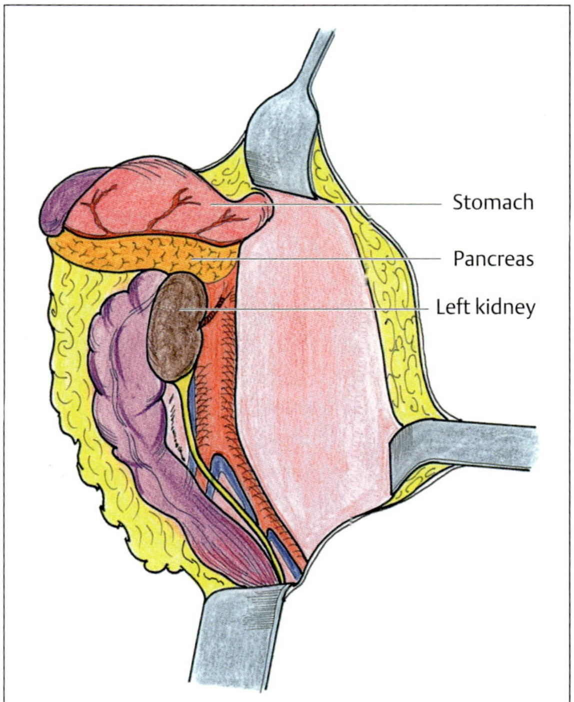

Fig. 3.**20** Mattox maneuver to expose retroperitoneum from left side.

Mattox maneuver (Fig. 3.**20**):

- Step 1 Incise the lateral peritoneum along the splenic flexure, descending colon, and upper sigmoid.
- Step 2 Divide the white line of Toldt.
- Step 3 Carefully mobilize the spleen, including the pancreatic tail, stomach, and left colon.
- Step 4 Gently push all left-sided anatomic entities anteromedially

Capelouto et al.[72] stated that safe and reliable primary retroperitoneal access can be performed for laparoscopy and laparoscopic surgery. Hulbert,[73] Gaur et al.,[74] and Chiu and Babayan[75] also reported on the "*laparoscopic*" approach to the retroperitoneal space.

Anatomic Complications

The anatomic complications of retroperitoneal surgery are the complications of the organs located in the several compartments of the retroperitoneal space.

We quote from Foster and Skandalakis[56]:

- The most commonly reported major complications of resection of retroperitoneal sarcomas are intraabdominal abscess, enterocutaneous fistula, and intraabdominal bleeding. Specific structures that can be injured include the pancreas, small and large bowels, ureter, retroperitoneal lymphatic vessels, including the cisterna chyli and retroperitoneal nerves.
- Manipulation of the pancreas may induce pancreatitis. Injury to or partial resection of the pancreas that opens up the ductal system may lead to a pancreatic leak and fistula.
- Entry into the intestine or compromise of the blood supply to the bowel that is not recognized and satisfactorily repaired can lead to abdominal sepsis of fistula. Sepsis in the area of a major vessel, particularly if the vessel has been injured, may be accompanied by bleeding.
- If an extensive pelvic dissection interrupts the iliac and pelvic lymphatic vessels, permanent leg edema may develop. Dissection behind the aorta on or cephalad to L2 may injure the cisterna chyli or lymphatic trunk and, if unrecognized, lead to a lymphatic fistula. If necessary, these structures may be ligated with impunity.
- Injury to the ureter may lead to hydronephrosis or urinary fistula.
- Injury to any of six peripheral nerves coursing through the lumbar space (iliohypogastric, ilioinguinal, genitofemoral, lateral femoral cutaneous, obturator, femoral) can lead to dysesthesia or anesthesia over the cutaneous sensory distribution of the nerve. Injury to the femoral or obturator nerves may, in addition, result in motor loss in the anterior and medial thigh muscles, respectively.
- During extensive retroperitoneal dissection it is important to maintain the patient's body temperature to prevent the coagulopathy that can occur with hypothermia.

McDougall et al.[76] reported on retroperitoneal laparoscopic surgery and balloon dilatation of the retroperitoneal space through the inferior lumbar triangle. Among 12 patients (10 nephrectomies, one partial nephrectomy, and one nephropexy), there was minimal morbidity, no mortality, and only two complications (pneumothorax and right hip bruise).

References

1. Periureteric fibrosis. Editorial. *Lancet*. 1957;2:780–781.
2. Hinman F. *Atlas of Urosurgical Anatomy*. Philadelphia: Saunders; 1993.
3. Skandalakis JE, Celborn GL, Weidman TA, Foster RS Jr, Kingnorth AN, Skandalakis LJ. Surgical Anatomy: The Embryologic and Anatomic Basis of Modern Surgery. Athens, GR: Paschalidis Medical Publication; 2004.
4. Pack GT, Tabah EJ. Primary retroperitoneal tumors. *Intl Abstr Surg*. 1954;99:209–231.
5. Nunn CR, Cullinane DC, Morris JA Jr. Retroperitoneal injury. In: Cameron JL, ed. *Current Surgical Therapy*. 6th ed. St Louis: Mosby; 1998:964–969.
6. Falcone RA Jr, Luchette FA, Choe KA et al. Zone I retroperitoneal hematoma identified by computed tomography scan as an indicator of significant abdominal injury. *Surgery*. 1999;126:608–615.
7. Trerotola SO, Kuhlman JE, Fishman EK. Bleeding complications of femoral catheterization: CT evaluation. *Radiology*. 1990;174:37–40.
8. Chaffanjon P, Mollier S, Le Bas JF, Champetier J. Original oblique sections of the retroperitoneum: radio-anatomic basis. *Surg Radiol Anat*. 1995;17:319–324.
9. Meyers MA. *Dynamic Radiology of the Abdomen*. 5th ed. New York: Springer; 2000.
10. Oliphant M, Berne AS. Computed tomography of the subperitoneal space: Demonstration of direct spread of intraabdominal disease. *J Comput Assist Tomogr*. 1982;6: 1127–1137.
11. Oliphant M, Berne AS. Holistic concept of the anatomy of the abdomen: A basis for understanding direct spread of disease. *Contemp Diagn Radiol*. 1985;8:1–6.
12. Oliphant M, Berne AS, Meyers MA. Subperitoneal Spread of Intraabdominal Disease. In: Meyers MA, ed. *Computed Tomography of the Gastrointestinal Tract: Including the Peritoneal Cavity and Mesenteries*. New York: Springer; 1986: 95–136.
13. Oliphant M, Berne AS, Meyers MA. The subperitoneal space of the abdomen and pelvis: Planes of continuity. *AJR*. 1996;167:1433–1439.
14. Oliphant M, Berne AS, Meyers MA. The subserous thoracoabdominal continuum: Embryologic basis and diagnostic imaging of disease spread. *Abdom Imaging*. 1999; 24:211–219.
15. Santaella RO, Fishman EK, Lipsett PA. Primary vs. secondary iliopsoas abscess: presentation, microbiology and treatment. *Arch Surg*. 1995;130:1309–1313.
16. Nathanson SD, Sonnino R. An anatomic approach to tumors of the psoas major muscle. *Surgery*. 1987;101:763–766.
17. Last RJ. *Anatomy: Regional and Applied*. 5th ed. Baltimore: Williams Wilkins; 1972.
18. Reich P, Schreiber HW, Lierse W. The mesoduodenum. *Langenbecks Arch Chir*. 1988;373:182–188.
19. Raptopoulos V, Lei QF, Touliopoulos P et al. Why perirenal disease does not extend into the pelvis: the importance of closure of the cone of the renal fasciae. *AJR*. 1995;164: 1179–1184.

20. Love L, Meyers MA, Churchill RJ et al. Computed tomography of extraperitoneal spaces. *AJR.* 1981;136:781–789.
21. Meyers MA, Whalen JP, Peelie K, Berne AS. Radiologic features of extraperitoneal effusions. *Radiology.* 1972;104: 249–257.
22. Parienty RA, Pradel J, Picard JD et al. Visibility and thickening of the renal fascia on computed tomograms. *Radiology.* 1981;139:119–124.
23. Rubenstein WA, Whalen JP. Extraperitoneal spaces. *AJR.* 1986;147:1162–1164.
24. Dodds WJ, Darweesh RMA, Lawson TL. The retroperitoneal spaces revisited. *AJR.* 1986;147:1155–1161.
25. Korobkin M, Silverman PM, Quint LE, Francis IR. CT of the extraperitoneal space: normal anatomy and fluid collections. *AJR.* 1992;159:933–941.
26. Mindell HJ, Mastromatteo JF, Dickey KW et al. Anatomic communications between the three retroperitoneal spaces: determination by CT-guided injections of contrast material in cadavers. *AJR.* 1995;164:1173–1178.
27. Raptopoulos V, Kleinman PK, Mark S et al. Renal fascia pathway: posterior extension of pancreatic effusions within the anterior pararenal space. *Radiology.* 1986;158: 367–374.
28. Feldberg MAM, Koehler PR, van Waes PFGM. Psoas compartment disease studied by computed tomography. *Radiology.* 1983;148:505–512.
29. Kneeland JB, Auh YH, Rubenstein WA. Perirenal spaces: CT evidence for communication across the midline. *Radiology.* 1987;164:657–664.
30. Hopper KD, Sherman JL, Ghaed N. Aortic rupture into retroperitoneum. *AJR.* 1985;145:435–437.
31. Hureau J, Agossou-Voyeme AK, Germain M, Pradel J. The posterior interparieto-peritoneal or retroperitoneal spaces. 1: Normal topographic anatomy. *J Radiol.* 1991;72:101–116.
32. Hureau J, Pradel J, Agossou-Voyeme AK, Germain M. The posterior interparieto-peritoneal or retroperitoneal spaces. 2: Pathological X-ray computed tomographic image. *J Radiol.* 1991;72:205–227.
33. Basmajian JV, Slonecker CE. *Grant's Method of Anatomy.* 11th ed. Baltimore: Williams Wilkins; 1989.
34. Greig HW, Anson BJ, Coleman SS. The inferior phrenic artery: Types of origin in 850 body-halves and diaphragmatic relationship. *Quart Bull Northwestern Univ M School.* 1951;25:345.
35. Heberer G, van Dongen RJAM. *Vascular Surgery.* New York: Springer; 1989.
36. Alusio FV, Berens AS, Colborn GL et al. Examination of the collateral flow and anomalies of the left renal vein with clinical correlations. *J Med Assoc Ga.* 1991;80:429–433.
37. Grant JCB, Basmajian JV. *Grant's Method of Anatomy.* 7th ed. Baltimore: Williams Wilkins; 1965.
38. Williams PL, ed. *Gray's Anatomy.* 38th ed. New York: Churchill Livingstone; 1995.
39. Rhee RY, Gloviczki P. Lymphatic Disease. In: Dean RH, Yao JST, Brewster DC, eds. *Current Diagnosis and Treatment in Vascular Surgery.* Norwalk CT: Appleton Lange; 1995:391–404.
40. Healey JE Jr, Hodge J. *Surgical Anatomy.* Philadelphia: BC Decker; 1990.
41. Grossman HB, Belville WD, Faerber GJ et al. Male anatomy and physiology. In: Greenfield LJ, ed. *Surgery: Scientific Principles and Practice.* 2nd ed. Philadelphia: Lippincott-Raven; 1997:2199–2216.
42. Roussel F, Delaville A, Campos H et al. Retroperitoneal human dirofilariasis with a pseudotumoral presentation. *Acta Cytol.* 1993;37:980–981.
43. Nunn CR, Cullinane DC, Morris JA Jr. Retroperitoneal Injury. In: Cameron JL, ed. *Current Surgical Therapy.* 6th ed. St Louis: Mosby; 1998:964–969.
44. Khaw H, Sottiurai VS, Craighead CC, Batson RC. Ruptured abdominal aortic aneurysm presenting as symptomatic inguinal mass: report of six cases. *J Vasc Surg.* 1986;4:384–389.
45. Nobel W, Marks SC, Kubik S. The anatomical basis for femoral nerve palsy following iliacus hematoma. *J Neurosurg.* 1980;52:533–540.
46. Altemeier WA, Alexander JW. Retroperitoneal abscess. *Arch Surg.* 1961;83:512–524.
47. Edwards JD, Eckhauser FE. Retroperitoneal perforation of the appendix presenting as subcutaneous emphysema of the thigh. *Dis Col Rect.* 1986;29:456–458.
48. Paule AM, Le Dreff P, Nonent M et al. Retroperitoneal lymphocele: a rarely reported complication of abdominal aortic surgery. *Ann Radiol (Paris).* 1994;37:270–273.
49. Lie JT. Retroperitoneal polyarteritis nodosa presenting as ureteral obstruction. *J Rheumatol.* 1992;19:1628–1631.
50. Jayatunga AP, Caplan S, Paes TR. Survival after retroperitoneal necrotizing fascitis. *Br J Surg.* 1993;80:981.
51. Mokoena T. Survival after retroperitoneal necrotizing fascitis [letter]. *Br J Surg.* 1994;81:722.
52. Crepps JT, Welch JP, Orlando R III. Management and outcome of retroperitoneal abscesses. *Ann Surg.* 1987; 205:276–281.
53. Michel P, Pagliano G. Peritonitis caused by rupture of a retroperitoneal abscess. *J Chir (Paris).* 1993;130:240–246.
54. Leone JP, Ngyen-Minh NC, Lee DA et al. Retroperitoneal fibrosis: a report of complete colonic obstruction. *Am Surg.* 1997;63:475–477.
55. Dagradi AD, Mangiante GL, Serio GE, Musajo FG. Fetus in fetu removal in a 47-year-old man. *Surgery.* 1992;112: 598–602.
56. Foster RS Jr, Skandalakis JE. Retroperitoneum. In: Wood WC, Skandalakis JE, eds. *Anatomic Basis of Tumor Surgery.* St Louis: Quality Medical; 1999:762–781.
57. Singer S, Corson JM, Demetri GD. Prognostic factors predictive of survival for truncal and retroperitoneal soft-tissue sarcoma. *Ann Surg.* 1995;221:185–195.
58. Bautista N, Su W, O'Connell TX. Retroperitoneal soft-tissue sarcomas: Prognosis and treatment of primary and recurrent disease. *Am Surg.* 2000;66:832–836.
59. Levine MR, Kaye L, Mair S, Bates J. Multifocal fibrosclerosis: report of a case of bilateral idiopathic sclerosing pseudotumor and retroperitoneal fibrosis. *Arch Ophthalmol.* 1993;111:841–843.
60. Dohmen K, Mizukami Y, Tanaka K et al. Retroperitoneal fibrosis associated with scirrhous gastric cancer. *Gastroenterolog Jpn.* 1993;28:699–705.
61. Fromowitz FB, Miller F. Retroperitoneal fibrosis as host response to papillary renal cell carcinoma. *Urology.* 1991;38:259–253.
62. Gheysens B, Baste JC, Midy D et al. Retroperitoneal Castelman disease: apropos of a new case. *J Chir (Paris).* 1994: 131:492–495.
63. Mayashita T, Inamura T, Ishikawa Y et al. Primary retroperitoneal synovial sarcoma. *Intern Med.* 1994;33:692–696.
64. Hida K, Iwasaki Y, Abe H et al. Schwannoma in the psoas muscle removed by the retroperitoneal approach. *Br J Neurosurg.* 1993;7:213–215.

1

65. De Peralta MN, Delahoussaye PM, Tornos CS, Silva EG. Benign retroperitoneal cysts of muellerian type: a clinicopathologic study of three cases and review of the literature. *Int J Gynecol Pathol.* 1994; 13:273–8.
66. Lambruschi G, Tagliagambe A, Palla L et al. Ganglioneuroma: the diagnostic procedure in a case of retroperitoneal localization. *Radiol Med (Torino).* 1992;84:328–330.
67. Posner R, Saks AM, Leiman G. Diffuse retroperitoneal amyloidosis: further radiological observations. *Br J Radiol.* 1991;64:469–471.
68. Bach DB, Vellet AD. Retroperitoneal sarcoidosis. *AJR.* 1991; 156:520–522.
69. Foerster HM, Sengupta EE, Montag AG, Kaplan EL. Retroperitoneal bronchogenic cyst presenting as an adrenal mass. *Arch Pathol Lab Med.* 1991;115:1057–1059.
70. Flummerfelt PM, Karakousis CP. Combined extraperitoneal and transperitoneal dissection in removal of retroperitoneal tumors. *Contemp Surg.* 1998;52:407–411.
71. Malerba M, Doglietto GB, Pacelli F et al. Primary retroperitoneal soft tissue sarcomas : results of aggressive surgical treatment. World J Surg 1999; 23:670-5.
72. Capelouto CC, Moore RG, Silverman SG, Kavoussi LR. Retroperitoneoscopy: anatomical rationale for direct retroperitoneal access. *J Urol.* 1994;152:2008–2010.
73. Hulbert JC. Laparoscopic approach to the retroperitoneum. *Semin Urol.* 1992;10:227–231.
74. Gaur DD, Agarwal DK, Purohit KC, Darshane AS. Laparoscopic condom dissection: new technique of retroperitoneoscopy. *J Endourol.* 1994;8:149–151.
75. Chiu AW, Babayan RK. Retroperitoneal laparoscopic nephrectomy utilizing three-dimensional camera: case report. *J Endourol.* 1994:139–141.
76. McDougall EM, Clayman RV, Fadden PT. Retroperitoneoscopy: the Washington University Medical School experience. *Urology.* 1994;43:446–452.

Upper Gastro-intestinal Tract

2

4 Esophagus

Ronald F. Martin

Esophageal neoplasms pose a significant challenge to physicians, surgeons, and health-care workers of many types. They pose medical system challenges relating to the capacity to screen and identify them in patients and this challenge persists to the level of how to best palliate those patients who suffer from incurable lesions. At every step in the care of these patients there is a significant challenge to providing any service whether it is diagnostic or therapeutic. Epidemiologically, adenocarcinoma of the distal esophagus is among the neoplasms with greatest increasing incidence in North America over the past few decades.

The purpose of this chapter is to outline and discuss in some detail the considerations for resection of tumors of the esophagus. This chapter will not attempt to persuade or dissuade anyone into a belief of what is the "right" operation for any given patient. The primary reason for this is because there is no "right" answer that serves all patients in all places. Differences in available resources including physicians, equipment, and monetary resources as well as differing expectations of patients and the societies in which they live will surely play as large a role as anything in which choice will be best for a given patient. The goal of this chapter is to illustrate a basic framework of the problems as they present and the solutions that are available. Furthermore, some attempt to evaluate the nature and utility of these solutions is made, based on the data that is available to us as of the time of writing.

The histologic types of esophageal cancers that surgeons predominantly concern themselves with are squamous cell carcinoma and adenocarcinoma. Sarcomas (leiomyosarcoma, rhabdomyosarcoma, and synovial cell sarcoma), lymphomas (Hodgkin's and non-Hodgkin's) and lesions metastatic to the esophagus comprise a smaller subset of esophageal malignancies. Squamous cell cancer is the most common esophageal cancer on a worldwide basis but the incidence of adenocarcinoma of the esophagus surpassed that of squamous cell cancer in North American males during the 1990s. In patients who have squamous cell cancer of the esophagus, the primary tumor is located in the cervical portion in about 6% of patients, the upper thoracic esophagus in about 7% of patients, and 61 and 26% in the middle and lower portions of the esophagus, respectively. Esophageal adenocarcinomas are predominantly located in the distal third of the organ. The distinction between distal third esophageal cancers and "junctional" tumors of the esophagogastric junction is somewhat blurry at best. These tumors share characteristics of both esophageal and gastric tumors. As such, some of the issues that apply to more proximal esophageal tumors may be less relevant or not at all relevant to these "nearly abdominal" tumors.

Table 4.**1** TNM Staging of esophageal carcinoma

Tumor	
Tis	Carcinoma in situ
T1	Invades submucosa
T2	Invades muscularis propria
T3	Invades adventitia
T4	Invades adjacent tissue
Node	
N0	No lymph nodes involved
N1	Lymph node(s) involved
Metastasis	
Mx	Metastasis cannot be assessed
M0	No distant metastasis
M1	Distant metastasis

In determining which operation is best for potential curative resection of esophageal cancer, there are three main concerns: the radial margin of resection, the longitudinal margin of resection, and the extent of lymphadenectomy. Since many operations for esophageal cancer are unlikely to cure patients with esophageal cancer, there must also be proper consideration of palliative issues as well. The same concerns about resection apply to palliative procedures as to curative procedures but other factors such as involvement of adjacent organs must be considered as well. In the absence of metastatic disease, patients with direct extension of tumor into adjacent viscera remain in the Stage III category (Tables 4.**1** and 4.**2** for TNM Classification and Stage Groupings). While survival for patients with stage III disease is worse than for those patients with lower stage disease, there are still a significant percentage of survivors reported at 5 years.[1] Neither the stance of "nihilism" nor of "irrational exuberance" as regards the benefit, or lack thereof, of esophageal resection for cancer is supported by the literature. The series with the best reported outcomes show significant 5-year mortality for resection of all but Stage I disease and show some benefit to resection in all but the most advanced,

2

Table 4.2 Stage groupings for esophageal cancer

Stage	T	N	M
0	Tis	N0	M0
I	T1	N0	M0
IIA			
	T2	N0	M0
	T3	N0	M0
IIB			
	T1	N1	M0
	T2	N1	M0
III			
	T3	N1	M0
	T4	Any	M0
IV	Any	Any	M1

Stage IV, patients. So the truth would appear to lie somewhere in between unbridled optimism and pessimism. In many cases the difference in patient outcome will depend upon the skill of the people caring for the patient more than the disease of the patient; but the most important skill may be choosing the correct operation for the right patient and then performing the operation correctly.

Extent of Resection

The desired extent of resection is predominantly judged on one of two criteria: survival advantage or anastomotic recurrence/local failure. The most consistently recognized prognostic factor portending a good long-term outcome is an R0 resection. To qualify as an R0 resection, the specimen must include the primary tumor and adjacent lymphatic tissue and have microscopically clear proximal, distal, and radial margins.[2]

The longitudinal margin of resection must address removal of the primary tumor plus any tissue that is likely to harbor intramural metastatic neoplasm. Multifocal disease or intramural metastatic disease is estimated to occur in as many as 25–30% of patients.[3] Longitudinal clear margins of resection that are 10 cm or greater in length are associated with a chance of anastomotic recurrence that is less than 5%.[4]

Radial margins should also be microscopically free of tumor whenever possible. The ability to safely achieve this goal is somewhat dependent upon the location of the primary tumor. For those tumors located in the proximal portion of the esophagus, this may be achieved by en bloc resection of the proximal esophagus and the proximal airway structures with concomitant reconstruction.[5] Tumors located below the tracheal bifurcation can be resected en bloc with adjacent structures such as pericardium, pleura, lung, periaortic tissue, thoracic duct, and azygos vein.[6,7] Technical details of this will be discussed later in this chapter. For those tumors located in direct continuity to the trachea (unless superficial, T1 or T2) or in those with tumor penetration into the aortic wall or myocardium, R0 resections are unachievable. Therefore, proposed resection of these most locally aggressive of tumors is ill advised. Microscopic tumor involvement of any margin (R1) confers a significantly worse outcome probability with a higher likelihood of local failure.[6]

The last, and most controversial, factor in deciding extent of resection regards the degree of lymph node resection that is appropriate. This decision may also lead to discussion of which route of approach is best for esophageal resection as well. Lymphatic involvement in esophageal cancer is thought to happen early in the biological process. In patients in whom there is submucosal penetration of the primary tumor, lymphatic involvement is found in as many as 50% of patients. Involvement of the muscularis mucosae is associated with up to 30% lymph node metastasis.[8,9] Intramucosal tumors are rarely associated with lymph node involvement. As a result of this recognized high occurrence of lymph node involvement with relatively superficial tumors, much interest has been generated in the extent to which lymph node dissection should be carried out. The three fields that are generally considered are the cervical nodes, the thoracic nodes, and the abdominal nodes. A two-field dissection usually refers to the thoracic and abdominal nodes. There is little controversy over the extent of abdominal lymph node dissection as it is a technically straightforward endeavor and confers little morbidity. The thoracic lymph node dissection is certainly only performed via a transthoracic approach. DeMeester and colleagues favored this approach as a superior operation in part because of its purported improved nodal clearance.[10] While others, such as Orringer and colleagues, have suggested that the degree of lymphadenectomy may be more related to staging than prognosis and therefore have championed the transhiatal approach for esophageal resection.[11] The benefit of cervical lymph node dissection is a little more difficult to assess. In a report from Japan, surgeons found that cervical lymph nodes were involved by metastatic tumor in up to approximately 46% of patients with proximal cancers, 28% with middle third cancers, and 28% with distal third cancers.[9] These findings have generated a great deal of enthusiasm for three-field lymphatic clearance. Other Japanese studies have reported a survival advantage for three-field lymph node dissection over two-field lymphadenectomy.[8,12,13] While randomized trials have shown a survival benefit trend, no statistical significance was attained.[13,14] Nearly all of the patients in these reports had squamous cell carcinoma and whether or not this data correlates well with the population of patients who have adenocarcinoma of the esophagus is unclear.

Two western studies have been reported using three-field lymphadenectomy for adenocarcinoma of the esophagus. Both studies showed pathologic involvement of cervical lymph nodes (27 and 30%) and, in both series, the preponderance of tumors were located in the distal third of the esophagus.[15,16] Neither study showed a survival advantage of three-field lymphatic clearance over two-field.

The three-field lymphadenectomy also has some substantial potential for concern. The cervical field nodal dissection is associated with significant morbidity, in particular related to the high incidence of inferior laryngeal nerve injury leading to vocal cord paralysis. This associated morbidity has been reported in as much as 70% of patients undergoing a cervical node dissection as part of a three-field lymphadenectomy.[17] Given the profound negative effect on quality of life associated with vocal cord paralysis (especially if bilateral) in patients with either short- or long-term expectations for survival, one is faced with a potentially difficult ethical dilemma as a surgeon on whether to offer the additional nodal clearance. It would seem reasonable at this time to focus the efforts of three-field lymphadenectomy to centers with experienced operators and excellent ability to measure and track outcomes before widely recommending the adoption of this technique.

Lung and Airway Involvement

Invasion of the lungs or major airways by local extension of an esophageal cancer is frequently a harbinger of an ominous outcome. The more central the airway invasion the less likely that operative intervention will be associated with a satisfactory long-term outcome. Esophageal cancer can directly invade the major airways or the lung parenchyma itself. Pulmonary invasion by esophageal cancer must be clearly distinguished from metastatic disease to lung. Pulmonary or airway involvement may or may not be associated with fistulous communication between the esophagus and the bronchial system.

While direct extension of esophageal tumor to lung or airways is usually associated with imminent patient demise, there have been reports of operative management of patients in these precarious circumstances (Figs. 4.1, 4.2). In two reports from Japan, patients benefit from en bloc resection of esophagus with the affected lung tissue. In the first report, esophagectomy with concomitant resection of the affected lung was compared with esophageal resection without lung resection. The 5-year survival rates of the groups are 21.1 and 8.7%, respectively.[18] A subsequent report evaluated patients who had either undergone a previous significant pulmonary operation or had undergone a concurrent pulmonary resection with esophagectomy. The authors conclude that major concomitant or previous pulmonary operation was not a contraindication to esophageal resection on the basis of survival rates of 92 and 45% at 1 and 3 years, respectively.[19] The patient population in this study reflected only 18 patients and

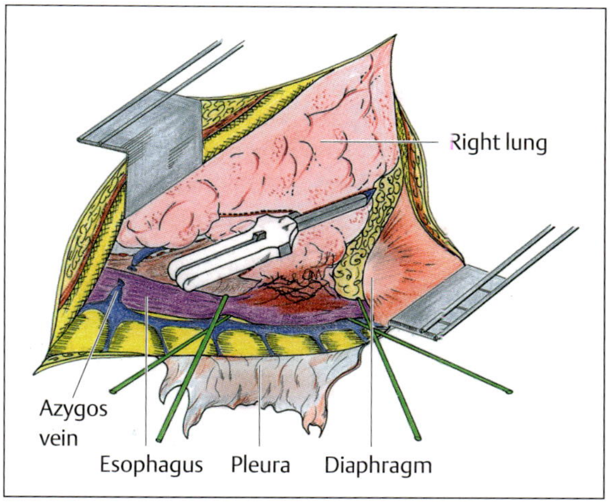

Fig. 4.1 Right posterolateral thoracotomy (see also p. 58). The parietal pleura has been removed and the azygos venous system is exposed. The azygos vein is tied and cut. The esophagus is dissected and encircled with 2 Penrose drains. The lower lobe of the right lung is invaded by the tumor. Before completion of the proximal esophageal dissection, the lung parenchyma is stapled. It will be removed with the esophagus.

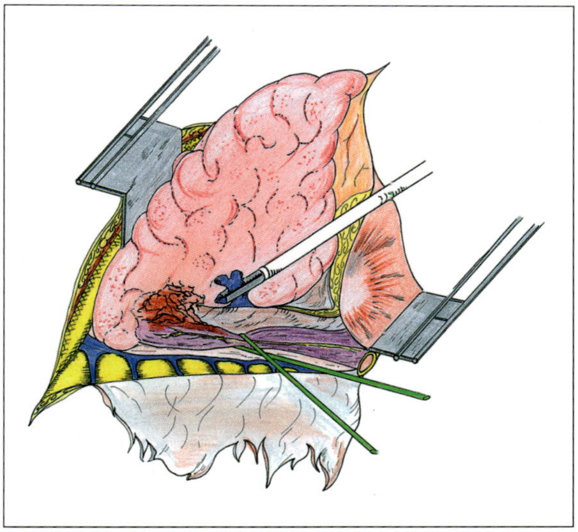

Fig. 4.2 En bloc right lower lobectomy and esophagectomy. The esophagus is exposed distal to the invasion of the lung parenchyma. The lower lobe is removed without opening the tumoral adhesions. After interrupting the right distal pulmonary artery, the pulmonary vein is here stapled. The lower lobe is then downward retracted and the proximal esophagus is prepared.

2

significant complications, though not fatal, were seen in 13 of these cases.

Matsubara and colleagues reported a series of 55 patients who were treated with esophagectomy and resection of a major airway structure over a 20-year period. Patients in whom resection was possible with clear margins and no lymph node involvement enjoyed the best results, 19% at 5 years.[5] Whether or not the patients who had responded to neo-adjuvant therapy garnered additional benefit from the ensuing resection remains uncertain. One study from the United States shows less favorable long-term results but also favors resection for local control when technically feasible.[20]

Nonresective Therapy

No current discussion of esophageal resection can be complete without some discussion of the nonoperative components for treatment of the patient with esophageal cancer. The use of a multimodality approach is widely employed in both adjuvant and neo-adjuvant settings although its exact benefit is not yet fully agreed upon.

Preoperative radiation therapy alone is possibly associated with decreased local failure rates but its overall survival advantage has not been demonstrated.[21–26] Postoperative radiation therapy has been suggested to reduce local failure in two trials but not to show survival advantage.[27,28] In another trial utilizing postoperative radiation therapy, increased early death and morbidity were seen secondary to injury to the esophageal replacement conduit.[29] Overall survival disadvantage was seen in the surgery plus radiation therapy group.

Neo-adjuvant chemotherapy has been shown to exert a significant downstaging effect on about 50% of patients with about 10% having a complete pathologic response.[25,30–33] It is not clear whether this will show a long-term survival advantage. The usual chemotherapeutic regimens include cisplatin and 5-fluorouracil.

Neo-adjuvant chemoradiation is currently the preoperative therapy that we most employ for a patient in whom there is evidence to suggest a T3 or greater tumor or high likelihood of nodal involvement. While results of many trials are still pending, at least one trial shows a survival benefit to neo-adjuvant chemoradiation plus operation as compared to operation alone.[34] However, some concerns have been raised about this study and the results of other studies will be needed to corroborate these findings.

At least one study may suggest that omission of operation, for squamous cell carcinoma, may be feasible. The Radiation Therapy Oncology Group Trial (85-01) evaluated cisplatin plus 5-fluorouracil given in adjunct with 50 Gy of radiation compared to 64 Gy of radiation alone.[35] Significant benefit was seen in the combined therapy group and the trial was stopped before its estimated completion date. In a subsequent report,[36] survival at 2 and 5 years was 36 and 27%, respectively. There were reductions in both local and distant failures. While toxicity from the treatment was high, 8% significant toxicity and 2% mortality, the group receiving chemotherapy and radiation fared far better than the group receiving radiation alone. We are, however, lacking in good randomized trials including chemoradiation and operative management at this time.

Operative Approach

The approach for tumors of the esophagus is variable. One can approach these tumors through the abdomen, the chest, or some combination. Open and videoscopically-assisted approaches are also possible. Determination of which approach is best depends upon the location of the tumor and the desired position of the enteric anastomosis. For distal esophagectomy with anastomosis below the inferior pulmonary vein, a left thoracotomy via the fifth or sixth intercostal space can be used. The left thoracoabdominal incision can be used or an isolated abdominal approach, although the last can present a challenging anastomosis. If it is preferred to place the anastomosis above the superior pulmonary vein, then one can choose from a superior mediastinal or a cervical position. This holds for either gastric or colonic anastomoses and for free jejunal transfers. For anastomoses in the superior mediastinal position, the right thoracotomy is generally preferred (Fig. 4.**3**). This can be accompanied by an abdominal incision (Ivor-Lewis) or by a laparoscopic approach. If one chooses the cervical position for anastomosis, the approach will include a cervical incision accompanied by either a right thoracic approach or abdominal approach or both. There are reports of either videoscopic-assisted thoracic or abdominal components.

Transhiatal Approach

For tumors of the distal esophagus, we prefer the transhiatal approach utilizing an abdominal and cervical incision (Fig. 4.**4**). We prefer to use the stomach as the replacement conduit for the resected esophagus and create a cervical esophagogastrostomy to restore enteric continuity. Although leak from these anastomoses is uncommon, if it were to occur, it is thought to be less consequential and easier to treat if the leak occurs in the neck rather than the mediastinum. We have tended to avoid the temptation for limited resection of the distal esophagus and proximal stomach with lower thoracic esophagogastrostomy to avoid the postoperative problems associated with gastroesophageal reflux

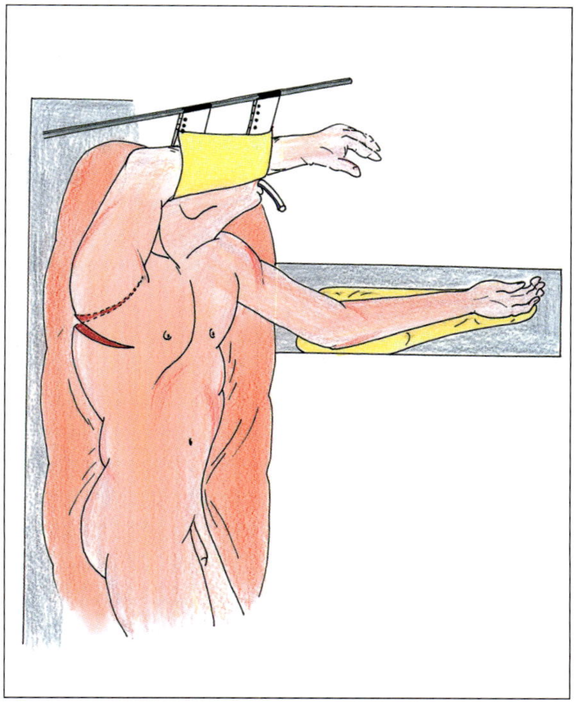

Fig. 4.**3** The patient is suitably positioned on the left side for a right posterolateral thoracotomy in the sixth intercostal space. The patient is here in a semi-lateral position allowing both abdominal and thoracic exposure and approach.

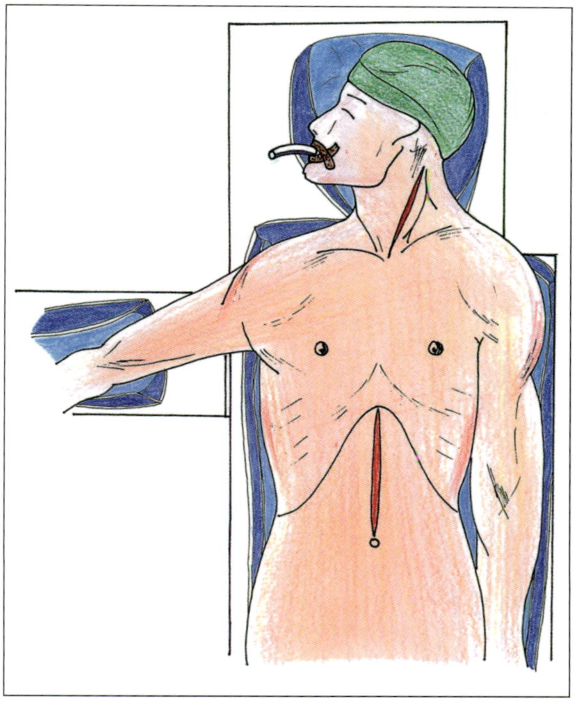

Fig. 4.**4** The left pre-sternocleidomastoid muscle and upper abdominal approach for the transhiatal esophagectomy.

that frequently ensue. One of the advantages of this last technique is that it also avoids well the postoperative pain commonly associated with the thoracotomy incision. A disadvantage of this technique is that it does require that the middle portion of the esophagus be resected "blindly" and this does, on occasion, prove technically challenging. We do not suggest this approach for middle and even less so for upper third esophageal cancers. Our operative approach for the transhiatal esophagogastrectomy is described.

We recommend placing epidural catheters for postoperative pain control prior to induction of general anesthesia. Additionally, we strongly advocate the use of continuous blood pressure monitoring via an arterial line during the operation. The patient is positioned supine on the operating table with a roll under the back to elevate the shoulders and extend the neck. The head is positioned with the neck rotated to the patient's right to facilitate access to the medial border of the left sternocleidomastoid muscle.

If there is any clinical question as to the presence of abdominal metastatic disease we begin with a laparoscopic evaluation of the abdomen unless there is compelling reason for laparotomy, such as gut obstruction or perforation. If laparoscopic evaluation is not required or is performed and does not demonstrate contraindication to proceeding, a longitudinal midline incision is utilized. This incision should extend from the costal margin to an inferior point of adequate size to facilitate excellent exposure of the upper abdominal structures as well as the hepatic flexure and duodenal sweep. Once the incision is made, the abdomen is again thoroughly explored to confirm the extent of disease. The liver, spleen, peritoneal surfaces, celiac and para-aortic nodes must all be evaluated.

After evaluation for distant disease has been completed, one must proceed to evaluate the local tumor. At this point, the falciform ligament is usually divided and ligated. The left lateral segment of the liver—segments II and III—are then mobilized using electrocautery to expose the medial aspect of the left hepatic vein or middle and left hepatic vein complex (Fig. 4.**5**). The xiphoid process is usually removed to facilitate superior exposure. A self-retaining retractor is placed to elevate and superiorly retract the costal margin.

Assessment of the esophagogastric junction must be performed at this point. We generally enter the lesser sac by means of dividing the gastrocolic ligament along the greater curve of the stomach. Great care must be taken to stay towards the colon to avoid injury to the gastroepiploic vascular arcade. This vascular bundle will be largely responsible for perfusing the gastric tube once it is pulled into its thoracic position later in the procedure. With the lesser sac opened (Fig. 4.**5**), the operating hands can be placed around the base of the esophagogastric junction to see if there is invasion of

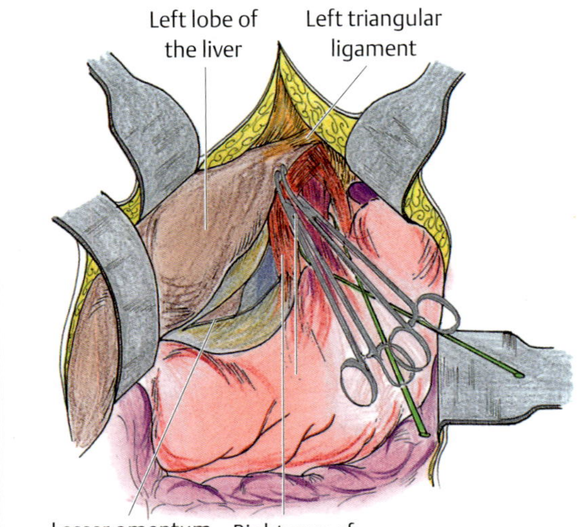

Fig. 4.**5** The segments II and III are mobilized (not represented here). The lesser sac is entered. The hiatus is opened anteriorly by dividing the right crus of the diaphragm.

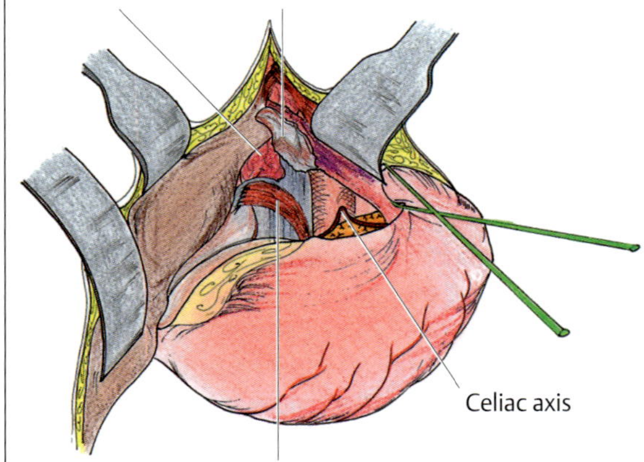

Fig. 4.**6** The distal esophagus with the tumor is cleared en bloc of the aorta. The celiac axis is exposed. The right diaphragmatic pleura is resected with periesophageal tissues and the lower lobe of the right lung is visible.

the superior border of the pancreas or the major vascular structures. Finding that these structures are intact, one then must open into the mediastinum.

The phrenoesophageal ligament is sharply incised to open into the inferior mediastinum. One must stay outside the tumor and be cognizant of the phrenic veins. The radial extent of tumor must be assessed and decision made as to the resectability of the lesion. If necessary pericardium and/or pleura can and should be included in the specimen if they are involved. Direct extension to cardiac muscle or aorta would be considered a contraindication to proceeding with resection in our judgment. If the esophageal hiatus is insufficient to allow for proper assessment of the distal esophagus, it should be enlarged anteriorly (Fig. 4.**5**). The esophagus and its adjacent tissue is then cleared en bloc to the level of the aorta posteriorly, to the parietal pleura laterally if necessary, and to the pericardium anteriorly (also if necessary) (Fig. 4.**6**).

At this point, attention should be returned to the abdominal portion of the case. The goals of this phase of the operation are to resect the proximal part of the stomach with its draining lymph nodes, create a viable gastric tube that will reach the neck for restoration of alimentary continuity and, optionally, performing enteric access for postoperative feeding. The first goal of this operation will require the proximal division of the left gastric arterial supply as well as the vasa brevia of the greater curvature of the fundus and cardia. Consequently, the stomach will eventually need to survive solely on its right-sided blood supply and its collateral vessels. This requirement will influence the steps required to produce a viable gastric tube.

As mentioned earlier, the lesser sac is first opened by division of the gastrocolic ligament close to the colon to avoid injury to the gastroepiploic arcade. The division of the gastrocolic ligament is then continued along the greater curve of the stomach to completely separate the stomach from the splenic flexure of the colon (Fig. 4.**7**). Care must be taken to avoid unnecessary traction on the short gastric vessels as this can be associated with unintended splenic injuries. We usually divide this ligament between clamps and ligate with absorbable ligatures although clips can also be used. As of late, we have increasingly employed the harmonic scalpel to facilitate dividing these vessels. The harmonic scalpel is particularly helpful in patients who are obese and in those patients with longer distances between their costal margins and the esophageal hiatus in whom knot tying is time-consuming and difficult. We have noted that the 10-mm harmonic scalpel appears to generate less heat than the 5 mm and, therefore, we prefer the 10-mm device. Division of the short gastric vessels then continue around the greater curve staying as far away from the stomach as is possible. This is done to preserve the gastroepiploic arcade and to minimize the potential tissue desiccation near the stomach from the dissipation of heat produced by the harmonic scalpel. The short gastric vessels will divide into two layers and each is taken independently until the esophagogastric junction is reached.

The hepatic flexure is carefully mobilized from its lateral peritoneal attachments. No attempt is made to separate it from the antrum or proximal duodenum. The duodenum is freed from its posterior attachments by a standard Kocher maneuver to facilitate medial and superior mobility of the stomach. The lesser omentum is then divided taking care to avoid any possible accessory or replaced hepatic arteries. Obviously there is no significant concern for protecting the hepatic branch of the vagus nerve. Dissection of the lesser omentum continues to the level of the esophagogastric junction.

With both curvatures of the stomach mobilized, the only remaining attachments of the proximal stomach are the pancreaticogastric fold and the left gastric blood supply. The arterial branches of the celiac axis are surrounded with a rich lymphatic network. Before the division of the left gastric artery, these lymph nodes must be cleared en bloc and remain attached to the lesser curvature. They will be resected with the specimen when the gastric tube is created. Thus, the left gastric vessels are the last abdominal attachments of the stomach (Fig. 4.**8**). Once the left gastric vascular pedicle is all that remains, it can be divided between clamps or with a vascular stapler. It is our preference to divide the bundle by separating the arterial and venous structures and ligating the proximal structures with ligature and suture ligature of nonabsorbable suture while using ligature alone for the specimen side of the bundles.

The number of teams that one employs for this operation will determine how to proceed next. If one is afforded the luxury of splitting into two teams at this point, one team can proceed to the neck while the other completes tasks in the abdomen. More commonly, we approach this via a single team. In this event, one can either proceed to the neck or perform a pylorus defeating procedure. Options at this time include pyloroplasty, pyloromyotomy, or no pylorus alteration at all. It is our preference to proceed with a Heineke–Mikulicz type pyloroplasty. This is performed in two layers using an absorbable running inverting inner layer and an external layer of interrupted nonabsorbable Lembert style sutures.

The neck dissection begins with an oblique incision oriented over the anteromedial border of the left sternocleidomastoid muscle. Dissection continues through the platysma muscle and the left sternocleidomastoid muscle is reflected laterally. Dissection continues to expose the lateral thyroid and the vascular bundle. The lateral thyroid veins are divided and the carotid artery and internal jugular vein are reflected laterally. Care must be taken to avoid an aberrantly positioned vagus nerve or a direct inferior laryngeal nerve branch (Fig. 4.**9**). Often, branches of the ansa cervicalis must be sacrificed to gain exposure to the posterior esophagus. The esophagus can now be palpated. It is helpful to have a nasogastric tube in place to facilitate this maneuver. Dissection is now kept close to the esophagus as one encircles it to minimize the risk of injuring the right inferior laryngeal nerve which is impossible to see from this approach. Once circumferentially freed from surrounding tissue, a Penrose drain is placed around the esophagus and secured with a clamp.

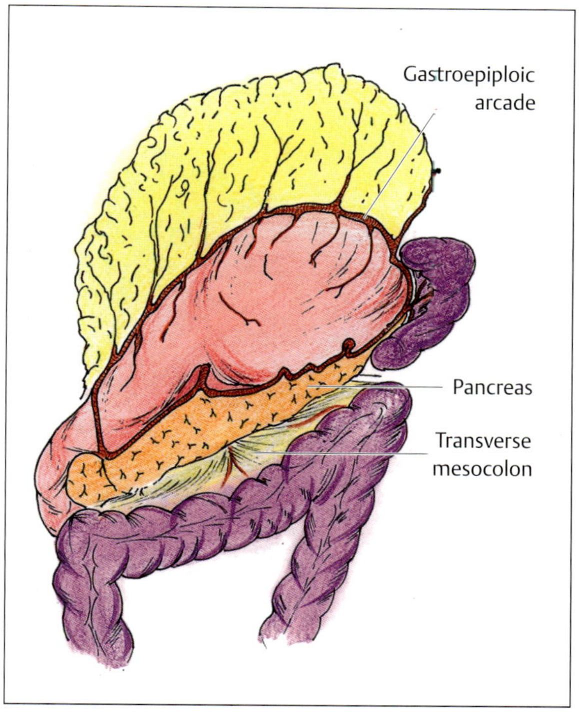

Fig. 4.**7** The gastrocolic ligament is divided with the gastroepiploic vascular bundle. The opening of the ligament ends with the separation of the greater curvature from the splenic flexure and the spleen.

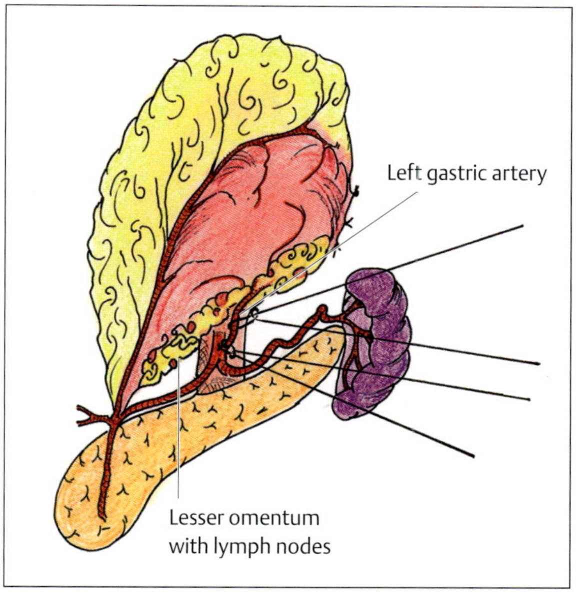

Fig. 4.**8** Division of the left gastric artery. The lymphatic tissue of the hepatic and splenic arteries is cleared. The left gastric artery is tied on the celiac axis.

Completion of the esophageal dissection can now be performed. If the opening in the esophageal hiatus of

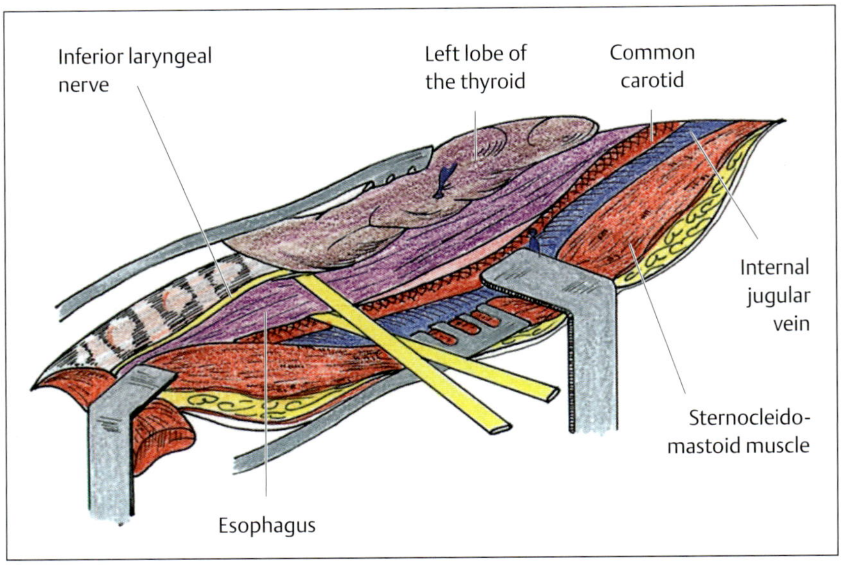

Fig. 4.**9** For the neck approach, the sternocleidomastoid muscle is retracted laterally. The thyroid veins are divided, the internal jugular vein and carotid artery are slightly reflected laterally. The omohyoid, sternocleidohyoid, and sternothyroid muscles are divided to allow distal cervical and high mediastinal dissection. The inferior laryngeal nerve is found in the tracheoesophageal groove.

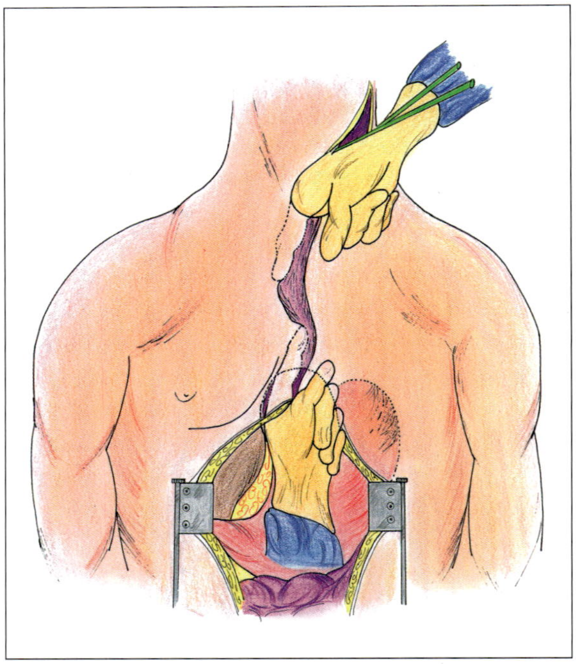

Fig. 4.**10** The esophagus is bluntly dissected. The hiatus is widely opened.

the diaphragm is not adequate to accept a fist, it must be enlarged. The distal esophagus is then mobilized bluntly (Fig. 4.**10**). Once one is well above the tumor, dissection needs to be carried out close to the esophageal tube. Vessels may be secured with surgical clips or divided using the harmonic scalpel where necessary. Eventually one will be able to reach his/her hand and forearm into the posterior mediastinum and the fingers of his/her other hand into the cervical incision. Circumferential dissection of the esophagus continues until the fingers of each hand meet.

While performing this "blind" portion of the operation, it is wise to keep one's eyes on the arterial blood pressure tracing on the monitors. The introduction of even a slim forearm will significantly impede venous return and subsequently decrease cardiac output. The patient will likely need frequent opportunities to "catch up" and improve systemic perfusion. Ensuring that the patient is well resuscitated during the case by maintaining adequate preload is imperative. We strongly advocate against the use of alpha-adrenergic agonists during the operation as they decrease mean systemic compliance and subsequently potentially decrease true preload. Furthermore, increased arteriolar tone may decrease intraorgan collateral flow within the stomach and increase the amount of gastric ischemia that may occur.

With the esophagus completely freed from its attachments, attention is turned to proximal division of the specimen. One should remember to withdraw the nasogastric tube to a safe location. The cervical esophagus is withdrawn from the incision and divided transversely using a 55 mm GIA stapler. The esophageal tube is then retracted along with the stomach through the esophageal hiatus. Inspection should be made to ensure that hemostasis is adequate in the mediastinum.

The stomach and esophagus are held with some firm retraction on the fundus of the stomach. This will allow for assessment for the boundaries of gastric resection. The blood supply of the lesser curve will need to be divided at the distal limit of resection. Creation of the gastric tube is performed using a 100 mm GIA stapler (Fig. 4.**11**). This will frequently require a second or third staple line to complete the division. The specimen should be pathologically evaluated to ensure that the gastric margin is free of neoplasm. We oversew the gastric staple line with a running nonabsorbable monofilament suture.

A final inspection for hemostasis in the mediastinum is now performed. Also, if either pleural cavity was

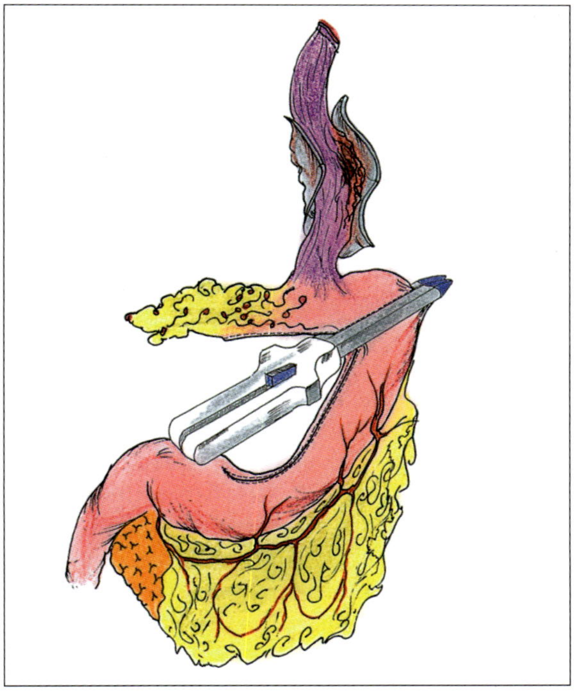

Fig. 4.**11** The gastric tube is created using a long GIA stapler. The specimen has also been stapled proximally. It is here presented with the tumor resected en bloc with periesophageal tissues and distal pleura. The lesser curvature is removed with the lymphatic nodes of the lesser omentum, of the hepatic and splenic vessels. The duodenum is Kocherized.

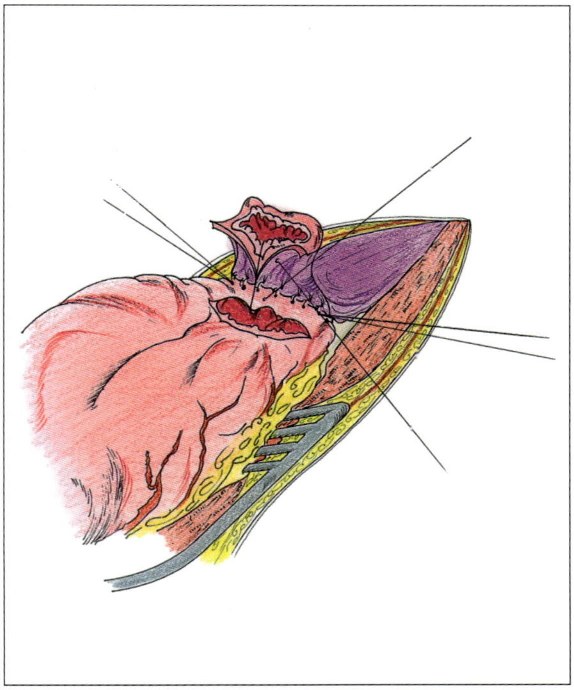

Fig. 4.**12** The esophagogastric anastomosis is performed in a two layers fashion. After the first posterior row, the esophagus is bevelled posteriorly and a full thickness absorbable second layer is carried out.

entered, tube thoracostomy should be performed in the affected hemithoracic cavity or cavities now.

The gastric tube is both pushed and pulled as gently as possible into the posterior mediastinum until it is brought into the cervical incision. Maintaining orientation of the gastric tube is mandatory to avoid twisting viscera. If the gastric tube cannot be adequately delivered into the cervical incision, it may be necessary to excise the medial clavicular head and a portion of the manubrium. This is usually not required. There may be as many methods of restoring alimentary continuity as there are surgeons who perform this operation. Technical options include a variety of hand-sewn methods to create an anastomosis as well as stapled techniques. It is our preference to perform a two layered hand-sewn anastomosis. Parenthetically, we would state that whichever technique works best for a given surgeon is the one that should be performed.

With the gastric tube positioned well in the posterior mediastinum, the cervical esophagus is reflected anteriorly and cephalad. This will expose the posterior proximal esophagus. A posterior row of interrupted Lembert style sutures of 3–0 silk are placed between the posterior proximal esophagus and the proximal anterior gastric fundus. An ellipse of stomach is then excised from the anterior wall. The posterior wall of the esophagus is divided such that a bevelled anastomosis will be created with the "long end" of the esophageal tube on the distal anterior surface. The inner layer of suture is created using interrupted absorbable suture incorporating the full thickness of esophagus and stomach (Fig. 4.**12**). Before the anterior row of sutures is complete it is advisable to guide the nasogastric back into the stomach under direct vision. Once in position, the nasogastric tube should be well secured to the patient's face. Completion of the anastomosis is performed with an anterior layer of interrupted 3–0 silk sutures in Lembert fashion incorporating the submucosal layer. The neck incision is then closed in layers. We rarely, if ever, place drains in the cervical position.

Returning to the abdomen, a final inspection for hemostasis is made. If necessary the hiatus in the diaphragm can be repaired although this is rarely required. The stomach can be secured to the diaphragm using a few interrupted sutures. It is our preference to place a jejunal feeding tube. An 18 French catheter is inserted in a standard Witzel fashion and secured to the anterior abdominal wall. We start enteric feedings at a low rate on the first postoperative day. The abdominal incision is closed using a running heavy nonabsorbable suture although absorbable sutures are also used on occasion. The patient is usually awakened and extubated in the operating room. Postoperative chest radiograph, hemogram, and serum electrolytes are routinely obtained.

Right Thoracotomy Approach

Circumstances for which the transhiatal approach to esophagogastrectomy will be sub-optimal will invariably arise. In the opinion of some that would include every situation of esophageal cancer. Our biases have been declared and subsequently described above regarding the transhiatal approach. For tumors that involve the middle or upper third of the esophagus or when en bloc resection of the esophagus and surrounding tissue in the upper mediastinum is desired the approach via the right thorax may be preferred (Figs. 4.**1**, 4.**2**). The approach can be undertaken via an open or videoscopic technique. We will describe, in brief detail, the procedure that we favor via an open technique though certainly the same principles should apply if the procedure were to be performed with videoscopic assistance.

The patient is positioned in the left lateral decubitus position with appropriate padding and protection of the extremities (Fig. 4.**3**) after induction of general endotracheal anesthesia has been given via a double lumen endotracheal tube. A standard posterolateral thoracotomy incision is made and the right hemithorax is entered through either the fourth or fifth intercostal space (if the operative plan is to perform the anastomosis in the cervical position, our preference, then the fifth space may be easier). The right lung ventilation is ceased and the lung is retracted. The mediastinal pleura are incised along the anterior border of the azygos vein and dissection is carried toward the adventitia of the aorta. The arch of the azygos vein is divided at its junction with the superior vena cava while preserving the main trunk of the azygos vein and the intercostal vessels. The thoracic duct is also divided superiorly at the level of the aortic arch. The esophagus and its surrounding tissue are elevated and dissection is continued inferiorly. The thoracic duct is divided inferiorly at the level of the aortic hiatus of the diaphragm.

Upon dissection of the cephalad portion of the esophagus one must take care to preserve the inferior laryngeal nerves after dividing the pleura along the tracheoesophageal groove. The esophagus is mobilized from the membranous portion of the trachea to the level of the carina. The subcarinal nodes and the pericardium along the pulmonary veins are included in the en bloc resection (Fig. 4.**13**). After freeing the specimen anteriorly, the bronchoesophageal arteries are ligated along the aorta until the left pleural space can be entered. Final division of the pulmonary ligament will fully liberate the specimen from its attachments with the mediastinum. This resection should contain the esophagus and its associated tissue with a surrounding layer of other tissue with the exception of the portion of the esophagus that was freed from the trachea.

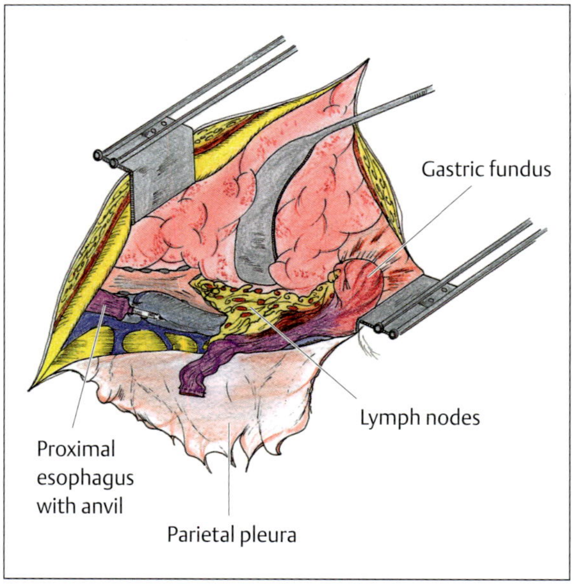

Fig. 4.**13** Right posterolateral thoracotomy. The esophagus has been dissected and interrupted proximally. The anvil of the circular stapler is inserted. The dissection takes en bloc the mediastinal and subcarinal lymph nodes. The hiatus is widely opened and the gastric fundus is delivered in the chest.

Conclusion

The management of the patient with esophageal carcinoma is anything but universally agreed upon. At its extremes we have a fairly congruous world opinion of what appears to be the right treatment from a surgeon's standpoint—with widespread disease resection offers little benefit and with limited cancer (or high grade dysplasia) operative management offers an extremely high probability of disease-free survival in technically capable hands. Once one intellectually wanders between the extreme boundaries of clinical presentation the data becomes less consistent and the interpretations of the data even more so. Some consistencies certainly exist; complete removal of the tumor is attended by better outcomes than either microscopically or macroscopically residual tumor, lack of involvement of lymph nodes is associated with better outcomes than when nodal disease is present, and long-term cure appears more likely when operative resection is possible than when it is not.

Inconsistencies, on the other hand, abound and include: the clinical benefit versus staging benefit of extended en bloc resection, the clinical benefit of extended three-field lymph node dissection versus lesser nodal clearance procedures, the value of adding operative management in patients who present with locally advanced disease and in whom apparent complete response to nonoperative management has been seen, the absolute value of neo-adjuvant chemoradiation and the risk-benefit analysis of cervical node clearance as it relates to the potential associated morbidity.

In our opinion, significant complications are unacceptable when performing palliative operations and are at best undesirable when performing potentially curative operations. We simply cannot tell prospectively in many cases when we are performing a palliative or curative operation. Therefore, our ultimate recommendations as to which procedure to perform is variable depending upon whom we are advising. The choice has to take into account the collective resources of the system in which one works. The ability to safely deliver chemotherapy or radiation therapy in either the adjuvant or neo-adjuvant must be considered. The operative and perioperative resources that the surgeon has at his or her disposal may also influence the best choice of procedure. In the final analysis, the true cancer surgeon must also well understand his or her own limitations dependent on and independent of the system in which he or she works for choosing advice that the literature may support but which cannot truly provide benefits and frequently harms the patient.

☐ References

1. Steup WH, De Leyn P, Deneffe G, Van Raemdonck D, Coosemans W, Lerut T. Tumors of the esophagogastric junction. *J Thorac Cardiovasc Surg.* 1996;111:85–95.
2. Hermanek P. pTNM and residual tumor classification: problems of assessment and prognostic significance. *World J Surg.* 1995;19:184–190.
3. Lam KY, Ma LT, Wong J. Measurement of extent of spread of oesophageal squamous cell carcinoma by serial sectioning. *J Clin Pathol.* 1996;49:124–129.
4. Siu KF, Cheung HC, Wong J. Shrinkage of the esophagus after resection for carcinoma. *Ann Surg.* 1986;203:173–176.
5. Matsubara T, Ueda M, Nakajima T et al. Can esophagectomy cure cancer of the thoracic esophagus involving the major airways? *Ann Thorac Surg.* 1995;59:173–177.
6. Sagar PM, Johnston D, McMahon MJ, Dixon MF, Quirke P. Significance of circumferential resection margin involvement after oesophagectomy for cancer. *Br J Surg.* 1993; 80:1386–1388.
7. Skinner DB, Little AG, Ferguson MK, Soriano A, Staszak VM. Selection of operation for esophageal cancer based on staging. *Ann Surg.* 1986;204:391–401.
8. Isono K, Sato H, Nakayama K. Results of a nationwide study on the three fields of lymph node dissection in esophageal cancer. *Oncology.* 1991;48:411–420.
9. Akiyama H, Tsurumaru M, Udagawa H, Kajiyama Y. Radical lymph node dissection for cancer of the thoracic esophagus. *Ann Surg.* 1994;220:364–373.
10. Hagen JA, Peters JH, DeMeester TR. Superiority of extended en bloc esophagogastrectomy for carcinoma of the lower esophagus and cardia. *J Thorac Cardiovasc Surg.* 1993;106: 850–859.
11. Orringer MB, Marshall B, Stirling MC. Transhiatal esophagectomy for benign and malignant disease. *J Thorac Cardiovasc Surg.* 1993;105:265–277.
12. DeMeester TR, Zaninotto G, Johansson KE. Selective therapeutic approach to cancer of the esophagus and cardia. *J Thorac Cardiovasc Surg.* 1988;95:42–54.
13. Nishihira T, Hirayama K, Mori S. A prospective randomized trial of extended cervical and superior mediastinal lymphadenectomy for carcinoma of the thoracic esophagus. *Am J Surg.* 1998;175:47–51.
14. Kato H, Watanabe H, Tachmimori Y, Iizuka T. Evaluation of neck lymph node dissection for thoracic esophageal carcinoma. *Ann Thorac Surg.* 1991;51:931–935.
15. Altorki NK, Skinner DB. Occult cervical nodal metastasis in esophageal cancer: preliminary results of three-field lymphadenectomy. *J Thorac Cardiovasc Surg.* 1997;113: 540–544.
16. Lerut T, Coosemans W, DeLeyn P et al. Reflections on three field lymphadenectomy in carcinoma of the esophagus and gastroesophageal junction. *Hepatogastroenterology.* 1999; 46:717–725.
17. Fujita H, Kakegawa T, Yamana H et al. Mortality and morbidity rates, postoperative course, quality of life, and prognosis after extended radical lymphadenectomy for esophageal cancer: comparison of three-field lymphadenectomy with two-field lymphadenectomy. *Ann Surg.* 1995;222: 654–662.
18. Kato H, Tachimori Y, Watanabe H, Itabashi M. Surgical treatment of thoracic esophageal carcinoma directly invading the lung. *Cancer.* 1992;70:1457–1461.
19. Matsubara T, Ueda M, Takahashi T, Nakajima T, Nishi M. Surgical treatment of cancer of the thoracic esophagus in association with a major pulmonary operation. *J Am Coll Surg.* 1997;185:520–524.
20. Altorki NK, Migliore M, Skinner DB. Esophageal carcinoma with airway invasion; evolution and choices of therapy. *Chest.* 1994;106:742–745.
21. Gignoux M, Roussel A, Paillot B et al. The value of preoperative radiotherapy in esophageal cancer: results of a study of the EORTC. *World J Surg.* 1987;11:426–432.
22. Launois B, Delarue D, Campion JP, Kerbaol M. Preoperative radiotherapy for carcinoma of the esophagus. *Surg Gynecol Obstet.* 1981;153:690–692.
23. Wang M, Gu XZ, Yin WB, Huang GJ, Wang IJ, Zhang DW. Randomized clinical trial on the combination of preoperative irradiation and surgery in the treatment of esophageal carcinoma: a report on 206 patients. *Int J Radiat Oncol Biol Phys.* 1989;16:325–327.
24. Arnott SJ, Duncan W, Kerr GR et al. Low dose preoperative radiotherapy for carcinoma of the oesophagus: results of a randomized clinical trial. *Radiother Oncol.* 1992;24: 108–113.
25. Nygaard K, Hagen S, Hansen HS et al. Preoperative radiotherapy prolongs survival in operable esophageal carcinoma: a randomized, multicenter study of preoperative radiotherapy and chemotherapy : the second Scandinavian trial in esophageal cancer. *World J Surg.* 1992;16: 1104–1110.
26. Huang GJ, Gu XZ, Wang LJ, Wang M, Zhang DW, Yin WB. Combined preoperative irradiation and surgery versus surgery alone for squamous cell carcinoma of the midthoracic esophagus: a prospective randomized study in 360 patients. In: Ferguson MK, Little AG, Skinner DB, eds. *Diseases of the Esophagus : Malignant Diseases.* New York, NY: Futura; 1992: 275–281.
27. Teniere P, Hay JM, Fingerhut A, Fagniez PL. Postoperative radiotherapy does not increase survival after curative resection for squamous cell carcinoma of the middle and

lower esophagus as shown by multicenter controlled trial. *Surg Gynecol Obstet.* 1991;173:123–130.
28. Zieren HU, Muller JM, Jacobi CA, Pichlmaier H, Muller RP, Staar S. Adjuvant postoperative radiation therapy after curative resection of squamous cell carcinoma of the thoracic esophagus: a prospective randomized study. *World J Surg.* 1995;19:444–449.
29. Fok M, Sham JS, Choy D, Cheng SW, Wong J. Postoperative radiotherapy for carcinoma of the esophagus: a prospective, randomized controlled study. *Surgery.* 1993;113: 138–147.
30. Schlag PM. Randomized trial of preoperative chemotherapy for squamous cell cancer of the esophagus. The Chirurgische Arbeitsgemeinschaft fuer Onkologie der Deutschen Gesellschaft fuer Chirurgie Study Group. *Arch Surg.* 1992;127:1446–1450.
31. Roth JA, Pass HI, Flanagan MM, Graeber GM, Rosenberg JC, Steinberg S. Randomized clinical trial of preoperative and postoperative adjuvant therapy with cisplatin, vindesine, and bleomycin for carcinoma of the esophagus. *J Thorac Cardiovasc Surg.* 1988;96:242–248.
32. Law S, Fok M, Chow S, Chu KM, Wong J. Preoperative chemotherapy versus surgical therapy alone for squamous cell carcinoma of the esophagus: a prospective randomized trial. *J Thorac Cardiovasc Surg.* 1997;114:210–217.
33. Kok TC, van Lanschot JJ, Siersema PD et al. Neoadjuvant chemotherapy compared with surgery in esophageal squamous cell cancer. *Can J Gastroenterol B.* 1998;12:297.
34. Walsh TN, Noonan N, Hollywood D, Kelly A, Keeling N, Hennessy T. A comparison of multimodal therapy and surgery for esophageal adenocarcinoma. *N Engl J Med.* 1996;335:462–467.
35. Herskovic A, Martz K, al Sarraf M et al. Combined chemotherapy and radiotherapy compared with radiotherapy alone in patients with cancer of the esophagus. *N Engl J Med.* 1992;326:1593–1598.
36. Cooper JS, Guo MD, Herskovic A et al. Chemotherapy of locally advanced esophageal cancer: long-term follow-up of a prospective randomized trial (RTOG 85-01): Radiation Therapy Oncology Group. *JAMA.* 1999;281:1623–1627.

5 Stomach

Martin S. Karpeh Jr and Murray F. Brennan

Stomach cancer continues to rank among the leading causes of cancer deaths worldwide. Although the incidence has decreased significantly in most western countries, epidemiologic studies have documented a rise in the percentage of adenocarcinoma of the gastric cardia and gastroesophageal junction. Overall survival is improving but the number of patients presenting with advanced stages of disease remains unacceptably high. A complete surgical resection (R0) of the primary tumor remains the cornerstone of curative treatment. Without an R0 resection, cure is not possible. The challenge in resecting an advanced tumor of the stomach is directly influenced by the number of vital structures surrounding the stomach, including the pancreas, spleen, liver, and colon that can be invaded by tumors arising in this organ. Resection of a portion or all of an adjacent organ may be necessary to achieve an R0 resection. In the absence of direct invasion, multiorgan resection is not a prerequisite for cure. However, distinguishing between adherent and invasive disease is often not possible and the surgeon should be prepared in these instances to perform an en bloc multiorgan resection if cure is the intent of the operation.

Indications

The vast majority of gastric resections for treating cancer can be done without the need to resect any of the adjacent organs. Past concerns regarding the surgeon's ability to achieve an adequate lymphadenectomy resulted in a policy of *en passant* resection of the pancreas and spleen regardless of the presence or absence of direct tumor invasion. Data from two large prospective randomized trials have documented an increase in morbidity and mortality associated with routine pancreaticosplenectomy.[1,2] Moreover, overall survival may actually be diminished by the morbidity associated with pancreaticosplenectomy.[2] It has been shown that distal pancreatectomy and splenectomy are not required procedures to achieve an adequate lymphadenectomy.[3,4] Therefore, an R0 resection can be accomplished without compromising the efficacy of the R0 resection.[1–3] In view of these data, the question is, who should undergo a gastrectomy with resection of an adjacent organ? Gastric tumors that invade an adjacent organ (clinical T4 tumor) in the absence of M1 disease will require resection of part or all of that organ in order to meet the requirements of an R0 resection.[5] Long-term survival has been documented following an R0 resection but the extent of such resections must be tempered by the potential associated morbidity and mortality for each individual patient. With proper patient selection and preoperative planning, multiorgan resections for treating gastric cancer can be accomplished with low mortality and acceptable morbidity.

Pretreatment Evaluation

If the patient is deemed an acceptable candidate for a major operation, the primary aim of the initial evaluation is to exclude the presence of M1 disease. The overall accuracy of computed tomography (CT) in staging primary gastric carcinoma has been reported in the range of 64 to 96%.[6] High-quality contrast-enhanced CT can provide a reasonable assessment of the extent of disease, particularly in the liver. However, distinguishing between invasion and adherence to adjacent organs remains a major weakness of CT scanning. Resectability is determined by defining the vascular relationships. Planning for a resection of this magnitude is done with data that are as current as possible. In general, imaging is performed within 4 weeks of the planned operation. CT scanning is still the most useful modality for treatment planning. The use of preoperative staging with F18-fluorodeoxyglucose positron emission tomography to rule out the presence of occult M1 disease has increased.

Proper evaluation of the liver to detect metastatic disease and to delineate vascular anatomy requires a CT scan with both oral and intravenous contrast. The CT should at least include the abdomen and pelvis. Scanning the chest is important when tumors involve the proximal stomach or gastroesophageal junction. Sarcomas of the stomach can metastasize to the lungs and patients with these sarcomas should have their chest scanned to avoid missing any multiple pulmonary metastases. Images captured with thin sections through the pancreas using a multidetector scanner enable the best assessment for gastric tumors invading the posterior wall and pancreas. Contrast-enhanced images of the arterial and venous phases highlight the celiac, splenic, and portal anatomy. Preservation of fat planes around these vessels suggests freedom from tumor encasement. With the help of modern spiral CT imaging, the potential for a multiorgan resection should be anticipated in most cases.[7] It is our practice not to proceed with laparotomy if M1 disease is discovered on CT. Therefore, high-quality CT is essential.

We routinely perform laparoscopy with peritoneal lavage prior to proceeding with laparotomy when planning a multiorgan resection. Patients with clinical T4 tumors are at very high risk for having peritoneal and/or occult hepatic metastases that can be identified prior to laparotomy. Since the goal of a multiorgan resection is to achieve an R0 resection, the finding of M1 disease is a relative contraindication to proceeding and the role of gastrectomy in this setting is at best undefined. We have found the need for prophylactic palliative gastrectomy with multiorgan resection to be exceedingly rare.[8]

☐ Material

Good preoperative preparation helps to minimize postoperative morbidity. Effective use of an epidural catheter can significantly reduce postoperative pain and enhance pulmonary toilet. The catheter is placed preoperatively and prior to the administration of deep venous thrombus prophylaxis. Once the epidural catheter has been inserted, 5000 units of subcutaneous heparin are given usually within an hour of the start of the procedure. Intraoperative measures used to avoid hypothermia include a warm air thermal device placed preferably over the patient's head, upper body, and/or lower body before performing the incision.

Adequate exposure is essential to the success of these operations. A self-retaining retractor greatly facilitates operative exposure and frees the hands of an assistant. To meet individual surgeon preferences, a number of different devises are on the market. Instruments need to be of sufficient length, particularly for the barrel-chested male patient. Strategic use of modern surgical staplers saves time. The endovascular 2.0-mm stapler is an example of a valuable instrument that can provide a secure and expeditious division of major vascular structures such as the splenic vein and artery once these vessels are adequately exposed.

☐ Positioning

Proper positioning of the patient makes a tremendous difference in exposure. Body habitus, the angle of the costal margins, and the location of the tumor are the primary determinants of the incision placement. In general, the supine position with a midline incision provides adequate exposure to the upper abdomen in most patients (Fig. 5.**1**). For the short barrel-chested patient with a broad costal margin, an oblique position facilitated by a rolled sheet under the left back is helpful. A subcostal incision with an extension across the midline provides excellent exposure to the left upper quadrant (Fig. 5.**2**). The left thoracoabdominal incision is the incision of choice for the patient with large tumors seated deeply in the left upper quadrant and involving the diaphragm (Fig. 5.**3**). This incision is also the best approach for the morbidly obese patient. In the case of the obese patient, a near-full left lateral decubitus position is preferred to access a tumor in the left upper quadrant, as it allows the mesentery and adipose tissue to be positioned out of the operative field.

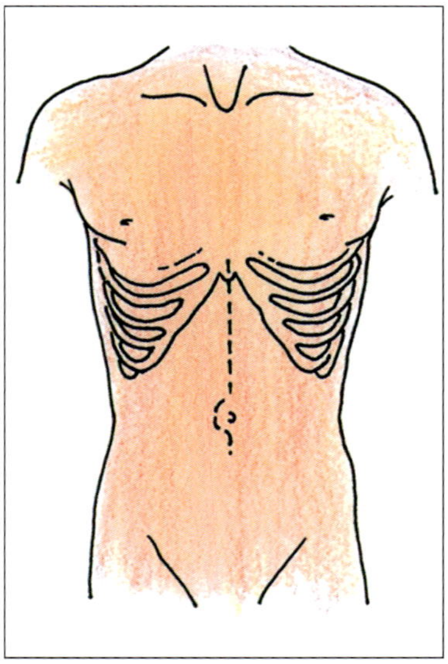

Fig. 5.**1** Midline incision.

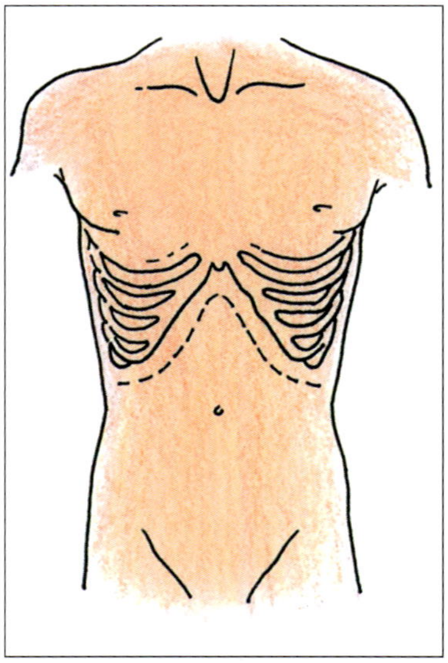

Fig. 5.**2** Bilateral subcostal incision.

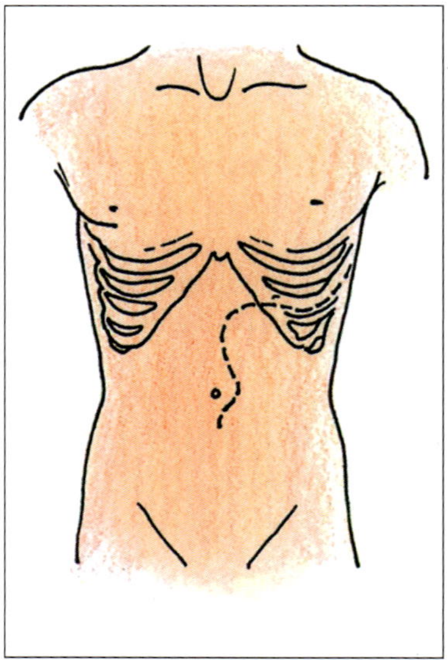

Fig. 5.**3** Left thoracoabdominal incision.

Technique

Total Gastrectomy with Pancreaticosplenectomy

Gastric cancers invading the body or tail of the pancreas can be a vexing problem for the surgeon. These tumors arise from the mid and proximal stomach and they can obscure the celiac axis, making the assessment of resectability a challenge. Common determinants of resectability include encasement of the celiac axis and encasement of the common hepatic artery. Following a negative laparoscopy, the laparotomy incision is extended from the xiphoid down to or just below the umbilicus, depending on the patient's build. For the large barrel-chested or obese patient, a thoracoabdominal incision is carried from a point in the upper midline of the abdomen and extended across the left 7th intercostal space into the left chest (Fig. 5.**4**).

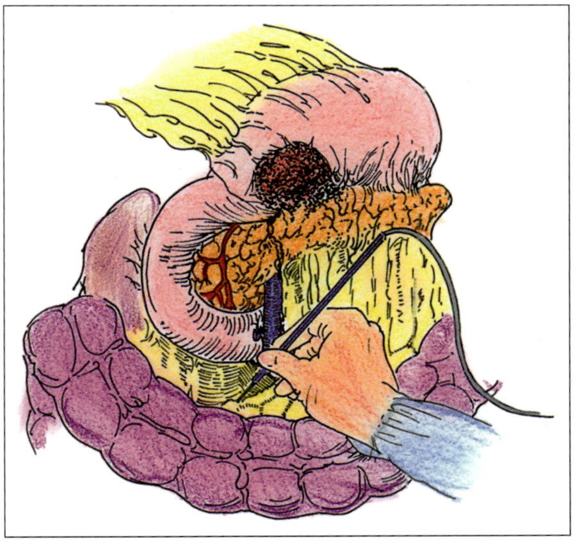

Fig. 5.**4** Gastric cancer invading the body of the pancreas. The posterior aspect of the gastric wall can be involved. Invasion of the celiac axis precludes a curative resection.

The gastrohepatic omentum is opened to assess the extent of local extension. If the tumor is clear of the celiac axis, the dissection begins with a left to right bursectomy, separating the omentum and anterior leaf of the mesocolon from the splenic flexure to the mid transverse colon. This is continued to expose the inferior border of the pancreatic body and tail (Fig. 5.**5**). Dissection continues beneath the pancreas and spleen.

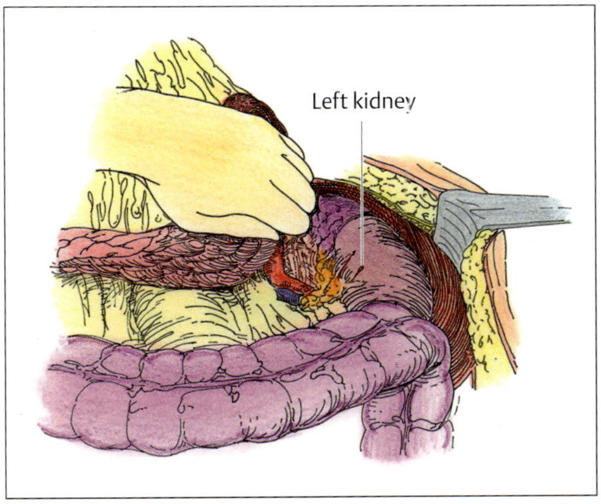

Fig. 5.**5** The stomach and tail of the pancreas are retracted from the left to the right. The retroperitoneum with the left kidney is exposed.

The pancreatic tail is fully mobilized, lifting the spleen and pancreas together from the left upper quadrant and sharply dividing the areolar tissue anterior to the left kidney. The next step is to divide the peritoneal attachments laterally and rotate the entire specimen medially to the left crus of the diaphragm. Some tumors may invade the diaphragm in this location, necessitating a wider dissection taking a portion of the diaphragm. Two packs are placed in the left upper quadrant behind the spleen to support the specimen in the operative field and provide hemostasis. The distal stomach and duodenum are then prepared for division of the duodenum.

Continuing the omental bursectomy across the transverse mesocolon to the right gastroepiploic vessels and separating the omentum from the transverse colon and hepatic flexure mesocolon completes the bursectomy. The right gastroepiploic vein will course across the plane of dissection often as a branch of the middle colic vein or come directly from the superior mesenteric vein. Once the vein is divided, the inferior border of the pancreas is then identified by dissecting along the anterior surface of the neck of the pancreas toward the head of the gland. The gastroduodenal artery will be visible along the anterior surface of the pancreas, coursing behind the gastric pylorus where it gives rise to the right epiploic artery. The epiploic is then ligated and divided in the standard fashion. All areolar tissue along the duodenum is swept cephalad toward the pylorus to be included within the specimen. The posterior wall of the duodenum is cleared of areolar tissue. Dissection is continued along the gastroduodenal artery cephalad to the common hepatic artery. Once the hepatic artery is visualized, this dissection is discontinued. Occasionally, the origin of the right gastric artery is identified from this approach and it can be ligated and divided.

Next, the gastrohepatic omentum is incised. The right gastric artery is typically identified at this time, ligated and divided. Once the superior border of the duodenum has been cleared of the surrounding areolar tissue, the duodenum is divided. A single fire of a stapling device (Endo-GIA 80 or 75; U.S. Surgical, Norwalk, CT) is sufficient. The duodenal stump can be oversewn, but this is not necessary.

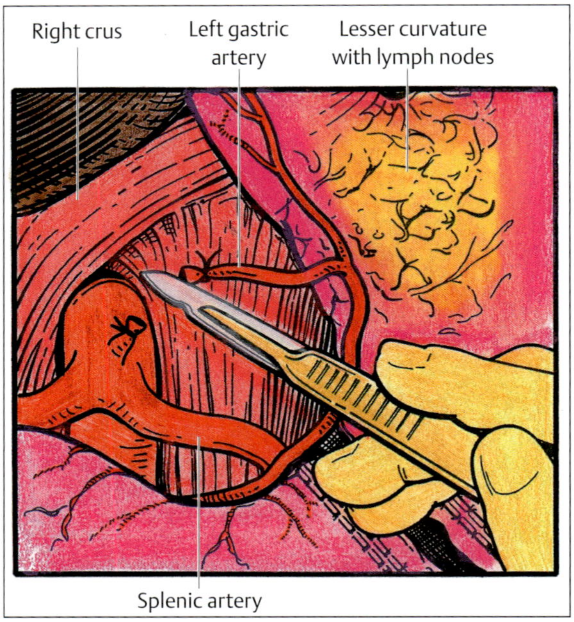

Fig. 5.6 The lesser omentum with nodal tissue altogether with hepatic artery and celiac axis lymph nodes are proximally reflected with the specimen. The left gastric artery is divided.

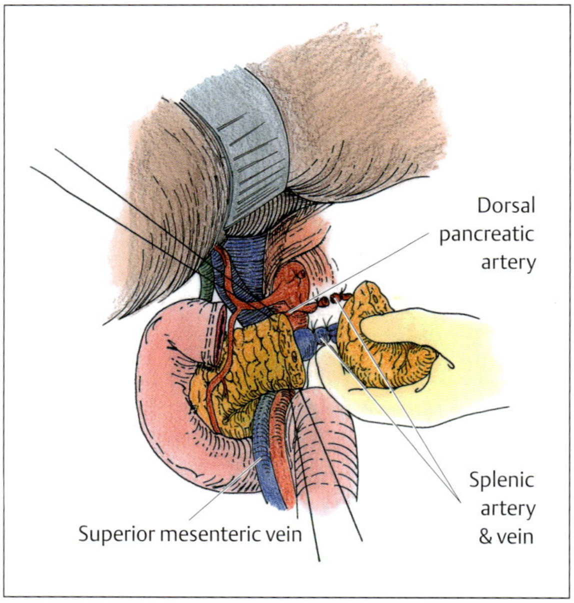

Fig. 5.7 The splenic artery is dissected beyond the dorsal pancreatic artery. The pancreas is transected between stay sutures. The splenic vessels are divided.

The stomach is further mobilized in a distal to proximal direction. A lymph node dissection is then carried along the proper hepatic artery toward the celiac origin. The area between the hepatic artery and superior border of the pancreas is cleared of nodal tissue, often exposing the portal vein. Nodal tissue along the celiac axis is carefully swept anteriorly and included with the specimen. The dissection is continued in a cephalad direction toward the origin of the left gastric artery. The left gastric artery is ligated in standard fashion at its origin and divided (Fig. 5.**6**).

The splenic artery is then identified at its origin and dissection is carried out laterally to the site of planed transection. If possible, the dissection is typically carried beyond the take-off of the dorsal pancreatic artery. Once the proximal splenic artery has been isolated, attention is turned to dividing the pancreas. Hemostatic stay sutures are placed in the superior and inferior borders of the pancreas and the pancreas is divided. The pancreatic parenchyma is then transected using a combination of cutting and coagulating current on the electrocautery. This allows for identification of the pancreatic duct, which is then ligated. In cases where the pancreas is atrophic, a stapler can be used as an alternative instrument to transect the gland. Once the pancreas had been transected, the proximal stump is oversewn with an interrupted 3–0 polydioxanone (PDS) or Prolene suture if the pancreas is divided sharply. If a stapler is used on a smaller gland, then no additional sutures are needed. The splenic artery and vein are identified. The artery is ligated followed by the vein (Fig. 5.**7**). Use of the endovascular stapler is an efficient means of individually transecting the splenic portal vein confluence.

The esophagus now tethers the specimen to the patient. The phrenoesophageal ligament is taken down from the diaphragm and skeletonization of both the right and left crura is completed. Once the esophagus, the specimen, and the surrounding paracardial nodes and areolar tissue have been freed circumferentially, an anterior and posterior vagotomy is performed and the nasogastric tube is withdrawn. The purse string applier is placed above the line of transection. An atraumatic bowel clamp is placed on the specimen side and the esophagus is sharply divided.

Following removal of the specimen, a stapled end-to-side esophagojejunostomy is performed. In brief, a Roux limb is brought through the mesentery in a retrocolic fashion. The anvil of a #28 end-to-end anastomosis (EEA) stapler (U.S. Surgical) is placed within the distal esophagus and secured with a purse string. The stapler is inserted through the jejunal limb and about 15 cm distally the spike is brought through the jejunal wall. An end-to-side stapled EEA anastomosis is then created. The resulting tissue rings are inspected and the anastomosis is checked to be sure there is good blood supply and no tension. Following this, a GIA stapler can be used to join the afferent and efferent limbs together to create a jejunal pouch about 10 cm in length. Once this has been completed, the edges of the enterotomy are approximated with fine Allis clamps and closed with a TA 90 stapling device (U.S. Surgical). The Roux-en-Y anastomosis is completed 45 to 55 cm distal to the esophagojejunostomy. This is performed in an end-to-side fashion. After firing the GIA stapling device, the TA 90 stapler is again used to close the jejunal enterotomy.

This can be closed by a single-layered hand-sewn technique as well.

Once the enteroenterostomy has been completed, the opening in the mesentery of the transverse mesocolon is closed with a 3–0 absorbable suture. The nasogastric tube is then advanced and properly placed just distal to the passage of the jejunum through the transverse mesocolon.

Alternative

An alternative to the above approach to resecting a bulky gastric cancer invading the body of the pancreas is to divide the duodenum and pancreas earlier in the procedure before mobilization of the distal pancreas and spleen. This will allow for early vascular control of the proximal splenic artery and vein. Dividing the pancreas over the superior mesenteric vein exposes the proximal splenic vein and artery for a safe division and early control of the major vasculature.

Distal Gastrectomy with Pancreaticoduodenectomy

Invasion into the head of the pancreas from gastric carcinoma often indicates an incurable situation and is a harbinger of systemic disease. Occasionally tumor invasion is limited to the duodenum and head of the pancreas where, in a fit patient, a pancreaticoduodenectomy results in an R0 resection (Fig. 5.**8**). When contemplating the pros and cons of proceeding with such a resection, one must ask whether extension of the gastrectomy to include the pancreas will result in a clear R0 resection. The main determinant of resectability is the presence of vascular encasement and the extent of pancreatic involvement. Tumors of the posterior gastric wall involving the head and neck of the pancreas define the limits of resectability. Signet ring tumors in particular can present with extensive periportal lymphatic involvement without gross adenopathy. Encasement of the middle colic and superior mesenteric vein or extension into the porta hepatis, directly by the primary or confluent nodal disease, should be apparent on a well-done CT scan.

Mobilizing the hepatic flexure to expose the duodenum followed by a full Kocher maneuver will facilitate assessment of resectability. With a finger in the foramen of Winslow, one can assess the porta hepatis for disease extension into the portal vein. The decision to proceed is often made after exposing the hepatic artery and demonstrating that the mass can be elevated from the portal vein on the superior border of the pancreas. Encasement of the hepatic artery and celiac axis defines unresectable disease.

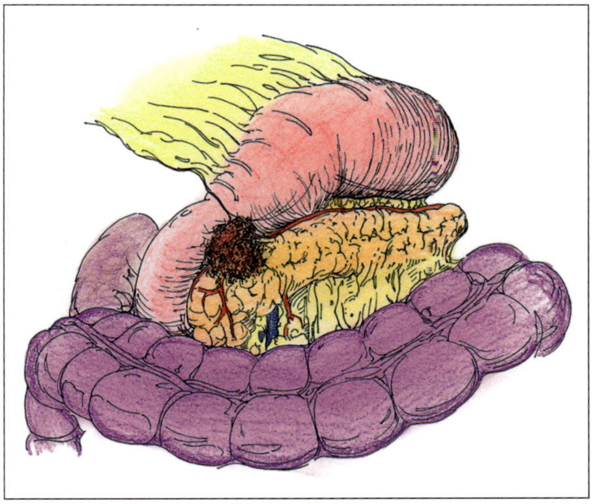

Fig. 5.**8** Distal gastric cancer invading the head and neck of the pancreas. A curative resection can be considered.

To assess the inferior border of the pancreas, the omentum is elevated from the hepatic flexure, which is retracted caudally to expose the second and third portions of the duodenum and uncinate process of the pancreas. The superior mesenteric vein (SMV) is exposed as it courses over the uncinate process of the pancreas toward the neck of the gland. The epiploic vein can be divided at this point to expose the inferior border of the pancreas. If the anterior surface of the pancreas is free at this level, resection can proceed.

Once the decision is made to proceed, exposure of the celiac axis and portal vein is improved by transecting the stomach early. The omental bursectomy is carried out, separating the transverse colon from the omentum. The plane of dissection is between the anterior and posterior leaves of the mesentery down to the inferior border of the pancreas. This plane is extended across the pancreas to elevate the pancreatic capsule to the splenic artery and the associated nodes. The distal stomach is then transected across the greater curve (Fig. 5.**9**). The line of transection is angled cephalad to include all of the lesser curvature nodes. Nodes along the splenic artery are dissected toward the celiac axis to expose the origin of the left gastric artery.

With the left gastric artery divided, the distal stomach can now be reflected to the right and the dissection is continued along the superior border of the pancreas, elevating the nodal tissue and unroofing the portal vein. The gastroduodenal artery (GDA) is then isolated and temporarily occluded. The proper hepatic artery is checked to insure that a pulse is maintained prior to ligating the GDA. After the GDA is divided, attention is then turned to the inferior border of the pancreas and the SMV. The pancreas is separated from the vein and stay sutures are placed in the pancreas prior to transection (Fig. 5.**10**). Once the pancreas is divided, the operation continues along the SMV, ligat-

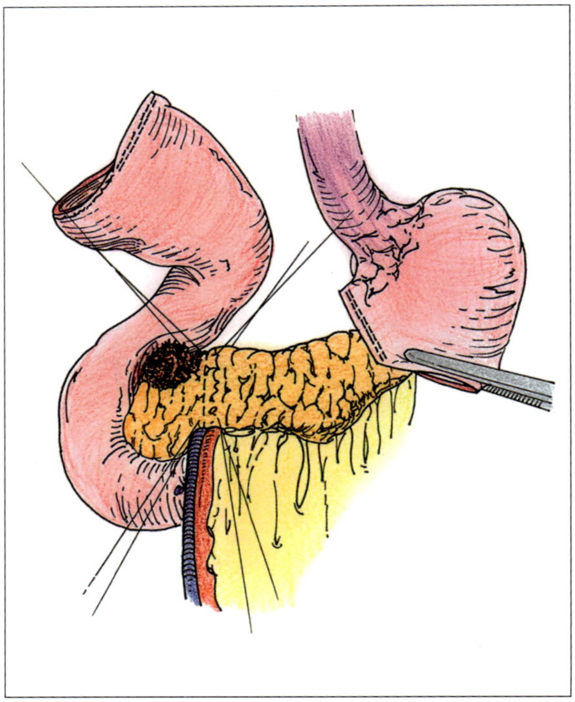

Fig. 5.**9** The stomach is stapled allowing exposure of the celiac axis. The nodes of the splenic artery are removed from the left to the right.

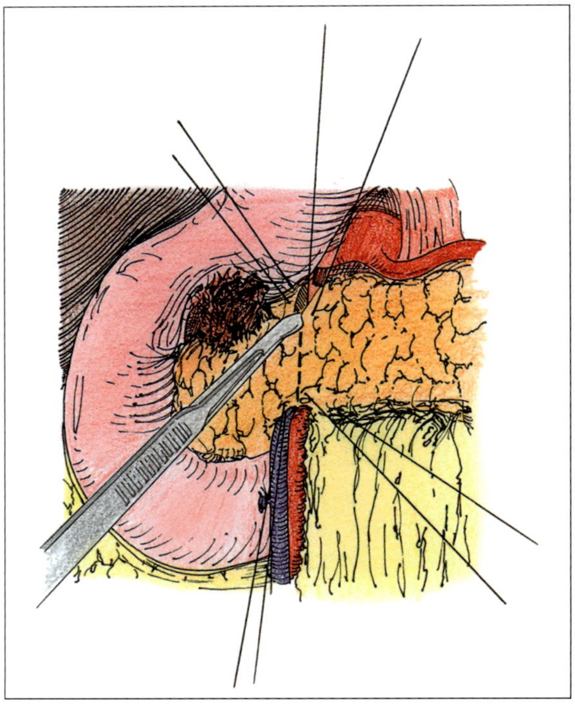

Fig. 5.**10** The distal stomach is reflected to the right. The neck of the pancreas is separated from the venous mesentericoportal axis and the pancreas is divided.

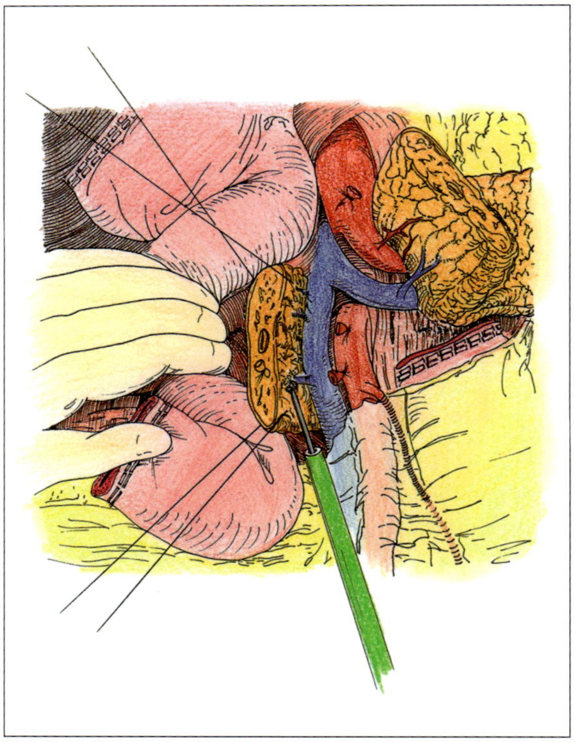

Fig. 5.**11** Small venous tributaries from the head of the pancreas to the portal vein are ligated and divided.

ing small venous tributaries and branches of the superior mesenteric artery as the head of the pancreas, tumor, and distal stomach are retracted to the patient's right (Fig. 5.**11**). Finally, the gallbladder is taken down from its bed and the common bile duct is divided. Separating the soft tissues from the proximal portal vein completes the dissection.

□ Gastrectomy with Combined Colon Resection

Tumors of the greater curvature of the stomach can extend into the omentum and invade the colon directly or encase the middle colic artery and vein, necessitating a partial colonic resection. This situation is encountered more often when resecting gastric remnant cancers where a prior anticolic Billroth II anastomosis has been created. Resecting a portion of the transverse colon early in the procedure can greatly facilitate resection.

The operation proceeds much like that described above with mobilization of the omentum and its bursa from the hepatic flexure to expose the pancreatic head and uncinate process. Once the epiploic vein is divided, dissection is continued onto the inferior border of the pancreas. With the omentum elevated from the uninvolved portion of the colon, one can evaluate the extent of tumor involvement. With the omental bursa opened, one can better evaluate the pancreas, which may also be involved. If the pancreas is invaded distal to the SMV, it can be included in the resection (see above). Invasion of a significant portion of the pancreatic body and head is a reason to abort the procedure. With less extensive tumors involving the colon, early transection of the involved segment of colon greatly facilitates the operation. The middle colic vein can be identified draining into the SMV. For tumors invading the transverse mesocolon, the middle colic vein and artery are generally uninvolved at this level. Once these vessels have been secured, the mesocolon can be divided proximal and distal to the involved colon, sparing much of the uninvolved vascularized transverse colon (Fig. 5.**12**). In the case of a prior Billroth II anastomosis, the afferent and efferent limbs of the gastrojejunostomy will have to be divided first in order to get to the involved colonic segment. Dissection is then directed along the inferior border of the pancreas to the origin of the middle colic artery and vein. The colonic segment is left attached to the tumor and removed en bloc with the gastrectomy. The operation proceeds, as described above, as either a distal or a total gastrectomy, depending on the available proximal margin.

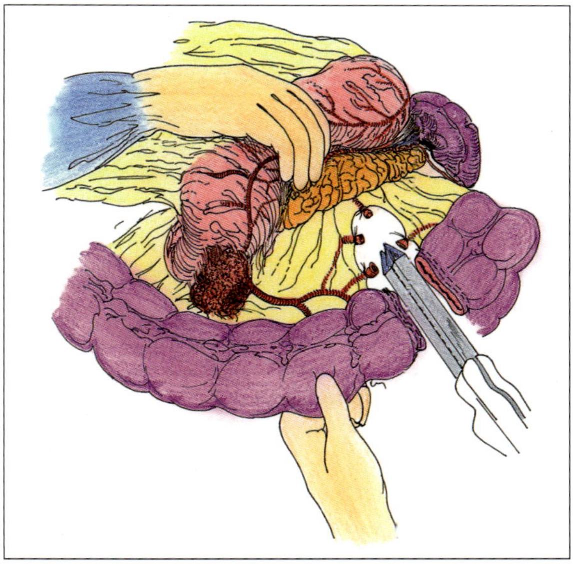

Fig. 5.1**2** The mesocolon and transverse colon are divided. The middle colic vessels can generally be respected.

Gastrectomy with Combined Liver Resection

Direct hepatic invasion is uncommon. Occasionally a bulky tumor of the body or proximal stomach invades the overlying segments II or III of the liver. The options for resection include wedging a portion of the liver or dividing the liver, leaving the lateral half of segments II and III on the tumor. Extensive parenchymal invasion of the liver is rare. When invasion is extensive, a more formal resection of the lateral segments is indicated. More often, a plane is preserved either above or below the gastrohepatic omentum between the liver and the stomach. In case of a proximal tumor it is important to be aware of the left hepatic vein as tumoral clearance may be close to the vena cava (Fig. 5.**13**). If possible, the left hepatic vein can be isolated and/or divided early, but more often access to the vein is obscured until the liver parenchyma is divided. The extent of hepatic resection is limited and the resection can be accomplished with the aid of a Pringle maneuver.

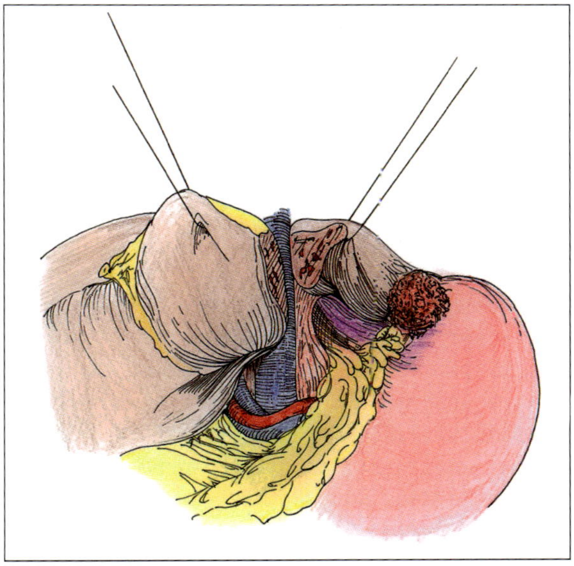

Fig. 5.**13** En bloc total gastrectomy and left hepatic lobectomy (segments II and III).

Postoperative Care

The principles of postoperative care are the same as for any major abdominal surgery. Hemodynamic monitoring with central venous monitoring is standard for a procedure of this magnitude and most patients have an arterial line placed during the procedure. Patients are kept in an intensive care setting for 12 to 24 hours depending on their hemodynamic parameters. The use of blood products during the perioperative course is minimized and transfusions are guided by hemodynamic parameters rather than by the absolute hematocrit. Deep venous thrombosis prophylaxis is continued with subcutaneous heparin.

The use of drains is limited to the difficult duodenal stump or pancreatic closure. When drains are used, only closed drainage systems are employed. There is an increasing volume of data supporting a selective rather than routine use of drains, but ultimately the final decision must be based on clinical judgement.[9,10] The nasogastric tube is usually placed overnight after total gastrectomy and after a day in the case of a distal subtotal gastrectomy.[11–13]

Good analgesia without over sedation is essential for early ambulation and to maximize pulmonary toilet.

Most centers use some form of patient-controlled analgesia given by intravenous injection or with an epidural catheter used to administer a bupivacaine/narcotic combination. Use of an epidural catheter to administer 0.2% bupivacaine with or without morphine has been shown to reduce the incidence of postoperative ileus.[14] These catheters are routinely placed preoperatively. The catheter can be left in place for up to 5 days or longer, by which time patients can begin to get adequate mobility as oral analgesia is introduced. Antibiotics are given prophylactically to cover skin and enteric bacteria. In general, antibiotics are discontinued after one or two postoperative doses and long-term "prophylactic" antibiotic use is discouraged.

Given the high morbidity rates associated with multiorgan resections, procedures of this magnitude should be performed in centers where nursing and ancillary support are accustomed to this magnitude of surgery.[15]

□ Complications

The risk of having a postoperative complication is high following a polyvisceral resection procedure. This population of patients is typically older and tends to harbor multiple co-morbidities. With proper vigilance and early intervention postoperative mortality can be held to a minimum. The morbidity and mortality following multiple organ resections performed at Memorial Sloan-Kettering Cancer Center (MSKCC) were reviewed in an effort to identify factors associated with an increased morbidity risk.[16] Four hundred eighteen patients underwent primary resection with one or more additional organs resected. Morbidity and mortality were compared to that of 826 patients who underwent gastrectomy alone during the same time period. Complications were segregated and analyzed based on their severity, ranging on a scale from 0 (no complication) to 5 (death). In this study, 580 complications occurred among 404 patients for an overall morbidity rate of 33% (404/1283). The majority of complications were successfully managed without the need for invasive therapy. Infection was the most common type of complication encountered, with pneumonia, anastomotic leak, abscess, and wound infections accounting for 47% of the complications. Cardiac complications accounted for another 15%. Analysis by number of organs resected revealed that complications requiring the need for invasive intervention increased significantly as the number of organs resected increased. Skilled interventional radiology and early operative intervention was essential to minimize the severity of the complications that did occur. Aggressive identification and treatment of infection is a major component for the successful management of postoperative complications following polyvisceral resections. With proper precautions, careful vigilance, and early intervention, postoperative mortality rates should be more than acceptable.

In the Memorial experience perioperative mortality was 4% (48 patients). Serious complications resulting in chronic disability combined with death occurred in 10%. Anastomotic leak was the most common reason cited as the primary cause for mortality. The number of organs resected was the most significant predictor of postoperative complications with a relative risk of 2.0. When minor complications (severity 1 and 2) were excluded, the relative risk increased to 3.8 for developing a severe complication (severity of 3, 4, or 5). Early intervention, in the majority of these cases, avoided mortality. The importance of careful surveillance and the ready availability of skilled interventional radiology cannot be overemphasized.

□ Results

High morbidity and mortality combined with poor prognosis have traditionally tempered enthusiasm to perform extended gastric resections. However, with improvements in surgical instruments and technique, a decrease in postoperative morbidity and mortality has been observed. In the MSKCC experience, gastrectomy with multiple organ resection accounted for 24% of all curative resections, which include organ resection for iatrogenic injury (i. e., splenic bleeding) in addition to clinical T4 tumors. The incidence of actual histologically proven pT4 tumors was low. In an analysis of 268 extended gastric cancer resections of one or more additional organs, Martin et al. found that 14% (38/268) had pT4 cancers.[17] Multiorgan resections most commonly involve just a single organ, with the spleen being the most common organ resected (n = 179) followed by the pancreas (n = 50). Compared to tumors resected by gastrectomy alone, the multiorgan resected tumors were significantly larger in size (median, 5 cm) and had greater degree of serosal invasion (57% pT3/T4 vs. 40%). The incidence of advanced N2 nodal disease was also higher in the multiorgan resection group (21 vs. 15%). It is reasonable to assume that survival, following resection of this advanced disease, would be poor.

Overall, the 5-year survival for all 268 patients undergoing polyvisceral resection was a respectable 32% with a median 32 months. The 5-year survival for patients with proven T3 and T4 tumors combined was 27%. Median survival decreased with the number of organs resected reflecting a greater tumor burden and observation that supports previous results.[18,19] Survival following resection of actual pT4 tumors is predicated on the presence or absence of lymph node metastases.[20,21] Thirty-five percent of all multiorgan resections in the report by Martin et al. were node negative.[16] A third of the T4 tumors were N0, identifying an opportunity to improve selection of a subset of patient with a better prognosis following polyvisceral resection. Median survival decreased as depth of invasion increased. In a multivariate analysis of significant factors identified by univariate analysis, advanced T stage (T3 or greater) and nodal stage (N1 or greater) emerged as the only adverse predictors of survival.[16] Multiorgan resection did not influence survival, further emphasizing the importance of stage of disease. The histopathologic characteristics of the tumor may also prove to be an important factor to consider. Kodama et al. found resection of Borrmann type IV tumors to be poor regardless of the R classification of the resection.[18] Polyvisceral resections for gastric cancer can be performed safely in experienced centers with the proper support staff but selecting who will benefit from this type of resection continues to be a major challenge. Invasion into multiple organs, the presence of distant peritoneal disease (p2 or p3), or separate visceral metastases has consistently been shown to be an unyielding impediment to cure.

References

1. Bonenkamp JJ, Hermans J, Sasako M, van de Velde CJ. Extended lymph-node dissection for gastric cancer. Dutch Gastric Cancer Group. *N Engl J Med*. 1999;340:908–914.
2. Cuschieri A, Weeden S, Fielding J et al. Patient survival after D1 and D2 resections for gastric cancer: long-term results of the MRC randomized surgical trial. Surgical Co-operative Group. *Br J Cancer*. 1999;79:1522–1530.
3. Maruyama K, Sasako M, Kinoshita T, Sano T, Katai H, Okajima K. Pancreas-preserving total gastrectomy for proximal gastric cancer. *World J Surg*. 1995;19:532–536.
4. Griffith JP, Sue-Ling HM, Martin I et al. Preservation of the spleen improves survival after radical surgery for gastric cancer. *Gut*. 1995;36:684–690.
5. Yong WS, Wong WK, Chan HS, Soo KC. Extended resection of locally advanced (T4) stomach cancer. *Ann Acad Med Singapore*. 2000;29:723–726.
6. Miller FH, Kochman ML, Talamonti MS, Ghahremani GG, Gore RM. Gastric cancer. Radiologic staging. *Rad Clin Am*. 1997;35:331–349.
7. Davies J, Chalmers AG, Sue-Ling HM et al. Spiral computed tomography and operative staging of gastric carcinoma: a comparison with histopathological staging. *Gut*. 1997;41: 314–319.
8. Burke EC, Karpeh MS, Conlon KC, Brennan MF. Laparoscopy in the management of gastric adenocarcinoma. *Ann Surg*. 1997; 225:262–267.
9. Conlon KC, Labow D, Leung D et al. Prospective randomized clinical trial of the value of intraperitoneal drainage after pancreatic resection. *Ann Surg*. 2001;234:487–494.
10. Fong Y, Brennan MF, Brown K, Heffernan N, Blumgart LH. Drainage is unnecessary after elective liver resection. *Am J Surg*. 1996;171:158–162.
11. Yoo CH, Son BH, Han WK, Pae WK. Nasogastric decompression is not necessary in operations for gastric cancer: prospective randomised trial. *Eur J Surg*. 2002;168: 379–383.
12. Wu CC, Hwang CR, Liu TJ. There is no need for nasogastric decompression after partial gastrectomy with extensive lymphadenectomy. *Eur J Surg*. 1994;160:369–373.
13. Nathan BN, Pain JA. Nasogastric suction after elective abdominal surgery: a randomised study. *Ann R Coll Surg Engl*. 1991;73:291–294.
14. Jorgensen H, Fomsgaard JS, Dirks J, Wetterslev J, Andreasson B, Dahl JB. Effect of epidural bupivacaine vs combined epidural bupivacaine and morphine on gastrointestinal function and pain after major gynaecological surgery. *Br J Anaesth*. 2001;87:727–732.
15. Begg CB, Cramer LD, Hoskins WJ, Brennan MF. Impact of hospital volume on operative mortality for major cancer surgery. *JAMA*. 1998;280:1747.
16. Martin RC, Jaques DP, Brennan MF, Karpeh M. Achieving R0 resection for locally advanced gastric cancer: is it worth the risk of multiorgan resection? *J Am Coll Surg*. 2002;194: 568–577.
17. Martin RC, Jaques DP, Brennan MF, Karpeh M. Extended local resection for advanced gastric cancer: increased survival versus increased morbidity. *Ann Surg*. 2002;236: 159–165.
18. Kodama I, Takamiya H, Mizutani K et al. Gastrectomy with combined resection of other organs for carcinoma of the stomach with invasion to adjacent organs: clinical efficacy in a retrospective study. *J Am Coll Surg*. 1997;184:16–22.
19. Yonemura Y, Kawamura T, Nojima N et al. Postoperative results of left upper abdominal evisceration for advanced gastric cancer. *Hepatogastroenterology*. 2000;47:571–574.
20. Kitamura K, Tani N, Koike H et al Combined resection of the involved organs in T4 gastric cancer. *Hepatogastroenterology*. 2000;47:1769–1772.
21. Saito H, Tsujitani S, Maeda Y et al. Combined resection of invaded organs in patients with T4 gastric carcinoma. *Gastric Cancer*. 2001;4:206–211.

6 Pancreas

Valery Usatoff and Robin C. N. Williamson

☐ Abbreviations

CBD: common bile duct
CT: computed tomography
ERCP: endoscopic retrograde cholangiopancreaticography
IMA: inferior mesenteric artery
IMV: inferior mesenteric vein
MRI: magnetic resonance imaging
PD: pancreaticoduodenectomy
PPPP: pylorus preserving proximal pancreaticoduodenectomy
PTC: percutaneous transhepatic cholangiography
PV: portal vein
SMA: superior mesenteric artery
SMV: superior mesenteric vein
SV: splenic vein
TP: total pancreatectomy
US: ultrasound scan

Approximately 6000 people die from pancreatic cancer in the UK each year. Second to colorectal carcinoma, it is the commonest cancer of the gastrointestinal tract and the fourth leading cause of cancer-related death at all sites. The incidence in Europe is 10–15 per 100 000 population per year. In the United States every year, 112 000 people die of gastrointestinal cancer and carcinoma of the pancreas accounts for 22% of these, making it the fifth leading cause of cancer death in the USA (1–3). Surgical resection offers the only chance of long-term survival, but the overall prognosis is poor. Pancreatic cancer accounts for the majority of pancreatic tumors (80%) but can be difficult to distinguish from other types of periampullary tumors on the basis of preoperative investigations and from unusual pancreatic primaries such as neuroendocrine neoplasms. Most of these other tumors have a much better prognosis than pancreatic cancer and the surgeon is usually faced with deciding about resection without definitive histologic guidance. Most pancreatic cancers (80%) are located in the head of the pancreas, but only 10–20% of these lesions are resectable at presentation and even fewer if the tumor arises outside the head. At the time of diagnosis, only 10% of patients have disease confined to the pancreas, while 40% exhibit local spread, and 50% distant disease.[4]

Surgery of the pancreas presents many technical challenges and is associated with a high morbidity rate for several reasons: (1) Patients are often elderly (80% between the ages of 60–80 years) and many have concomitant medical problems. (2) Despite substantial improvements, preoperative imaging may still leave doubt about the histologic nature of the tumor and the exact extent of the disease. (3) The pancreas is relatively inaccessible in its retroperitoneal location, being closely related to major vessels and other important viscera, which makes the approach and mobilization difficult. (4) The frequent presentation with obstructive jaundice results in potential problems with hepatic insufficiency, renal impairment, and coagulopathy. (5) Resection of the head of the pancreas requires a complex reconstruction with potentially disastrous complications if leakage occurs, particularly from the pancreatic anastomosis. (6) Patients have often lost a substantial amount of weight before operation and are consequently malnourished, which compromises their surgical recovery.

The treatment of pancreatic cancer has been dictated by the underlying philosophy of the physician/surgeon involved.[5] Nihilists recommend a palliative approach for all patients, suggesting that the high operative mortality and morbidity rates cannot justify the dismal long-term outcome. Realists recognize the value of a resection when this can be achieved in a limited fashion but see no role for extending the operation beyond the pancreas. At the other end of the spectrum, activists recommend an extended pancreatectomy in the belief that they can achieve a curative resection. The nihilistic view is highlighted by claims that the overall number of five-year survivors is not significantly influenced by operation at all and that the number of those surviving without resection is similar to the number of those surviving with a resection.[6]

Patients with known hepatic or peritoneal disease are clearly incurable and resection of the primary tumor is of little or no value.[7] No difference in survival times exist between patients with gross metastases detected at laparoscopy and those with positive cytologic test results but no visible metastatic disease.[8] In the absence of symptoms such as gastric outlet obstruction, these patients are best palliated by nonsurgical means. On the other hand, patients in general good health who have a tumor that appears resectable on imaging should undergo exploratory laparotomy and possible resection since this represents the only chance of cure.[9] The situation is more complex when the imaging suggests borderline resectability or when a less aggressive histologic type of tumor is suspected. A similar problem can arise during laparotomy when the surgeon finds that a previously considered "resectable" tumor is closely applied to adjacent structures and it is very difficult to differentiate tumor invasion from inflammatory adhesion.

The extension of pancreatectomy to include adjacent structures is controversial and detailed argument in support of the case is beyond the practical nature of this text, but situations may arise in which even conservative surgeons encounter tumor extension at a late stage of the operation and an extended resection becomes a reasonable option.

Preoperative Diagnosis and Staging

The appropriate diagnostic work-up of patients with suspected pancreatic carcinoma is a matter of debate, particularly the role of percutaneous biopsy in obtaining a histologic diagnosis before surgical intervention. Factors likely to influence this work-up include: the patient's age and general health, the clinical presentation, the site of the tumor in the pancreas, the local expertise with various imaging modalities and the patient's wishes. Spiral CT scanning is replacing angiography and even ERCP in many centers. The morbidity and mortality rate of major pancreatic resection is low today and most experienced surgeons will be comfortable with performing a resection without histologic confirmation. The potential complications associated with percutaneous biopsy of the pancreas are numerous, but in reality they occur very infrequently and the main disadvantage is the false-negative rate. This rate is higher with smaller lesions and these are the ones that are most likely to represent "curable" tumors. The occasional resection for benign pathology needs to be balanced against the tragedy of not resecting a potentially curable lesion. The old adage of not performing an investigation unless the result is likely to influence management holds true in the imaging of potentially resectable pancreatic tumors.

Somewhat paradoxically, a histologic diagnosis is more desirable in patients in whom operation is not likely to be an option, whether for tumor reasons or patient reasons. One always needs to be suspicious of very large or unusual pancreatic tumors, particularly those that are hypervascular or calcified on imaging. Pancreatic lymphoma is rare but eminently treatable, while neuroendocrine tumors of the pancreas also have a much better prognosis than that associated with adenocarcinoma. Biopsy of these large tumors should be straightforward and should yield an accurate diagnosis. If potentially toxic treatments are to be considered such as chemotherapy or radiotherapy, then a tissue diagnosis is essential.

Even small tumors of the pancreas will cause a surrounding area of inflammation and fibrosis that can lead to "sampling errors" when percutaneous biopsy is attempted. Thus, a negative biopsy for cancer certainly does not exclude cancer. In a resectable tumor, the occasional complication from percutaneous biopsy such as hemorrhage or pancreatitis can increase the technical difficulty of operation or even delay the procedure long enough for the tumor to progress to an irresectable stage. Percutaneous needle biopsy of the pancreas is a relatively safe and sensitive technique for establishing a histologic diagnosis, but it should generally be limited to patients with unresectable or metastatic tumors, many of which are sited in the body or tail of the pancreas. Percutaneous biopsy of pancreatic tumors potentially results in release of malignant cells and may affect the prognosis adversely as well as cause seeding along the biopsy tract.[10,11] We would support percutaneous biopsy only in the setting of unresectable disease to confirm diagnosis or to determine whether a major resection would be worthwhile in the context of a large tumor that may have a less aggressive histologic pattern than "ordinary" ductal carcinoma of the pancreas.

The objective of imaging in pancreatic neoplasms is both to diagnose and stage the tumor and also to assess resectability. Tumor markers CA19-9 and CEA can be helpful to confirm clinical suspicion but are usually unhelpful in the context of patients with small and resectable tumors.[12] Ultrasound scanning (US) is very good at detecting larger pancreatic neoplasms, but for lesions less than 1 cm in diameter computed tomography (CT) has a sensitivity of 79% compared to a sensitivity of 50% for ultrasound (13).[13] Endoscopic retrograde cholangiopancreaticography (ERCP) has a sensitivity of 96%,[9] but the combination of clinical presentation, US and CT (without ERCP) allows an accurate preoperative diagnosis in more than 96% of patients.[14] It is likely that ERCP will be required to make the diagnosis in a minority of patients, but it may clearly be helpful in relieving jaundice preoperatively; however, the placement of an endoscopic stent early in the patient's work-up may impair the quality of CT images obtained with the stent in place. The role of angiography is debated: some authors report a greater accuracy in the detection of vascular involvement on CT than by angiography,[15] while others suggest that angiography will detect vascular invasion in up to 31% of patients reported as having negative CT scans.[16] Angiography will detect vascular abnormalities in 30–45% of patients, but these can usually be identified during operation. Our policy is to perform angiography if the CT scan indicates a lesion lying close to the mesentericoportal venous trunk. Endoscopic US is reported to have 85% accuracy in assessing tumor resectability, but it is highly operator-dependent and is not yet widely available. Although magnetic resonance imaging (MRI) does not appear to improve on CT findings,[17] the additional benefit of providing cholangiopancreaticographic and angiographic information from the single investigation promises an expanding role over the next few years. If involvement of adjacent organs such as stomach or colon is suspected, upper or lower gastrointestinal endoscopy helps to exclude full-thickness invasion, which may affect the decision to operate.

Role of Laparoscopy

Advocates of laparoscopic staging suggest that more than 40% of patients with pancreatic cancer whose CT scan shows no evidence of distant disease will have metastases detected by this means.[18] The incidence of peritoneal disease detected by laparoscopic staging of left-sided pancreatic carcinomas is reported to be as high as 53%.[19] This technique is uniquely valuable at identifying peritoneal nodules. Others suggest that left-sided cancers are generally unresectable because of mesenteric axis infiltration; since this infiltration is not detected by routine laparoscopy, only 7% of patients will benefit from laparoscopy.[9] We perform laparoscopy only if clarification is required for suspicious CT findings regarding distant metastases.

Preoperative Preparation

In patients with deep jaundice, particularly those with renal impairment or any suspicion of sepsis, we advocate a period of preoperative biliary drainage. The preferable route is with ERCP, but percutaneous transhepatic cholangiography (PTC) can successfully achieve internal drainage of bile in most cases. In patients with mild, uncomplicated jaundice it is reasonable to proceed to operation without decompressing the biliary tree, although in practice a stent has often been inserted before surgical referral at the time of diagnostic cholangiography.[20]

All patients for pancreatectomy should receive intravenous broad-spectrum antibiotics on induction of anesthesia and all will have subcutaneous low molecular weight heparin perioperatively. Jaundiced patients receive parenteral vitamin K and operation is usually delayed until the prothrombin time has normalized. Patients with tumors located in the body or tail of the pancreas, in whom splenectomy may be anticipated, are vaccinated prophylactically 2 weeks before operation against *Streptococcus pneumoniae*, *Haemophilus influenza-B*, and *Neisseria meningitidis*. If a colonic resection is suspected, particularly a left-sided resection, then osmotic bowel preparation is also given on the day before operation. Patients with recent jaundice are rehydrated on the night before operation with intravenous fluids. Cross-matched blood is made available with a minimum of four units for a major pancreatic resection.

Materials

We use a general surgical instrument tray during the procedure but have available a vascular tray with a selection of straight and side-biting vascular clamps. The operating theatre is stocked with a range of prosthetic vascular grafts and appropriate vascular sutures. Our choice of incision is a bilateral subcostal or "gable" one and we prefer to use a fixed retractor system for displacing the costal margin.

Positioning

The patient is placed in the supine position. Operation is commenced with a right subcostal incision for initial assessment. In the absence of gross signs of irresectability, the incision is extended to the left as necessary in a "gable" or "rooftop" fashion.

Technique

Basic Operative Approach

Although the major components of a pancreatic resection are traditionally described as "assessment," "resection," and "reconstruction," in reality the first two steps are closely interwoven and a good deal of mobilization may be needed to complete a full assessment. Sometimes towards the end of the resection it becomes clear that a curative excision is not possible, yet so much of the resection has been performed that the operator is committed to completing what then becomes a palliative resection. Alternatively, the surgeon may elect to perform an extended resection in an attempt to clear all macroscopic disease.

The following description of operative technique will be based upon our "standard" pylorus-preserving proximal pancreaticoduodenectomy (PPPP) for tumors located in the head of the gland and will highlight the stages of the procedure at which further radicality/extension may be considered.[21,22] These maneuvers will then be discussed in more detail. A later section will discuss the approach to pancreatic tumors located to the left of the portal vein. Underlying the overall approach to pancreatic surgery is the surgeon's philosophy regarding the appropriate degree of radicality. Some surgeons set out to be very radical and will plan extended resections from the outset, while others will find themselves doing extended resections infrequently only after reaching the "point of no return" mentioned above. We acknowledge that all surgeons, regardless of their philosophy, may find themselves in the position to consider extension of the standard approach in certain situations and it is with this assumption that we proceed to describe how this might safely be accomplished.

☐ 1. Standard Pylorus-Preserving Proximal Pancreaticoduodenectomy

Assessment

The first step is a detailed search for metastatic disease: hepatic metastases, lymph node deposits, peritoneal seedlings, and nodules in the omentum. The transverse colon and greater omentum are retracted upwards to expose the base of the transverse mesocolon and the area of the duodenojejunal flexure. Both are potential sites of tumor extension that will often suggest encasement of the superior mesenteric artery and irresectability. The dorsal surface of the stomach and the peritoneal surface of the lesser sac are also carefully palpated. In the case of neuroendocrine tumors, it is particularly important to examine the small bowel in some detail as the primary tumor may be identified, particularly in gastrinoma. The presence of metastatic disease is not necessarily a sign of irresectability. Some groups have advocated resection of liver metastases in patients with pancreatic adenocarcinoma,[7,23] despite the generally poor prognosis in this group of patients. While noting this difference in surgical attitudes towards pancreatic tumors, we would not advocate resection of liver metastases in the setting of adenocarcinoma of the pancreas but certainly support this procedure in selected patients with neuroendocrine tumors.

Mobilization of the head of the pancreas starts with the performance of a Kocher maneuver by incising the peritoneum along the lateral edge of the second part of the duodenum (Fig. 6.**1**). The hepatic flexure of the colon will sometimes need to be mobilized to achieve this step, but complete mobilization is usually only achieved once the lesser sac is fully opened. With the fingers of the left hand behind the pancreatic head and duodenum, the tumor is elevated to determine size, fixity, and invasion of contiguous structures, notably the portal and superior mesenteric veins (Fig. 6.**2**). At this point it may be possible to identify posterior fixity to the preaortic fascia, which is often heralded by back pain. It may be possible to develop a plane between the tumor and aorta in the case of peritumoral inflammation, but frank posterior invasion of the tumor precludes this step and makes the tumor irresectable. Pancreatic cancer spreads first along the nodes of the anterior and posterior duodenopancreatic grooves and then either along the hepatic artery to the nodes of the celiac

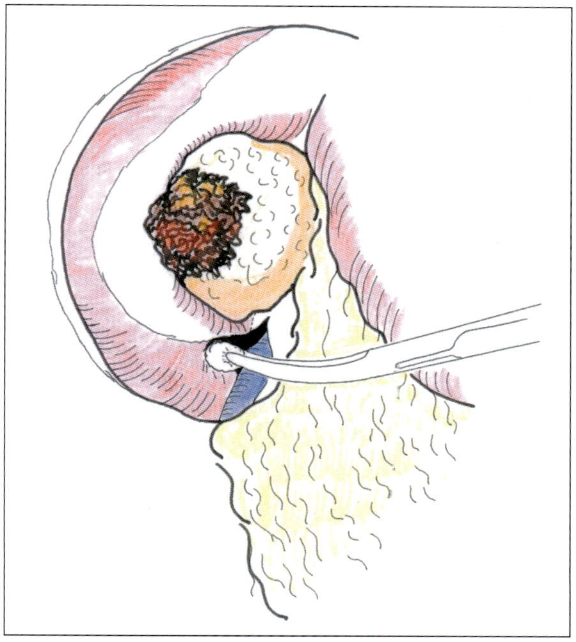

Fig. 6.**1** Incision of the posterior peritoneum and blunt dissection of the second duodenum.

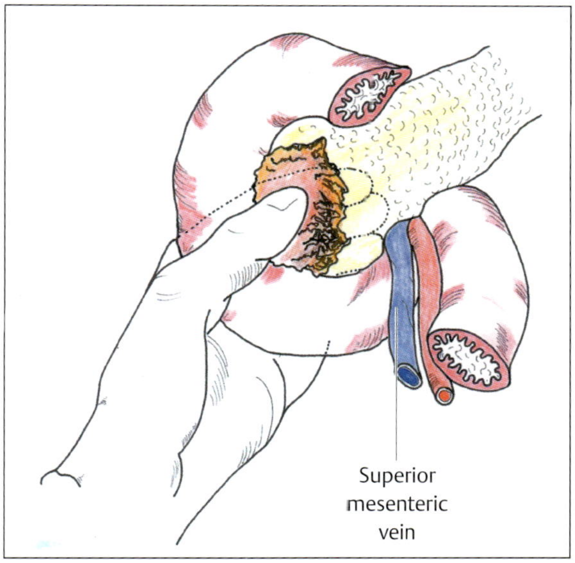

Fig. 6.**2** The head of the pancreas is mobilized by incising the peritoneum along the lateral edge of the second part of the duodenum (Kocher maneuver). After full mobilization of the duodenum and head of the pancreas it is possible to palpate the periampullary area to assess the relationship of the tumor to the portal and superior mesenteric veins and the superior mesenteric artery.

axis or to the superior mesenteric nodes or both, depending on the position of the primary. Nodes adjacent to the pancreas can be resected en bloc and are generally included in a "standard" resection. The inclusion of distant nodes is controversial and is covered below as one possible type of extension.

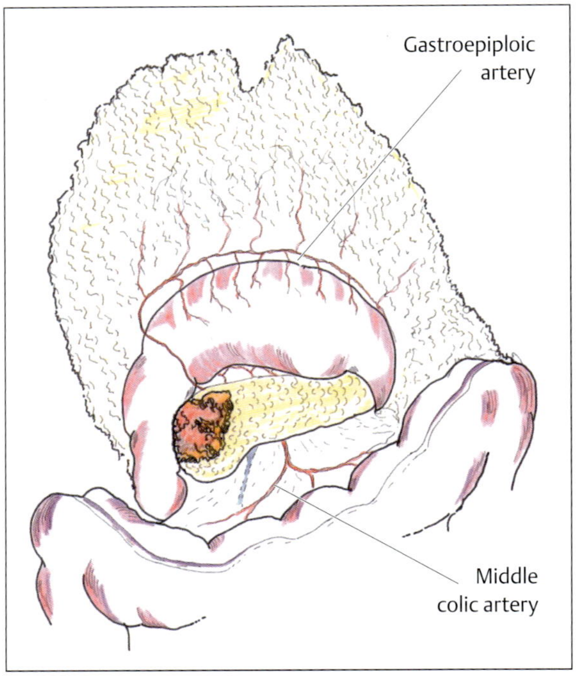

Fig. 6.**3** The lesser sac is entered by elevating the greater omentum and developing the avascular plane between it and the transverse colon, thus exposing the body of the pancreas.

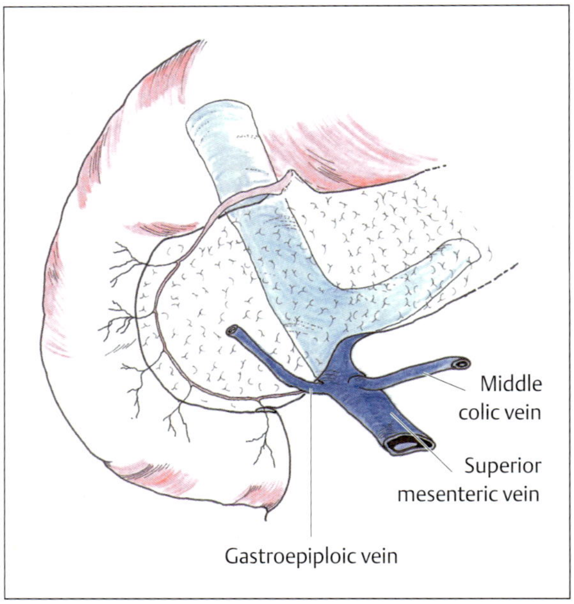

Fig. 6.**4** The superior mesenteric vein is identified at the inferior border of the pancreas. Care must be taken not to damage the middle colic and gastroepiploic veins that enter the superior mesenteric vein at this point.

Once obvious signs of irresectability have been excluded in the form of extensive local invasion or remote metastases, further assessment takes the form of a trial dissection. Much of the necessary mobilization can be achieved without irreversible commitment to a resection. At this point the lesser sac is widely entered by developing the avascular plane between the transverse colon and the greater omentum, keeping well clear of the gastroepiploic vascular arcade (Fig. 6.**3**). Infrequently sizeable veins cross this "avascular" plane and require formal ligation, but most of the dissection can be usually performed with diathermy. Dissection of the greater omentum is continued to the right to mobilize the hepatic flexure of the colon and to the left as far as necessary to expose the neck and body of the pancreas. The tumor may occasionally involve the right colon or its mesocolon by direct tumor invasion or inflammatory adherence. The nature of this involvement may be difficult to determine and en bloc resection of the right colon may then be required (see below).

The stomach and attached greater omentum are retracted upwards and the transverse mesocolon is drawn downwards to expose the lower edge of the pancreatic neck. The middle colic veins are identified and followed as a guide to the superior mesenteric vein below the neck of the pancreas and the peritoneum over the vein is carefully incised to expose the vessel wall (Fig. 6.**4**). Gentle blunt dissection is employed to develop the tunnel between the portal vein and the neck of the pancreas. It may help to divide the right gastroepiploic vein and artery on the pancreas and below the first part of the duodenum to facilitate this exposure, but this step has no adverse consequence if resection is not in fact performed. In some instances it may be quicker and safer to identify the portal vein by approaching it in the lateral groove between the uncinate process and the third part of the duodenum as an extension of Kocher's maneuver (Figs. 6.**5**, 6.**6**), but often it is the clearance of the right lateral border of the portal vein that is most in doubt and a plane may be difficult to develop (Fig. 6.**7**).

If the portal vein tunnel is difficult to develop from below, it may be safer to expose it from above. The peritoneum of the lesser omentum/gastrohepatic ligament is divided to enter the lesser sac from above. The hepatic artery is located, being usually marked by a lymph node or nodes at this site. The artery is traced proximally and distally for a short distance to identify the origin of the gastroduodenal artery, which arises from a "genu" or right-angled bend on the hepatic artery. The gastroduodenal artery is ligated and divided at this point. The hepatic artery is now slung and retracted cephalad to expose the portal vein below. This maneuver is facilitated by dissecting the common bile duct (CBD) and passing a sling around this structure to retract it laterally (Fig. 6.**8**). The plane between the portal vein and the neck of the pancreas is further developed. No major tributaries enter the anterior surface of the portal vein in this area and as long as the dissection does not stray from this plane, bleeding is not usually a problem. At this stage it should be becom-

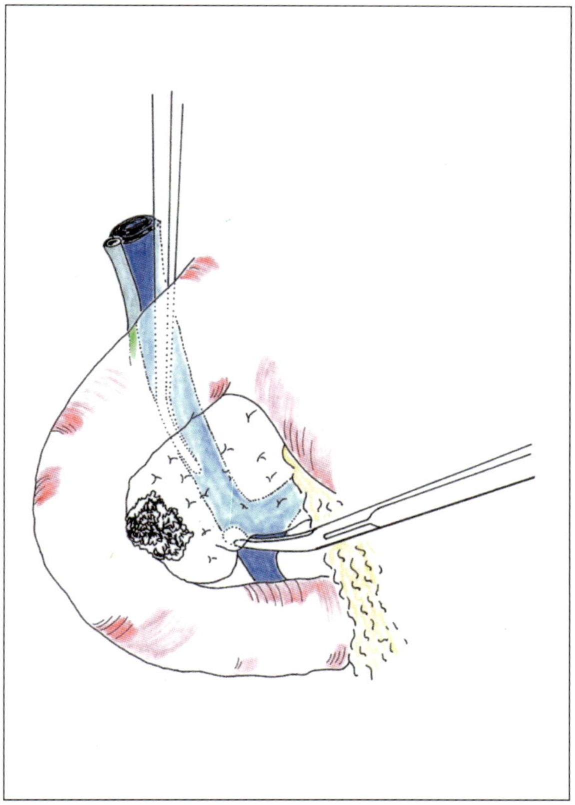

Fig. 6.**5** The superior mesenteric vein is approached between the uncinate process and the third duodenum.

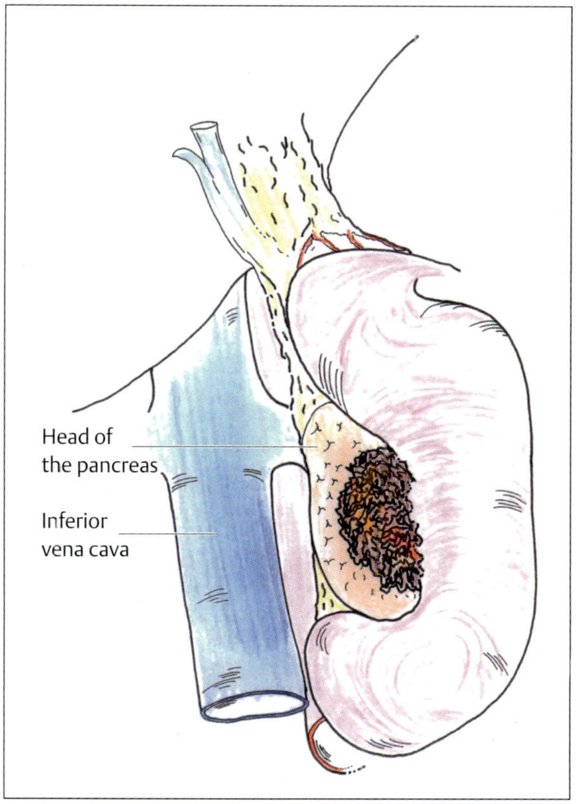

Fig. 6.**6** Complete mobilization of the duodenum and head of the pancreas is shown (Kocher maneuver).

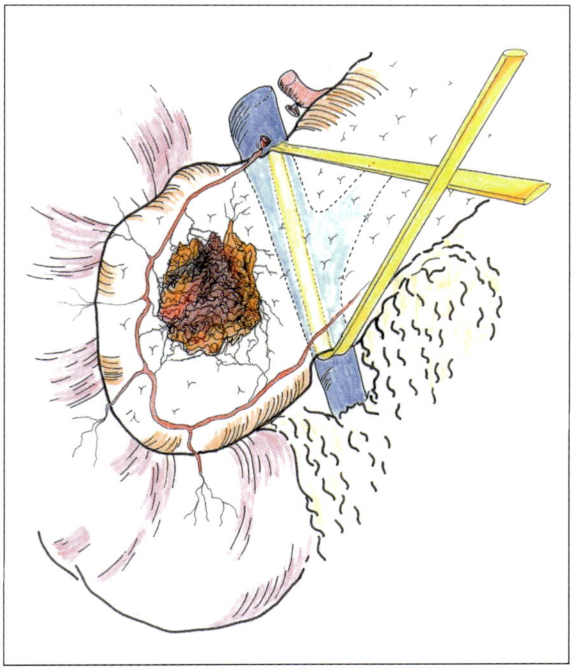

Fig. 6.**7** Gentle blunt dissection is employed to develop the tunnel between the portal vein and the neck of the pancreas. The tunnel between the portal vein and the neck of the pancreas is established and the passage of a sling often aids further dissection.

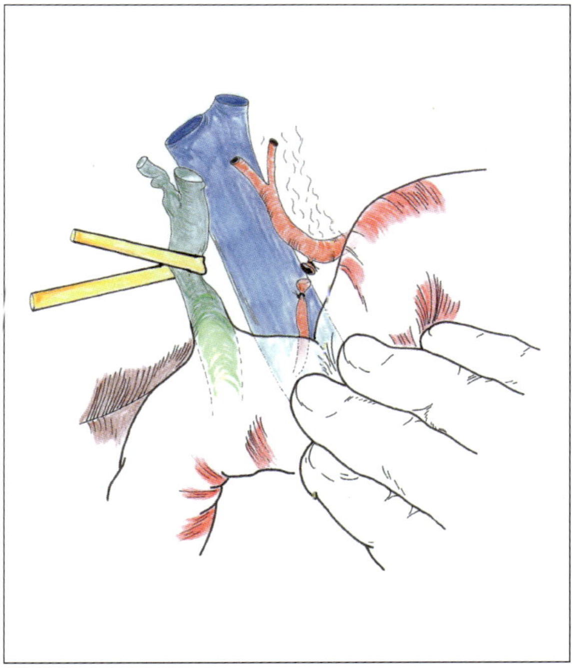

Fig. 6.**8** The gastroduodenal artery is securely ligated before division. As the bile duct is retracted laterally, the suprapancreatic portion of the portal vein is exposed.

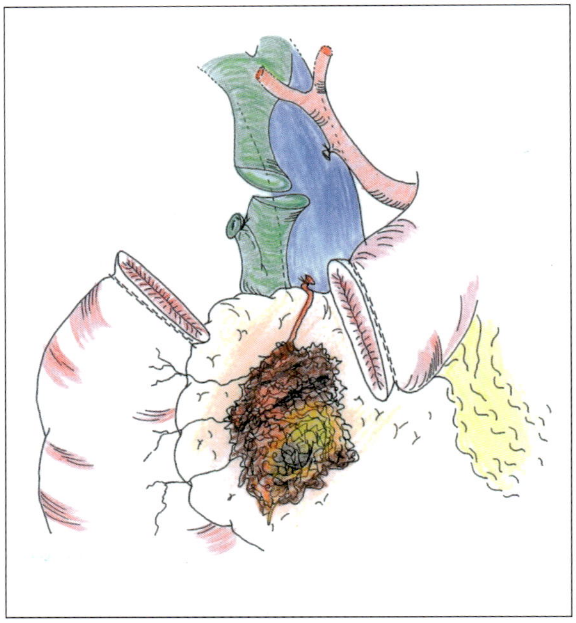

Fig. 6.**9** The bile duct is divided just above the entry of the cystic duct. The duodenum is stapled after the pylorus.

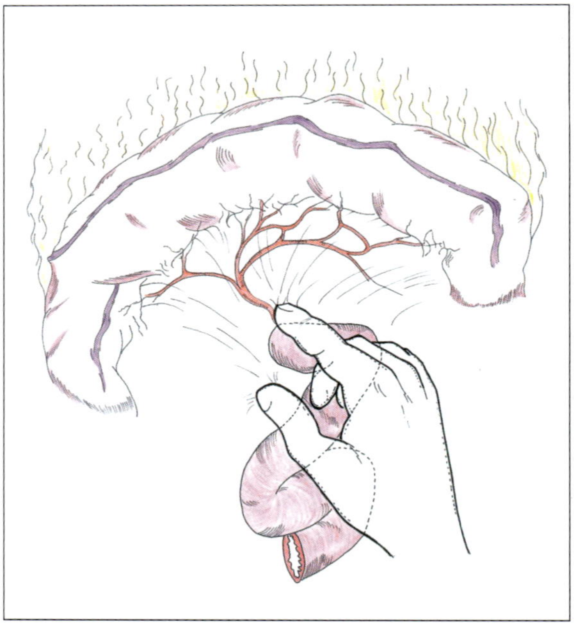

Fig. 6.**10** The root of the transverse mesocolon and the area around the duodenojejunal flexure are further assessed for tumor invasion.

ing clear how the portal vein is related to the tumor and thus whether resection is a possibility. If a surgical palliative bypass is to be completed in any case, then it may be appropriate to divide the CBD at this point to improve access and allow further assessment of the relationship between the tumor and the portal vein. A swab of bile is taken for culture and any indwelling stent is removed and also sent for microbiological examination.

Although there is no clear oncological benefit in removing the uninvolved gallbladder, we generally complete a retrograde cholecystectomy and divide the bile duct at the point of entry of the cystic duct (Fig. 6.**9**). Removing the gallbladder should allow for a higher division of the bile duct, thus clearing more nodal tissue, avoiding the problem of an ischemic stump and future potential problems with gallstones and cholecystitis due either to tumor invasion of the cystic duct or as a consequence of any adjuvant chemotherapy. In practice, however, experience with preservation of the gallbladder in pancreaticoduodenectomy for chronic pancreatitis or less aggressive periampullary tumors has shown little or no ill effect from such a maneuver.[22]

Attention is now turned to the duodenojejunal flexure, where the fourth part of the duodenum is further mobilized by dividing the ligament of Treitz to assess the tumor relationship to the SMA (Fig. 6.**10**). If resection looks feasible, then it is reasonable to divide the first part of the jejunum and begin mobilization of the proximal portion by dividing the jejunal and duodenal branches of the SMA close to the bowel wall, taking care not to damage the main vessel or the adjacent inferior mesenteric vein. This maneuver represents an irreversible step as the jejunum quickly becomes ischemic and will need to be resected in any case. Jejunal transection can be delayed until after division of the pancreas, but in reality the resectability or otherwise of the tumor is usually evident by this stage of the assessment. We tend to mobilize the jejunum and fourth part of the duodenum as much as possible from below the transverse mesocolon as the access and exposure allow this to be achieved more easily than from above, although the dissection can proceed from both aspects according to satisfactory progress.

Resection

The boundary between assessment and resection becomes blurred at this stage of the procedure, but it is now that a decision needs to be made on the resectability of the tumor and whether the antrum and/or portal vein are to be resected. For a carcinoma arising in the upper head of the pancreas close to the pylorus or duodenal cap, a formal Whipple procedure incorporating distal gastrectomy will be needed. For lesions of the lower pancreas head or uncinate process, we generally favor a pylorus-preserving resection but perform frozen section histology of the duodenal resection margin. Should the result (exceptionally) be positive for carcinoma, or should we feel that tumor clearance might be compromised in any way, we have little hesitation in resecting the antrum of the stomach (see below). The first part of the duodenum is mobilized from the pancreas by securing several small vessels

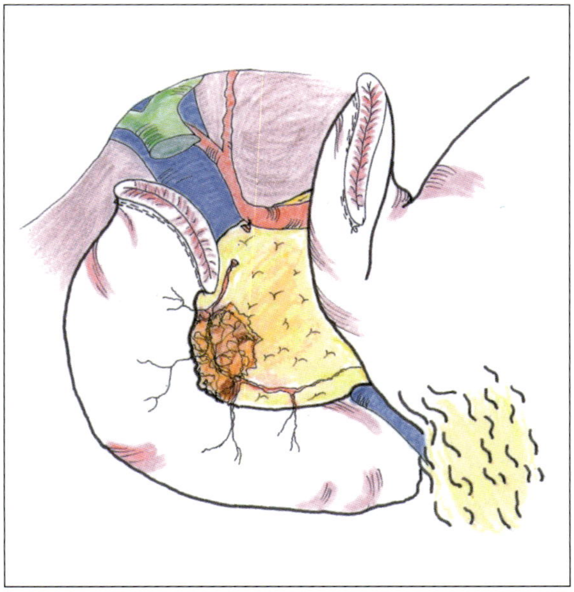

Fig. 6.**11** The bile duct is divided at a convenient point, usually above the cystic duct. This provides further access to the portal vein.

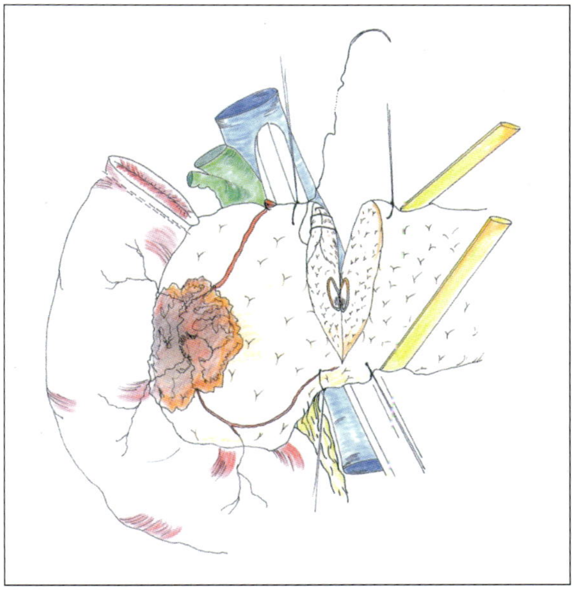

Fig. 6.**12** The neck of the pancreas is divided between hemostatic stay sutures. Care is taken to protect the portal vein at this point.

that run between the two organs thereby allowing division of the duodenum by stapling or between fine clamps about a few cm distal to the pylorus (Fig. 6.**11**). The distal end is oversewn and the proximal end is tucked away into the left upper quadrant, taking care not to damage the spleen. The stomach is emptied by suction and the duodenal cap is then surrounded by a swab soaked in antiseptic solution if occluded by tissue forceps. If stapled the duodenal stump is simply rubbed with an antiseptic swab. It is important to maintain an adequate blood supply to the pylorus and in the absence of the gastroduodenal artery, the blood supply is dependent on the gastroepiploic arcade which should be preserved on the greater curve of the stomach. This is another reason for elevating the greater omentum off the transverse colon rather than entering the gastrocolic omentum directly.

Our standard approach is now to divide the neck of the pancreas, which has been clearly exposed by retracting the stomach to the left (Fig. 6.**12**). In some instances the portal vein can be resected at this point and this maneuver is described below. A Kocher's grooved director is inserted along the portal vein tunnel and stay sutures are inserted into the inferior and superior margins of the neck of the pancreas on either side of the line of anticipated division partly to enclose small arteries running on the surface of the gland and partly to facilitate retraction. The neck of the pancreas is now divided. We prefer to use a scalpel as it allows clear visualization of the pancreatic duct and makes frozen section examination of the cut surface easier to interpret without diathermy artefact. If frozen section is positive, then we consider extending the pancreatectomy or completing a total pancreatectomy (see below). Frozen section is used in this way by other groups.[24–27]

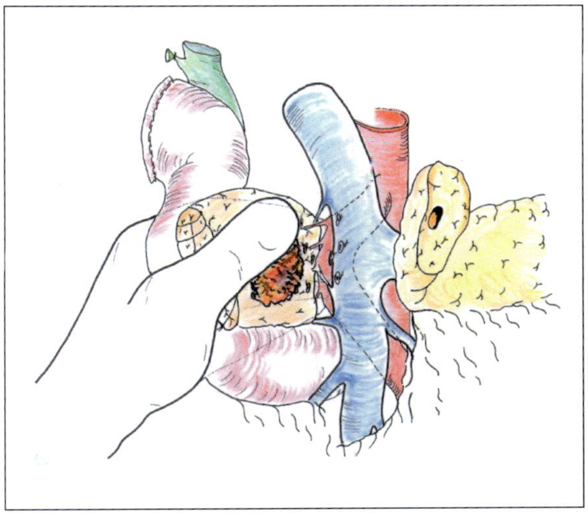

Fig. 6.**13** With the operator's left hand behind the head of the pancreas, the plane between the pancreas and portal vein is gently developed, ligating any vessels that are encountered. Excessive traction may pull the superior mesenteric artery to the right of the portal vein and place it at risk during dissection.

The head of the pancreas and duodenum are now supplied only by a few tributaries of the portal vein and the duodenal branches of the second/third part of the duodenum. With the operator's left hand behind the head of the pancreas and with aid of a small swab, the right hand is used to sweep the portal vein gently off the pancreas, ligating any vessels that are encountered (Fig. 6.**13**). The venous drainage is relatively constant and comprises an upper pole vein and two-to-three

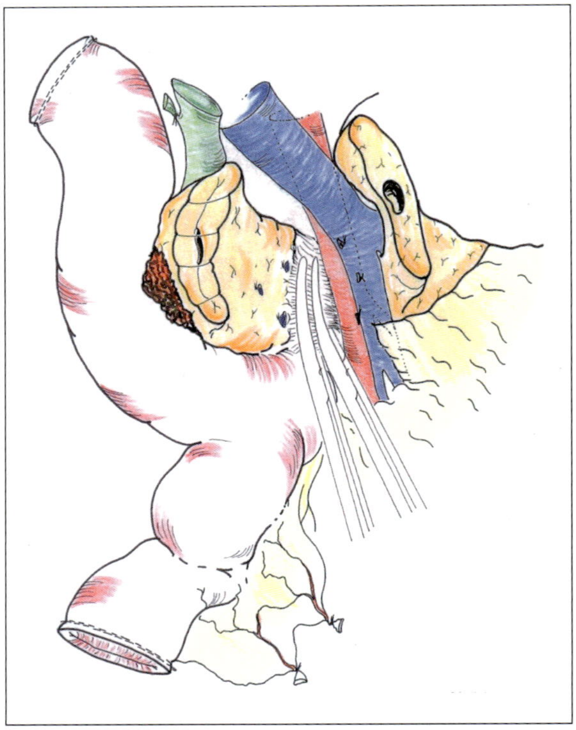

Fig. 6.**14** The deep part of the pancreas is bound down by fascia surrounding the aorta and superior mesenteric artery. This usually needs to be divided between ligatures.

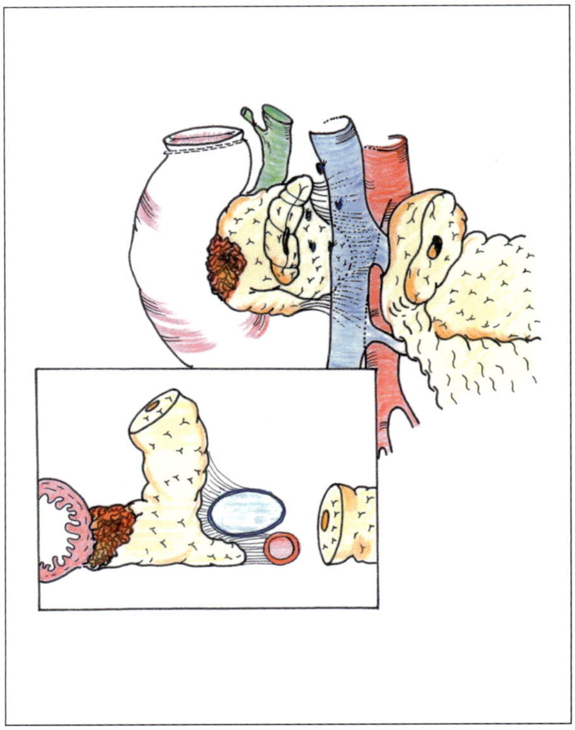

Fig. 6.**15** The frontal view and cross-section show how the deep part of the pancreas is closely bound to the superior mesenteric artery by tough connective tissue and requires retraction of the margin of the portal vein for full exposure.

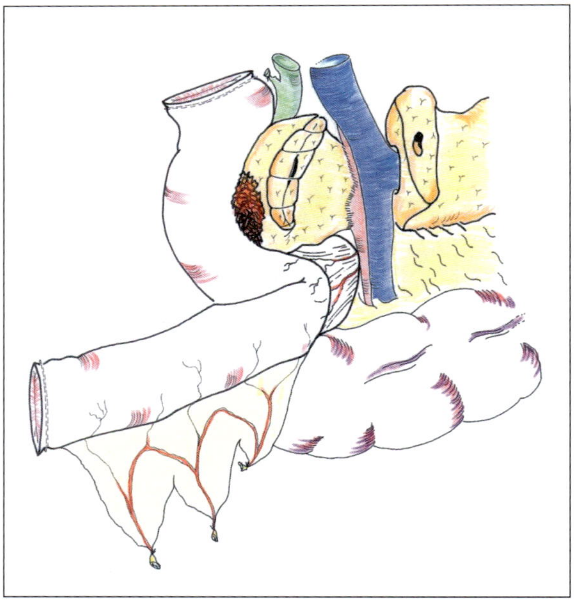

Fig. 6.**16** The first jejunal loop is passed through the mesocolic window on the right of the superior mesenteric vessels.

inferior pancreatic veins; they are fragile and need to be encircled and ligated with care. The left hand in this position allows palpation of the SMA to make sure it is not included in ligatures and it also allows for control of the portal vein if hemorrhage is encountered. It is necessary to divide the roots or "crura" of the pancreas, i.e., the tough connective tissue that binds its deep surface to the preaortic fascia (Figs. 6.**14**, 6.**15**). Leashes of tissue are encircled with a right-angled forceps and are ligated and divided. One or more of these tissue leashes will include SMA branches, i.e., inferior pancreaticoduodenal artery or arteries, but if they are all ligated then bleeding should not occur. The dissection is carried out just beyond the border of the pancreas (which is recognized by its lobular appearance) unless the tumor appears to be infiltrating in this region or a decision is taken to skeletonize the SMA. Pulling the mobilized proximal jejunum through the congenital mesocolic window into the supracolic compartment often helps orientation and clarifies the appropriate place for jejunal division, which is usually 20–30 cm beyond the duodenojejunal flexure (Fig. 6.**16**). It is during this final dissection that the detailed relationship between tumor and portal vein becomes apparent. A degree of "adhesion" often exists and it can be difficult to decide between tumor invasion and inflammatory change. This part of the operation is time-consuming

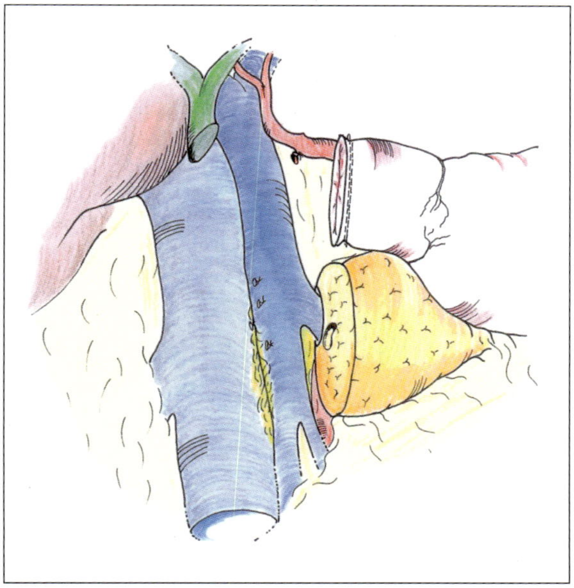

Fig. 6.**17** Once the specimen is resected the deep attachments of the pancreas head can be inspected for final hemostasis.

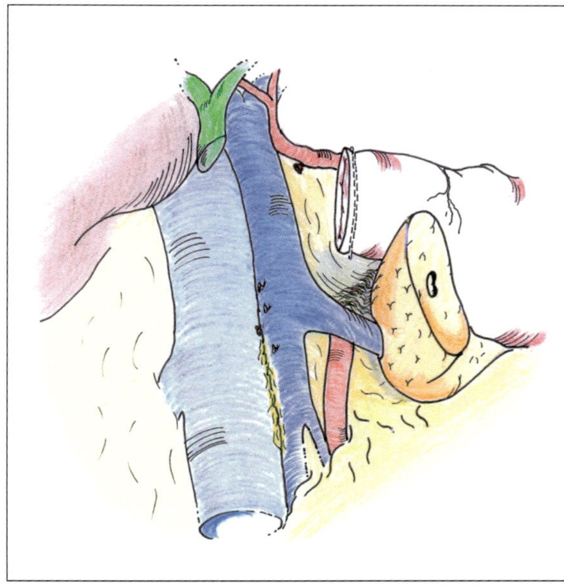

Fig. 6.**18** The pancreatic anastomosis is facilitated by mobilizing the posterior surface of the proximal body of the pancreas off the splenic vein for a distance of 3–4 cm.

and care must be taken to achieve hemostasis (Fig. 6.**17**). The indication and technique for resection of the portal vein are described below if this maneuver is to be included.

Reconstruction

Several methods of reconstruction are possible, each with its own advocates and none of proven superiority. The most important points are technical skill in creating the several anastomoses and adherence to surgical principles of good blood supply, freedom from tension, and careful hemostasis. The pancreatic anastomosis is the Achilles' heel of pancreaticoduodenectomy and a greater impact on postresection survival can be made by reducing the operative mortality rate than by the application of extended resection or adjuvant treatments. Our preference is to commence by joining the pancreatic neck to the upper jejunum, end-to-end, followed by the bile duct anastomosis, and finally the duodenoenterostomy, as described previously.[28] The jejunum is usually delivered to the supracolic compartment through the congenital tunnel behind the superior mesenteric vessels but in certain cases, for example a tumor of the uncinate process, it may be better to use a separate right-sided mesocolic window.

The two-layer pancreaticojejunostomy is facilitated by mobilizing the posterior surface of the proximal body of the pancreas off the splenic vein for a distance of 3–4 cm, carefully dividing between ligatures one or more tributaries of the splenic vein (Fig. 6.**18**). The exact technique employed depends on the disease process and consequently the calibre of the pancreatic duct and the nature of the pancreatic parenchyma: soft glands with small ducts require an invaginating or "dunking" type of anastomosis with a supporting stent, while glands with dilated ducts and firm parenchyma can be sutured directly mucosa-to-mucosa with the jejunum. However, in every case it is appropriate to have at least some of the sutures incorporate ductal mucosa and to include an outer layer of invaginating sutures.

The end-to-end invaginating anastomosis is carried out using two layers of interrupted nonabsorbable (3–0 silk) sutures. However, some authors perform the entire anastomosis with 4–0 or even 5–0 PDS absorbable sutures. Initially, a few anterior sutures are placed through the pancreatic parenchyma so as to emerge from the duct and these are held in hemostats; if the duct is small this may be the only opportunity to suture its mucosa anteriorly (these sutures are represented on Fig. 6.**19a,b**). Then a first posterior row of inner sutures is placed between the pancreatic duct (and pancreatic parenchyma outside the duct) and the seromuscular layer of the jejunum. When meeting the duct, the full thickness of the jejunum is taken (Fig. 6.**19a**). In this posterior row, the sutures are first inserted then tied up. The second inner layer incorporates the pancreatic parenchyma and the full thickness of the small intestine (Fig. 6.**19b**). The sutures must be tied with great care to avoid them cutting through the pancreatic tissue and causing troublesome bleeding halfway through construction of the anastomosis. The anterior inner layer then unites the cut surface of the pancreas and its duct to the full thickness of the jejunum (Fig. 6.**19c**) and the

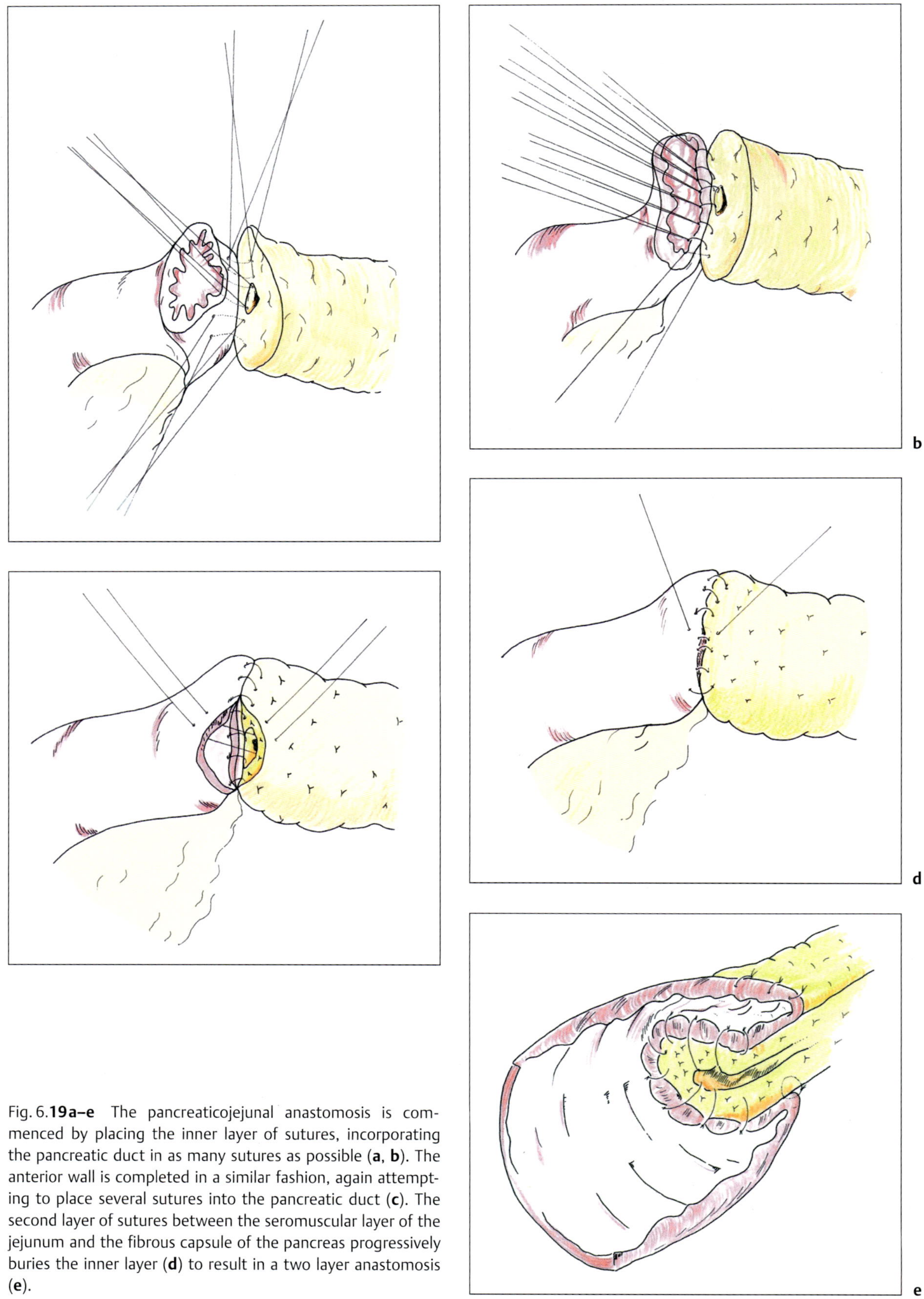

Fig. 6.**19a–e** The pancreaticojejunal anastomosis is commenced by placing the inner layer of sutures, incorporating the pancreatic duct in as many sutures as possible (**a**, **b**). The anterior wall is completed in a similar fashion, again attempting to place several sutures into the pancreatic duct (**c**). The second layer of sutures between the seromuscular layer of the jejunum and the fibrous capsule of the pancreas progressively buries the inner layer (**d**) to result in a two layer anastomosis (**e**).

outer layer of sutures is placed between the seromuscular coat of the bowel and the fibrous pancreatic capsule, drawing the jejunum over the inner anastomosis like a sheath; this second layer should be placed approximately 1 cm beyond the first layer so as to ensure sufficient tissue for invagination (Fig. 6.**19d**). Although each individual outer suture only draws the jejunum over by a small amount, with care and progressive suturing, it is eventually possible to "bury" the inner layer 1.5–2 cm within the outer layer (Fig. 6.**19e**). We attempt to incorporate the duct mucosa in as many inner sutures as possible and even in very small ducts find that 3–4 sutures can be placed in this fashion both anteriorly and posteriorly. When concerned about patency of the pancreatic duct, we place a trans-anastomotic stent in the form of a pediatric feeding tube (6 or 8 Fr) across the anastomosis (Fig. 6.**20a,b**). The tube is first passed through the abdominal wall and then along the jejunum, entering some 30 cm distal to its cut end. The tube is passed up the pancreatic duct, if possible for 5–10 cm. The stent is anchored within the pancreatic duct using an absorbable suture (4–0 PDS) before completing the anastomosis. The stent is pierced by one needle of a double-ended suture and each needle is brought out through the duct and the pancreatic tissue so the suture can be tied over a small buttress of muscle taken from the rectus abdominus (Fig. 6.**20c**). Using this technique we have reported a pancreatic leak rate of 4%.[21] The stent is then exteriorized and the jejunum around the stent exit point is ultimately sutured to the peritoneum of the anterior abdominal wall. The stent can be clamped (with or without tubography) after the early postoperative phase and it is removed before the patient's discharge or at an early outpatient follow-up visit.

The biliary anastomosis is now fashioned at a point 10–15 cm distal to the pancreatic anastomosis. We perform an end-to-side hepaticojejunostomy using a single layer of interrupted absorbable sutures (4–0 Vicryl). Again some authors use 4–0 or 5–0 PDS sutures. We place all the posterior wall sutures before tying them on the inside (Fig. 6.**21a**). The anterior wall is completed in a similar fashion with sutures being tied on the outside (Fig. 6.**21b**). We rarely use a stent or T-tube for this anastomosis.

Finally, the duodenoenterostomy is completed a further 30–40 cm distally.

The viability of the duodenum is assessed once the clamp is removed and usually 1–2 cm of the duodenum is trimmed. We aim to leave 2–4 cm of duodenum beyond the pylorus and carry out a two layer end-to-side anastomosis (Fig. 6.**22**). Soft drains are placed in the region of the pancreatic and biliary anastomoses before the abdomen is closed. A 14 Fr T-tube is frequently placed well below the duodenoenteric anastomosis for use as a feeding jejunostomy.

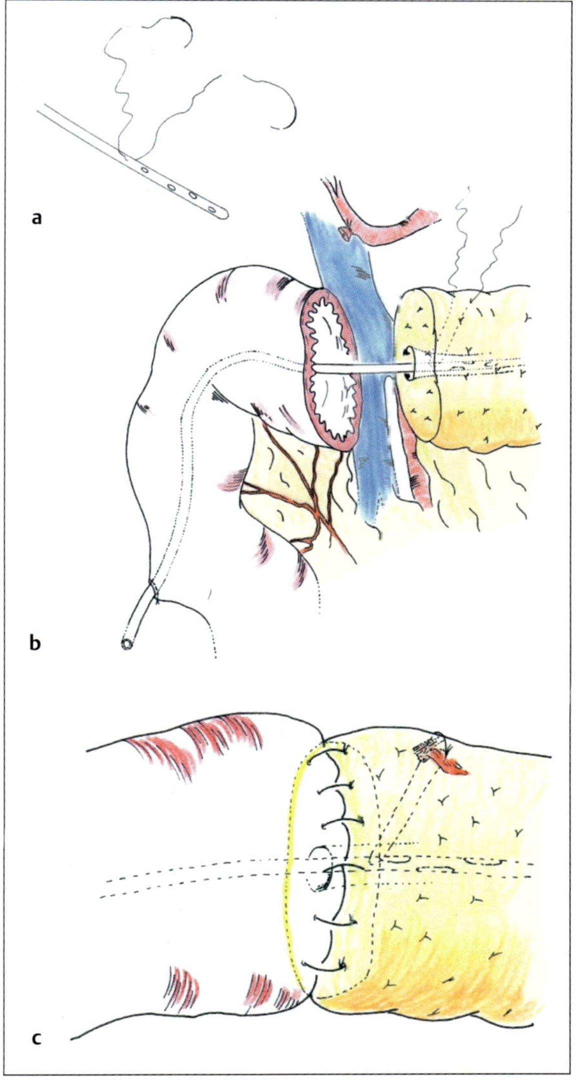

Fig. 6.**20a–c** To secure the transanastomotic stent we firstly transfix the stent with a double-ended, fine absorbable suture (**a**). Each needle is then brought out through the pancreatic parenchyma via the pancreatic duct (**b**) before the suture is tied over a small buttress of abdominal wall muscle (**c**) to prevent it cutting through the parenchyma.

This is the description of our "standard" technique, but we accept that there are many variations to the basic pancreaticoduodenectomy procedure, many of which have been widely published. The rest of this chapter will focus on aspects of the procedure that may be "extended" in some way, describing the indications, technique, and the results that are being achieved in different centers.

2. Distal or Total Pancreatectomy with Splenectomy

Tumors of the pancreas located to the left of the portal vein and tumors of the stomach may occasionally re-

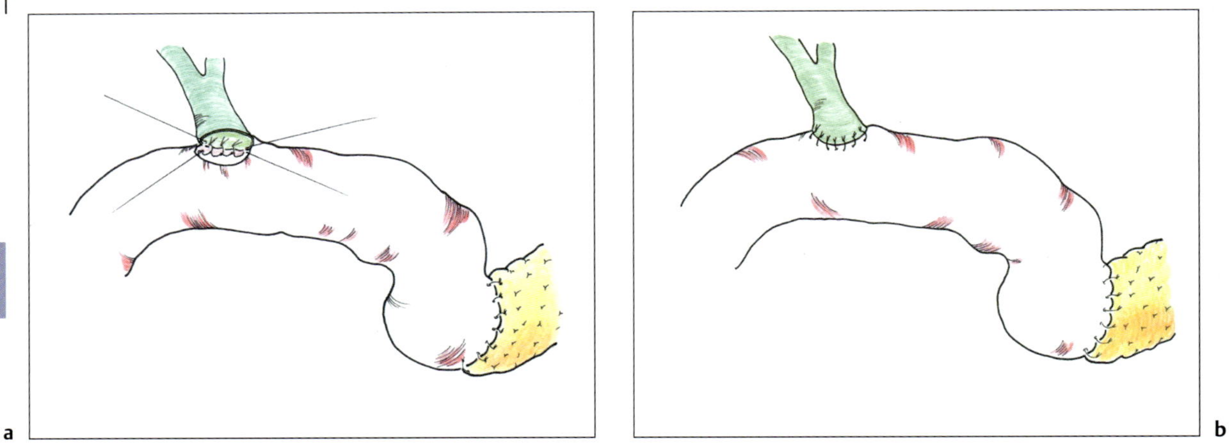

Fig. 6.**21 a,b** The hepaticojejunostomy is completed with the interrupted posterior full thickness row of fine absorbable sutures tied on the inside (**a**) and the anterior similar row tied on the outside (**b**).

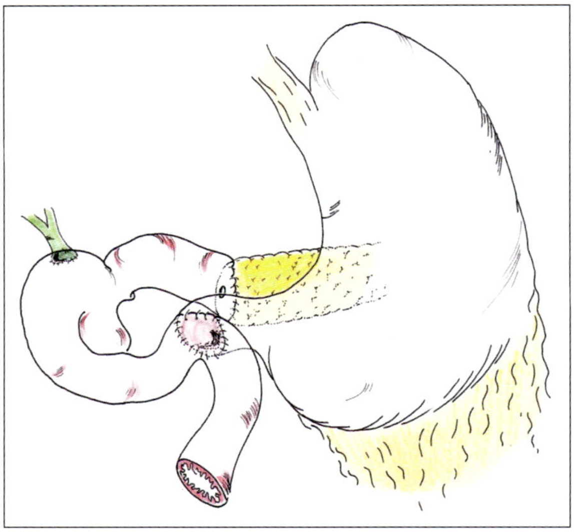

Fig. 6.**22** Once the end-to-side anastomosis between the duodenum and jejunum is carried out, the "standard" pylorus preserving proximal pancreaticoduodenectomy (PPPP) is completed.

quire an en bloc resection of both organs (see below). Although it is unlikely that pancreaticosplenic resection in combination with gastric carcinoma adds any survival advantage,[29] it may sometimes be required to achieve a curative resection. The present chapter is concerned with distal pancreatectomy either as a stand-alone procedure or as the second half of a total pancreatectomy in situations in which the gland has already been divided. Despite several small reports of encouraging results for left-sided pancreatic tumors, nihilism still prevails in ductal carcinoma. One paper advocated that "resection of pancreatic cancer of the body or tail should only be performed for those rare, small tumors not extending outside the pancreas."[30]

Distal pancreatectomy can sometimes be achieved with splenic preservation and we have described this technique elsewhere for benign disease,[31] but in the setting of pancreatic adenocarcinoma of the body or tail, conservation of the spleen is surely inappropriate. Others have suggested that because the long-term outcome after splenectomy in this setting is worse, splenectomy should only be performed if there is direct tumor extension, vascular invasion, or the need for nodal clearance.[19,32] In a nonrandomized study, the group that required splenectomy had significantly larger tumors and a higher rate of vascular involvement.[32] Cystic neoplasms of the pancreas and neuroendocrine tumors have a different biologic behavior to that of adenocarcinoma and preservation of the spleen may therefore be appropriate.[33]

Although the benefit of staging laparoscopy for tumors of the pancreatic head is debatable, the yield from this investigation for tumors of the body or tail would certainly justify its performance. A prospective study has shown a higher rate of detection of liver and peritoneal metastases in this situation.[34]

Early in the assessment of resectability of a left-sided tumor, it is essential to consider encasement of the celiac axis as nodal involvement can be present even in small tumors.[35] This step can be aided by intraoperative US. Although involvement of the vessels in this area does not preclude resection, it does substantially diminish the likelihood of long-term survival. Most authors believe that encasement is a sign of incurability and that resection should not be undertaken in such circumstances.[19,36]

At laparotomy for carcinoma of the neck, body, or tail of the pancreas, the lesser sac is opened further to the left than described above and the short gastric vessels are ligated and divided outside the gastroepiploic arcade. The portal vein tunnel is developed as before and a decision is made on where to transect the pancreas. Following transection, the distal end of the proximal pancreatic remnant is oversewn with interrupted 3–0 nonabsorbable sutures (Prolene or silk). The pancreatic duct should be identified and separately transfixed with a fine suture before closure of the parenchyma (Fig. 6.**23**). The posterosuperior surface of the pancreas is freed from the retroperitoneal tissue to identify the origin of the splenic artery, which is doubly ligated before division as it runs from the celiac trunk to gain the superior border of the pancreas. The splenic vein is then separated from the posterior aspect of the gland and divided immediately beyond its junction with the inferior mesenteric vein (IMV). The IMV can usually be spared because it joins the splenic vein very close to its termination, but if its junction is further to the left then it can also be divided without additional morbidity. Using the hemostatic stay sutures placed into the pancreas before division, the distal gland can be drawn upwards, facilitating the dissection of a margin of retroperitoneal, peripancreatic tissue with the gland. Once the distal dissection becomes difficult the spleen can be drawn medially and division of the lienorenal and lienocolic ligaments at this stage will complete the resection.

Total pancreaticoduodenectomy has certain specific indications but is not routinely performed. A one-stage procedure may be performed in patients in whom pancreatic head tumors reach too close to the plane of division of the pancreas for a standard pancreaticoduodenectomy (PD) or similarly if large tumors of the body of the pancreas reach across to the right side of the portal vein.[37] A total pancreatectomy (TP) may be considered in patients who present with tumors in the head of the pancreas but have preexisting insulin-dependent diabetes mellitus. A two-stage procedure may be performed at the time of the initial resection of the pancreatic head if frozen section of the resection margin confirms positive margins or alternatively at a later date, usually for a dehiscence of the pancreatic anastomosis requiring salvage surgery.

The incision and initial phase of dissection and exploration are identical to those of the standard PD described above. If resection is to proceed, the whole of the greater omentum is freed from the transverse colon to expose the lesser sac. Dissection of the hepatoduodenal ligament, including Kocher's maneuver, cholecystectomy, division of the gastroduodenal artery, and mobilization of the pancreatic neck are performed as already described. The splenic artery is identified at its origin and doubly ligated before division. The ligamentous attachments of the spleen are divided taking care not to damage the splenic flexure of the left colon. The spleen and pancreatic tail are retracted medially and the pancreas is dissected from its retroperitoneal attachments in a plane deep to the splenic vein (Fig. 6.**24**). In cases of large tumors of the body of pancreas, there may be encroachment onto the transverse mesocolon and consideration can be given to en bloc resection of this structure, as described below. Once the splenic vein has

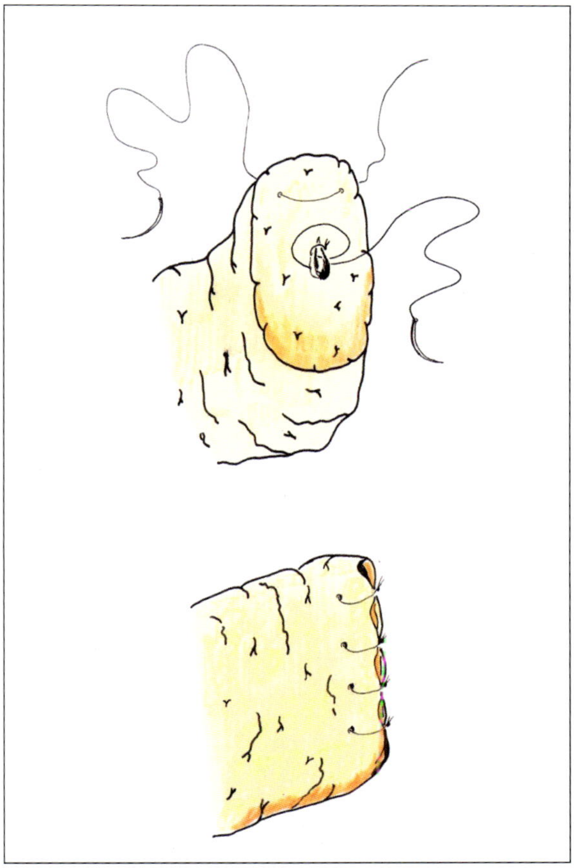

Fig. 6.**23** The pancreatic duct is identified within the bevelled cut surface of the distal pancreas and is specifically sutured before the parenchyma of the gland is closed with interrupted sutures.

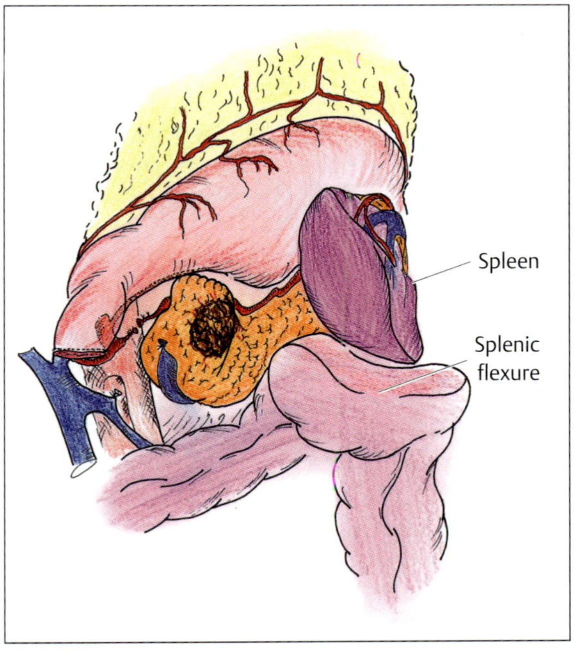

Fig. 6.**24** Total pancreatectomy: the splenic vessels are ligated. The splenic flexure of the colon is mobilized. The spleen and body of the pancreas are medially retracted.

2

2

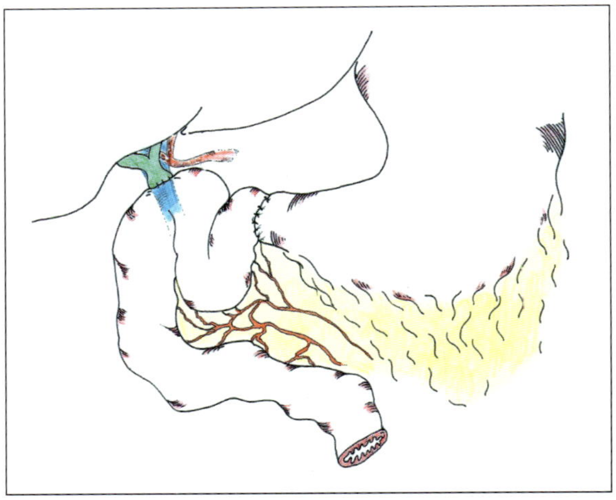

Fig. 6.**25** In the absence of a pancreatic anastomosis the reconstruction is simplified to two anastomoses.

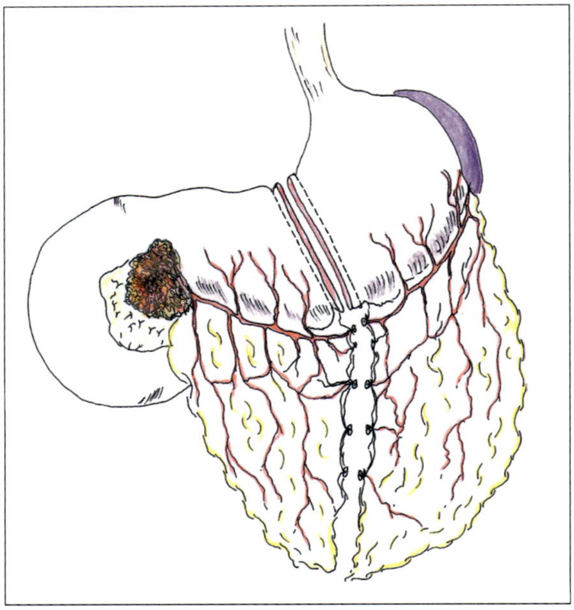

Fig. 6.**26** The greater omentum is divided between ligatures along the line of planned transection of the stomach if a partial gastrectomy is to be added to the resection.

been exposed on the posterior surface of the pancreas, it can be safely ligated and divided close to the SMV. Since all the short gastric vessels will have been divided the venous return of the stomach will be primarily through the left gastric vein (coronary vein) and this vessel should be preserved. Reconstruction is completed by formation of a two-layer end-to-end duodenojejunal anastomosis followed by an end-to-side hepaticojejunostomy some 10–15 cm distally (Fig. 6.**25**).

The argument in support of TP has been based on its being a safer procedure without a pancreaticojejunal anastomosis and a better cancer operation, dealing with multicentric carcinoma and allowing for a complete lymphadenectomy and a wider soft tissue resection. Although pancreatic cancer was thought to be multicentric in about 30% of cases,[38,39] this has not been borne out by histologic studies[25,40] suggesting that although tumors can spread widely (supporting the case for frozen section examination[24,41]), most are continuous with the primary focus and true discontinuous tumors are uncommon. With the operative mortality rate of PPPP at or below 5% in most larger centers, the case for TP being a safer operation is difficult to support. Earlier reports show that the operative mortality rate for TP was 15% with a mean survival of 14 months.[39] Thus, TP does not emerge as a superior treatment[38,42,43] and its routine use in pancreatic carcinoma is not recommended particularly considering reports of a worse outcome than compared to standard PD.[44]

□ 3. Gastrectomy

It may be necessary to remove the distal stomach in tumors related to the head of the pancreas or occasionally the body of the stomach in tumors related to the body or tail of the pancreas. It is also appropriate to resect the distal stomach when tumors of the upper part of the pancreatic head are closely applied to the pyloric area or in the setting of previous duodenal/pyloric surgery, or active peptic ulcer disease. This resection usually entails no more than an antrectomy, i. e., a distal 30–40% gastrectomy. Modern drugs to control gastric acid secretion obviate the need for routine vagotomy; stomal ulceration in the postoperative period is rare. The site of gastric division is identified, linking a convenient point on the greater curve and a point on the lesser curve distal to the left gastric artery and mobilization commences. The greater omentum is divided between ligatures to expose the greater curve of the stomach at the predetermined site and a similar clearance is achieved for the vessels on the lesser curve (Fig. 6.**26**). The lesser omentum close to the gastric wall can be separated into an anterior and posterior sheet and care is required to secure both leashes of vessels to avoid troublesome bleeding. We prefer to divide the stomach with a linear stapling device after withdrawal of the nasogastric tube into the proximal remnant. We oversew the staple line with a running 3–0 Vicryl suture primarily for hemostasis. It is now necessary to fashion a gastroenterostomy rather than a duodenoenteric anastomosis, but this is completed in the same sequence and the same position. A continuous double-layer anastomosis is created between the jejunum and posterior wall of the stomach at a point 2–3 cm proximal to the staple line (Fig. 6.**27**).

During a distal pancreatectomy (see above) it may sometimes be necessary to resect the posterior gastric wall[36] or be ready to undertake a complete a gastrectomy[45] because of tumor proximity, especially in the

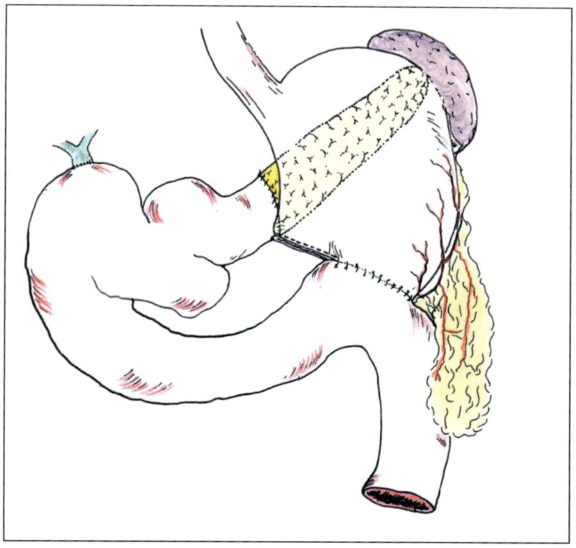

Fig. 6.**27** The reconstruction used in cases of resection of the distal stomach (Whipple's resection) is shown.

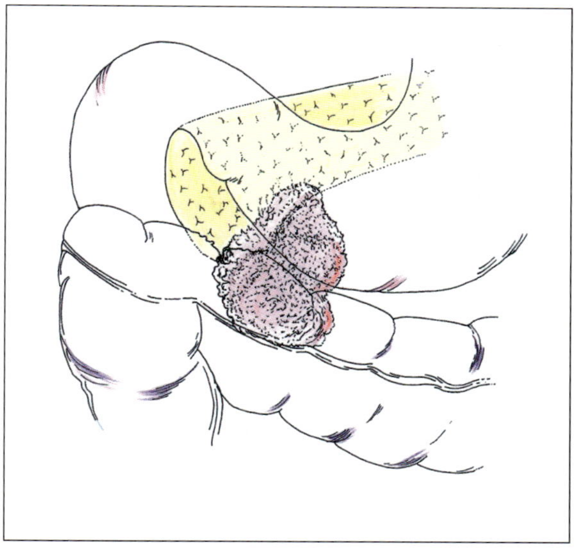

Fig. 6.**28** Tumors involving the mesocolon of the right colon (either originating from the colon or the pancreas/duodenum) may occasionally warrant a combined resection.

setting of a large neuroendocrine tumor. With adenocarcinoma of the pancreas, gastric invasion is seldom the only limitation to a curative resection. Once the lesser sac is opened widely to the left to include all the short gastric vessels, the posterior wall of the stomach is very accessible, particularly if a total pancreatectomy is being performed and the duodenum has already been divided. If the greater omentum is involved in the tumor mass, then this should be excised en bloc and a distal gastrectomy may be more appropriate than a partial excision of the posterior gastric wall. However, if the posterior wall of the stomach alone is involved, then it may be sufficient to "tent" this portion of the stomach and resect a disk of stomach wall with the aid of a linear stapling device.

□ 4. Colectomy

Combined resection of the pancreas and colon is occasionally performed for advanced colonic cancer but may also be appropriate in the context of pancreatic disease. Carcinoma of the head of the pancreas rarely invades the colon directly (in the region of the hepatic flexure) but quite commonly involves the mesocolon (Fig. 6.**28**). The decision to perform a resection in such circumstances is focused primarily on the relationship of the tumor to the superior mesenteric vessels and often involves a tumor of the ventral pancreas (uncinate process). In some instances it may be necessary to divide the middle/right colic vessels to delineate the SMV/PV junction and this maneuver can lead to ischemia of the transverse colon sufficient to require resection. If initial division of the vessels in such circumstances is performed close to the base of the mesocolon, then a sufficient arcade will often exist to sustain the transverse colon whether pancreatectomy is undertaken or ultimately abandoned.

The initial steps of the operation for a pancreatic carcinoma invading the mesocolon comprise mobilization of the duodenum and full mobilization of the right colon. As in any extended resection, it is generally easier to begin the dissection away from the site of tumor adherence and then move closer to it from many directions. In this situation the cecum and terminal ileum are mobilized from below to the level of the duodenum to allow full assessment of the superior mesenteric vessels. Careful exposure of the SMV below the tumor will give some indication of the length of PV/SMV involved and in some circumstances it may be possible to resect the PV as well (see below). The rate-limiting step in this setting is usually encasement of the SMA, but if this vessel seems to be clear of the cancer we proceed to divide the pancreas as above and to divide the transverse colon (beyond the affected segment) and the terminal ileum with the aid of a linear stapler. The upper part of the pancreas is then mobilized from the portal vein, further closing in on the area of maximal tumor involvement. This maneuver may expose an area of SMV that is involved and a decision regarding resection can now be made. Resection is completed taking particular care not to damage the SMA, which can be drawn a long way to the right with traction on the tumor mass. Despite this prolonged dissection it may become evident that the SMA is encased with tumor or nodal disease. Although not the initial aim, by now the surgeon is committed to completing a palliative resection. In patients with neuroendocrine tumors or cystic neoplasms of the pancreas, a palliative resection can provide useful symptom relief and is likely to prolong survival. Following combined colectomy and pancreaticoduodenectomy, reconstruction is carried out in the usual way leaving the ileocolic anastomosis to last. After thorough lavage of the abdominal cavity, an attempt can be made physically to separate the ileocolic anastomosis from the other anastomoses by using the remaining omentum as a barrier.

Tumors of the left pancreas tend to be larger than those of the right pancreas at the time of presentation and commonly involve the transverse mesocolon. Those tumors arising from the tail may lie at a distance from the PV/SMV area and may therefore be amenable to resection en bloc with an involved segment of left transverse colon and/or mesocolon, should adherence to these organs be the only limitation to a complete tumor excision (an unusual circumstance). Again, the initial assessment of resectability usually involves extensive mobilization of the left colon including the splenic flexure, transverse and descending colon. The critical area is again in the region of the superior mesenteric vessels or the celiac axis and suprarenal aorta, so a careful dissection is required to assess the tumor involvement in this area. If a colonic resection has been anticipated and appropriate bowel preparation performed then a segmental colonic resection may be appropriate, but alternatively an extended right hemicolectomy and an ileosigmoid reconstruction can be performed. Full mobilization of the right colon may improve access to the fourth part of the duodenum during this assessment phase. Resection is abandoned if aortic encasement is identified, but involvement of the renal vessels can be explored further and left nephrectomy may occasionally be considered. Function of the remaining right kidney must clearly be confirmed before contemplating such a procedure and excretion of the intravenous contrast used during the preoperative CT scan is a useful guide in such circumstances.

If a curative resection is felt to be a realistic possibility for an invasive tumor of the left pancreas, we proceed to divide the pancreas over the PV as for distal pancreatectomy (see above) and to secure first the splenic artery and then the splenic vein. Division of the middle and right colic vessels close to the base of the mesocolon may preserve the marginal arcade to the proximal left colon. The entire right colon or a segment of affected colon is isolated by means of a linear stapler. As the spleen is mobilized forward, the remaining area of tumor attachment may be seen to lie in the area of the celiac axis/aorta. These vessels should be spared even if the resection is to be incomplete as a consequence, but such extensive involvement should previously have been excluded. This type of radical distal pancreatectomy is completed by closing the proximal pancreatic stump and creating the colonic anastomosis.

□ 5. Major Vascular Resections

Several principles have been established with regard to major vascular resection at the time of PD: (1) Tumor involvement of the SMA/celiac axis indicates extensive disease and effectively precludes curative resection.[26,46,47] (2) Unlike arterial reconstruction, resection of the PV can be performed safely with mortality and morbidity rates similar to those of standard PD. (3) Tumor involvement of the PV in the absence of SMA involvement is generally not a predictor of poor prognosis but rather an indicator of tumor location.[48] (4) Involvement of the PV has not been shown to be associated with a higher rate of positive resection margins or lymph nodes.[26] An understanding of the three-dimensional relationship between the PV/SMV and the

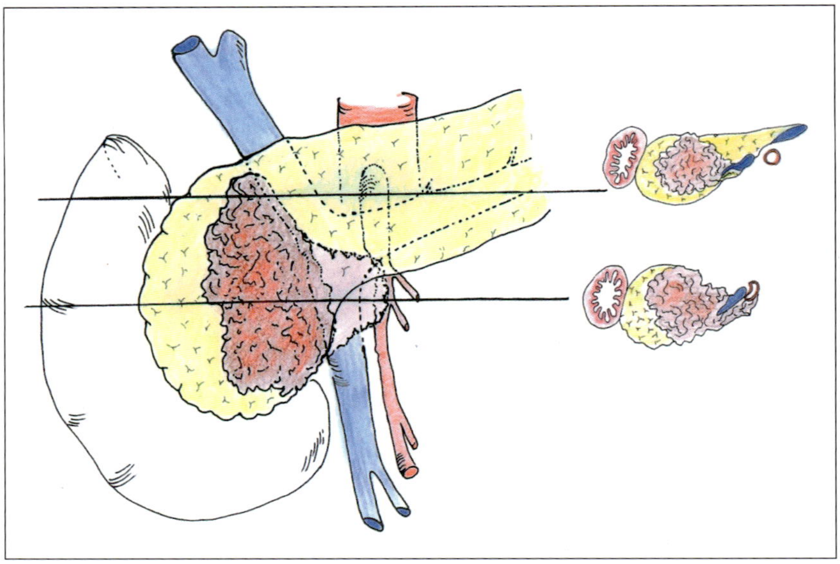

Fig. 6.**29** Understanding the three-dimensional relationship between the tumor and the mesenteric vessels is important in assessing tumor extent and potential resectability.

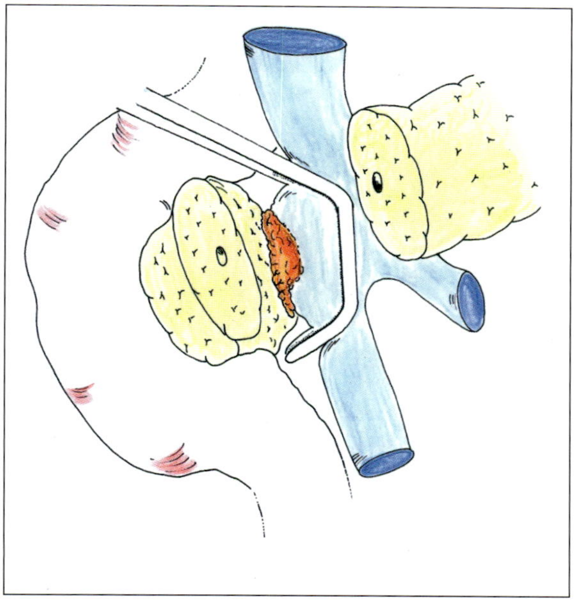

a

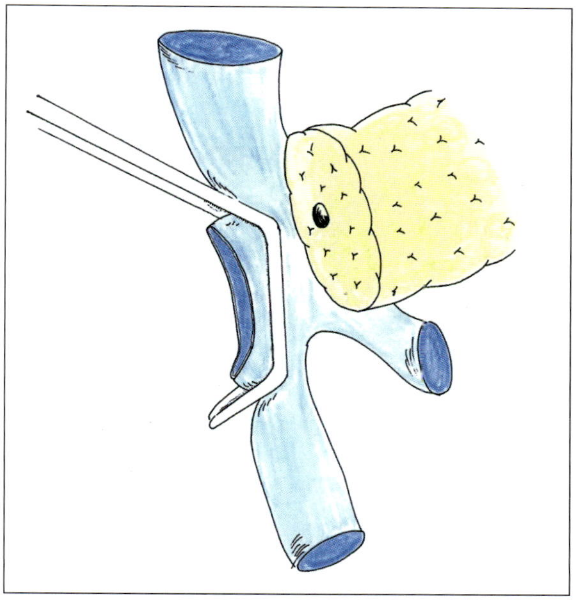

b

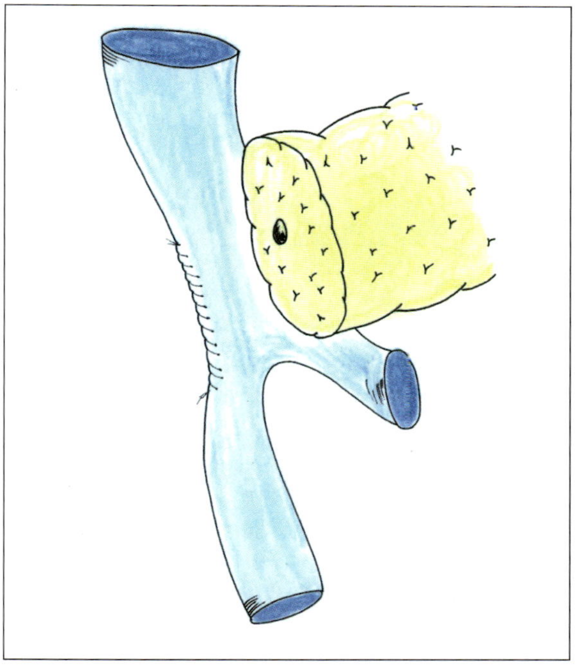

c

Fig. 6.**30a–c** Lateral excision of the portal/superior mesenteric vein is possible. The extent of tumor adherence is defined and the vein partially clamped (**a**). Once the specimen is resected (**b**) the vein is closed with a fine nonabsorbable suture (**c**). Care must be taken not to narrow the vein by this maneuver.

SMA is crucial in assessing these patients (Fig. 6.**29**). Tumors that extend to the left of the SMV will virtually always involve the SMA, the proximity of these vessels being a constant finding on contrast-enhanced CT images.

Some groups perform resection of the PV with all[49–51] or almost all (89%) pancreatic resections,[52] while others perform such resections rarely (2%).[53] We undertake this maneuver on a selective basis but more often for tumors other than ductal carcinoma. Once the pancreatic neck is divided, adherence between the uncinate process and the right lateral border of the PV becomes obvious. The nature of this adherence can be difficult to predict; resected specimens demonstrate a rate of tumor invasion into the PV that varies between 21–86%.[49,54] Cystic neoplasm of the pancreas rarely seems to invade the PV; in a report of four cases in which the PV was resected, there was no evidence of tumor invasion.[33] If there is no easily definable plane between pancreas and PV it may be appropriate to proceed to resection of the PV if suspected invasion of this vessel is the only factor limiting a complete resection. As much as possible of the standard mobilization for PD is carried out as described above, leaving the specimen attached only by the PV. This order of dissection has the advantage that it clarifies the area of tissue involvement of the vein and minimizes the dissection that needs to be carried out while the PV is clamped. However, exposure of the SMA is incomplete at this stage and subsequent dissection of this vessel should not be prolonged excessively because of the risk of venous congestion of the small bowel during the period of PV occlusion. One solution is to resect the PV segment at an early stage, leaving it attached to the pancreatic tumor and then proceed to immediate repair of the defect, thus allowing a more controlled approach to the posterior attachments of the uncinate process.

For a short partial circumference (25%) involvement of the vein, lateral excision may be adequate with the aid of a side-biting vascular clamp such as a Satinski (Fig. 6.**30a,b**). The defect is closed with a fine vascular suture (5–0 Prolene®; Fig. 6.**30c**). The clamp is released and hemostasis is checked. Care is needed to avoid excess narrowing of the PV during the repair. For longer

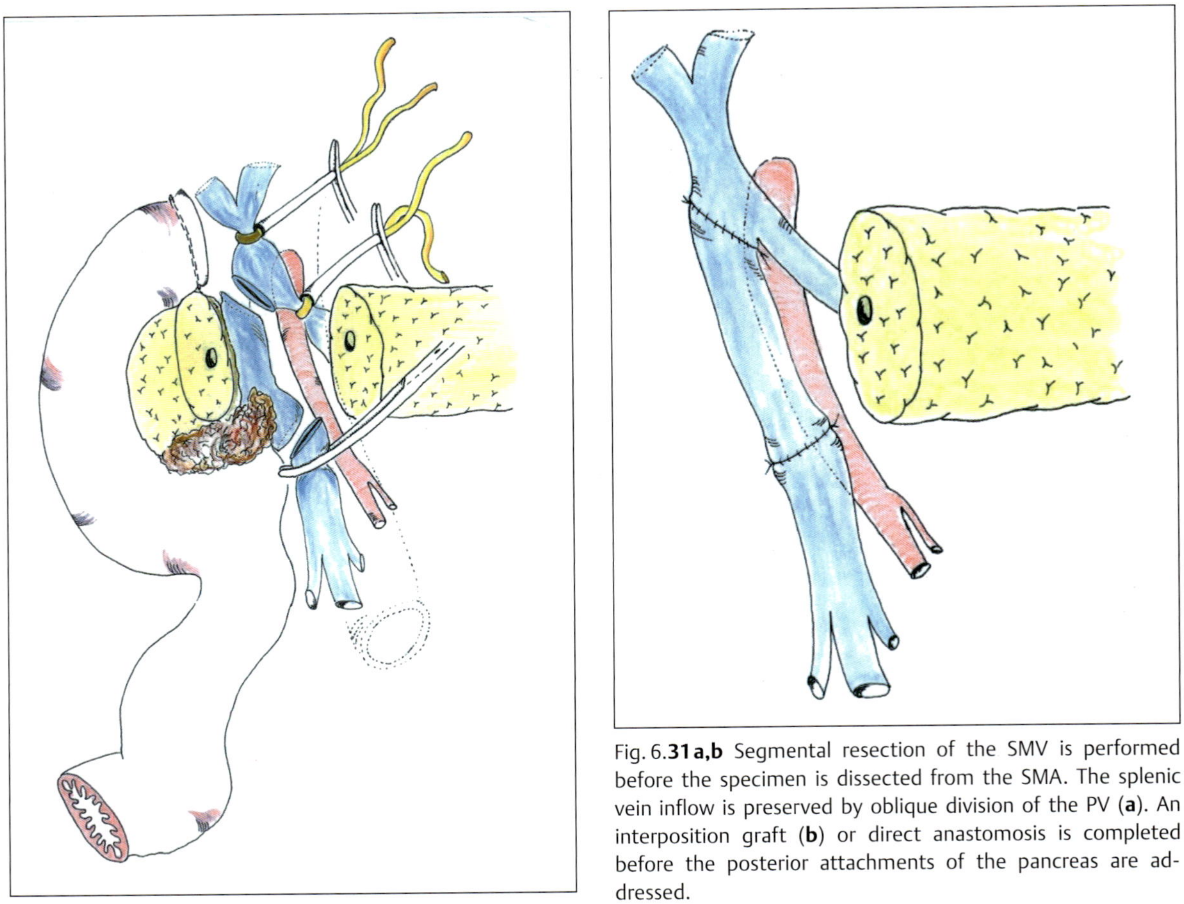

a

b

Fig. 6.**31 a,b** Segmental resection of the SMV is performed before the specimen is dissected from the SMA. The splenic vein inflow is preserved by oblique division of the PV (**a**). An interposition graft (**b**) or direct anastomosis is completed before the posterior attachments of the pancreas are addressed.

lateral resection of the PV, it is possible to patch the defect with autologous vein (e.g. saphenous) or prosthetic material (Gore-Tex patch). A long lateral defect can also be closed without a patch by a transverse venorrhaphy as described,[55] thus preserving splenic vein inflow. For more extensive involvement of the PV circumference it will be necessary to resect the portal vein. As for any vascular procedure, thorough exposure and vascular control are essential. The distal pancreas is carefully mobilized off the splenic vein and the PV/SMV junction is also cleared of peritoneal tissue. The PV, splenic vein, and SMV are all isolated with vascular slings or clamps. In most cases the PV can be exposed for a length of 7–8 cm and if 3–4 cm of vein is resected (i.e., the normal width of the pancreatic neck), a tension-free anastomosis can readily be completed. In 89 such resections, Nakao and colleagues have reported a mean length of PV resection of 3.5 cm (range 0.8–8.5 cm) with an end-to-end repair in all cases. Tension can be further reduced by bringing the liver down with the aid of several surgical packs above the right lobe and by elevation of the small bowel mesentery. If tension is still a problem, the gap can be bridged with autologous tissue (saphenous or internal jugular vein) or prosthetic grafts. Vascular clamps are placed on the three vessels and the specimen is resected along with the vein. The splenic junction can be preserved by oblique division of the PV at both ends, but the level of resection will be dictated by the site of the tumor (Fig. 6.**31 a**). Care is taken to mark the orientation of the specimen and the site of suspected venous involvement with a suture before sending the specimen to pathology. The end-to-end anastomosis is completed using a running fine vascular suture (5–0 Prolene) and tying the knot loosely to incorporate an expansion factor (Fig. 6.**31 b**).[56] Temporary occlusion of the PV for up to 60 minutes is usually well tolerated,[51] but longer periods may lead to severe congestion of the bowel and portofemoral extracorporeal bypass may be needed. Congestion may be reduced by inflow occlusion during PV clamping. Simple ligation of the splenic vein without reconstitution of flow to the portal system is an easy maneuver but one that can lead rarely to massive upper gastrointestinal bleeding from gastric varices.[57,58] Not all surgeons subscribe to the importance of preserving the SV inflow and claim that simple ligation causes little hazard.[47,48,54]

Although en bloc resection of major arteries such as the celiac axis[59] or superior mesenteric artery[45] is possible, the reports consist of small series of highly selected cases and long-term survivors are rare. Most surgeons would regard arterial involvement as a definite sign of incurability and a contraindication to resection.[36,60]

6. Lymphadenectomy

The extent of lymph node dissection is a greatly disputed facet of pancreatic surgery and one that is difficult to standardize.[41] Some centers include distal gastrectomy in the specimen as a way of resecting nodes along the right gastric and gastroepiploic arteries, while others complete a PPPP and concentrate on the retroperitoneal dissection. Lymphatic clearance is essentially aimed at dissecting loose, node-bearing tissue from around vessels, thereby skeletonizing them. Although we aim to complete much of this dissection en bloc with the specimen, it is usually necessary to perform a secondary "sweep" of the lymphatic tissue. Once the common hepatic duct is divided (usually above the entry point of the cystic duct), the gastroduodenal artery is divided between ligatures and the hepatic artery is encircled with a sling and retracted in a cephalad direction. The loose tissue is cleared from the hepatic artery back to the level of the celiac axis and one of the celiac nodes is sampled separately. Once the artery has been retracted, the PV is exposed and all lymphatic tissue can be cleared from around it. This dissection is continued down to the level of the SMV. With the pancreatic head removed, the SMA can be relatively easily identified. Tissue should be cleared from the right side only of this vessel so as to avoid the intractable diarrhea that is likely to follow a circumferential clearance. Attention then moves to the retroperitoneum where all lymphatic tissue is cleared from the hilum of the right kidney to the left lateral border of the aorta and from below the divided hepatic duct to the junction of the PV/SMV (Fig. 6.**32**). The gonadal veins enter the vena cava in this area and can be a source of troublesome bleeding if not carefully identified.

Some surgeons perform an even more radical resection to include the nodal tissue circumferentially around the celiac and SM arteries and along the aorta from the diaphragm to the IMA and laterally to both renal hila. On the other hand, many surgeons perform a "standard" dissection of the nodal tissue that is only incorporated in the PD specimen. The debate comparing these two approaches is considered below.

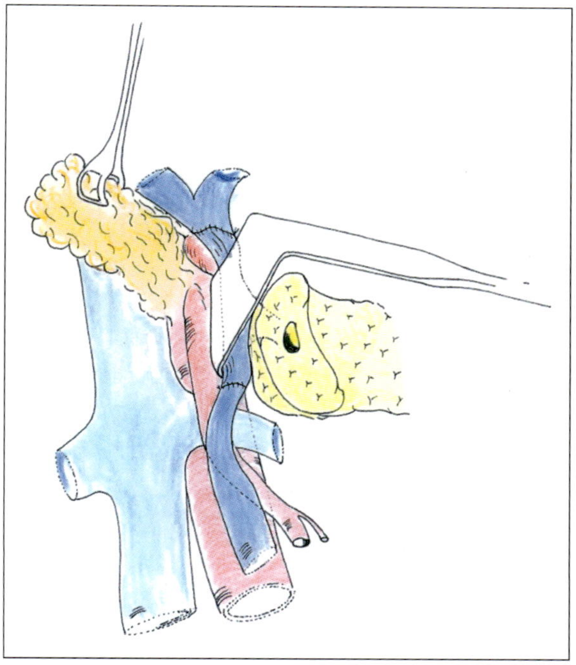

Fig. 6.**32** After the specimen is resected a clear view is obtained of the retroperitoneum. Excision of lymphatic tissue around the celiac axis, SMA, or aorta can be completed if necessary.

Postoperative Care

The postoperative care of the patients undergoing extended resections is similar to that of those having PD alone. Many of the complications stem from the pancreatic anastomosis and a careful watch is kept for this possibility. The first signs of a pancreatic leak can be subtle, namely fever, tachycardia, or an increase in abdominal pain. The use of epidural analgesia can mask the pain to some degree, but any adverse change in the patient's condition should always raise the possibility of a pancreatic leak. Minor leaks will often settle with conservative treatment including bowel rest, antibiotics, and octreotide. We have a low threshold for placing nasojejunal or direct jejunal feeding tubes at operation, especially in the elderly or those with a degree of malnutrition secondary to jaundice. Gradual jejunal feeding is commenced on the second postoperative day. This type of enteral access becomes an invaluable asset in the case of a complication, when prolonged enteric feeding is preferable to parenteral nutrition.

Nasogastric aspiration is maintained until the volume of aspirate is less than the oral intake, sips of water being allowed from the first postoperative day. Delayed gastric emptying can be a problem after Whipple resection as well as PPPP, but most patients are able to start on a light diet between 5–7 days after operation. Antibiotics are continued beyond 24 hours only if there is a specific indication. Patients are encouraged to mobilize early with the assistance of the ward physiotherapist and compression stockings and low-dose heparin are continued until discharge.

Although we do not use octreotide routinely, we do use it in patients who are considered to be at high risk of leakage from the pancreatic anastomosis, namely those with small ducts in combination with soft, friable parenchyma. A review of seven published randomized trials comparing octreotide to placebo in this setting showed a significant reduction in the incidence of postoperative complications in six of the seven studies, particularly complications related to pancreatic fistula, peripancreatic fluid collections, and leakage from the anastomosis.[61] A randomized study of the prophylactic use of octreotide however, reports no benefit in its use[62]; methodological differences may explain the discrepancy.

2

Delayed gastric emptying can prevent early patient discharge. In selected patients—those with high volume nasogastric aspirates or duodenal obstruction preoperatively and in whom complete obstruction and anastomotic leak have been ruled out with a contrast study—we prescribe intravenous erythromycin in low doses to promote gastric motility.[63]

Complications

When discussing complications in the setting of extended resections, the morbidity and mortality rates should be compared with those of "standard" PD. Morbidity rates of 20–40% are commonly reported, but the mortality rate is now 5% or less in many large centers. Exploratory laparotomy alone is associated with complications in 12% of patients.[64] In a review comparing 114 standard PD resections to 75 extended resections, Klempnauer and colleagues highlight the increased risk of the more major procedure which included 46 major vascular resections and 45 additional organ resections (overall 40% of the patients undergoing resection). Standard resections in this series were associated with a mortality rate of 6% and relaparotomy with a rate of 19%, compared to 13 and 32% respectively for extended resections. Resection of the PV alone increased neither the mortality nor the relaparotomy rate, while the resection of additional organs increased both of these significantly. Most of the additional deaths were associated with resection of the colon, whereas the relaparotomy rate increased substantially with arterial resection.[45]

Resection of the pancreas and/or spleen in combination with a gastric resection is associated with an increased rate of complications such as pancreatic fistula, anastomotic leakage, and intraabdominal abscess, without any survival advantage.[29] In a review of 590 cases of pancreatic cancer located in the body or tail of the pancreas, when lymph nodes are involved survival is not improved by "curative" resection compared to palliative bypass, though operative morbidity is higher with bypass than with laparotomy alone.[30]

It should be remembered that diabetes mellitus is occasionally present in patients undergoing pancreatic resection and has been reported to occur in 18% of patients with left-sided pancreatic carcinomas[30] but the incidence of postoperative diabetes is related directly to the amount of pancreatic tissue removed and the degree of chronic pancreatic damage in the remaining gland. The incidence of new-onset diabetes after distal resection has been given as 11%.[30]

Exocrine function can suffer after resection; patients undergoing resections for left-sided pancreatic cancers are reported to have postoperative exocrine insufficiency in 5%.[30] The results for proximal resections are often reported together with operations for chronic pancreatitis but nevertheless, in patients undergoing resections of the head of the pancreas for neoplasms, it is estimated that exocrine failure occurs in 23% on formal testing and frank diabetes in 3%.[22]

Radical clearance of tissue circumferentially from around the SMA/celiac axis results in a serious disturbance in nutrition mainly related to diarrhea, the degree of disturbance being related to the extent of nerve dissection. In centers that perform circumferential clearance in this manner, nearly all patients have troublesome diarrhea and nutritional disturbance.[25,65] Vessels that have been skeletonized in this fashion are at serious risk of bleeding in the setting of a pancreatic leak and this is often a lethal combination.

Delayed gastric emptying does occur after PPPP although it is probably not significantly more common than after standard Whipple's procedure.[66] Although the reported data on incidence are conflicting, there are several reasons why some delay in gastric emptying is observed. Firstly, the surgical trauma to the pylorus or nerves of Latarjet; second, moderate ischemia of the remaining duodenum; third, removal of the duodenal source of hormones involved in the regulation of gastric emptying[67]; fourth, hematoma or edema at the duodenoenteric anastomosis and lastly, loss of the supposed duodenal pacemaker.

Results

Extended Resections

Radical or extended pancreatectomy was initially popularized by Fortner but his series was associated with a 23% mortality rate and no 5-year survivors.[68,69] An important factor in resectability and ultimate survival is case selection. Those surgeons excluding patients on strict CT or angiographic criteria or further selecting patients with the aid of laparoscopic staging will obviously resect a higher proportion of patients with smaller, better prognosis tumors. These exclusion criteria are often not stated in reported data which makes comparisons between series very difficult.

Extended resections for pancreatic adenocarcinoma cover a wide range of procedures with various combinations of additional organs resected as well as different types of vascular and lymphatic resection. Once again, direct comparison of results is difficult. Enthusiasts may publish outstanding results that cannot necessarily be extrapolated to standard surgical practice. Dalton and colleagues[70] showed that extensive resection for pancreatic carcinoma of the body or tail involving adjacent organs resulted in a high rate (78%) of recurrence and only produced a modest gain in survival. A brief overview of the results available in the modern literature is presented below.

The incidence of distant metastasis increases in relation to tumor size either measured intraoperatively or judged from the operative specimen. The incidence was 11.3% for tumors 3 cm in size and 75.5% for tumors >3 cm in size.[9] Klempnauer reported resection of liver metastases in 22 patients with pancreatic adenocarcinoma. They achieved "curative" resections in 69% of patients with an operative mortality rate of 4.3%. The median survival time was 8.3 months after synchronous resection and 5.8 months after metachronous hepatic resection. The one-year survival rate was 40%.[23]

Left-Sided Cancer

Resection of carcinoma of the body or tail of the pancreas is only possible in 12% of patients[37] but when adverse prognostic factors are taken into consideration median survival is similar for pancreatic adenocarcinoma at any location.[30] Stage for stage, tumors of the body or tail of the pancreas are said to carry a similar survival prognosis to tumor of the pancreatic head, but they generally present much later and usually at an advanced and incurable stage.[35] It was previously held that survival beyond 1 year after resection was very rare indeed for carcinoma of the body and tail of the pancreas. Reviewing 45 years of literature on the subject, Moossa found only one survivor[71] but more recent reports offer greater hope. In a series of 26 patients who underwent resection for carcinoma of the body or tail, the median survival was only 10 months yet two patients survived 5 years.[70] In another series of 13 selected patients, seven survived beyond 1 year.[37] In a collected review of 590 patients with left-sided tumors undergoing resection, 28 patients had resections involving additional organs and only two (7%) survived beyond 2 years, with operative morbidity and mortality rates of 46 and 14% respectively.[30] Splenic vein thrombosis is an ominous sign but not an absolute indicator of inability to perform resection, although the tumors tend to be larger and extension of resection to other organs is usually required.[37] Provided the venous involvement is at some distance from the portal vein, resection may yet be possible.[19]

Colectomy

Combined colonic and pancreaticoduodenal resection for pancreatic cancer is not commonly reported in the literature. One of the largest series reports 17 such combined resections with a mixture of right, left, transverse, and subtotal colonic resections.[45] Direct tumor infiltration into the colonic wall was demonstrated in eight patients (47%), while the remaining nine patients had tumor infiltration of the mesocolon. Overall, there was a 35% 30-day mortality rate (6/17) and the survivors had a median survival of 6.2 months; there were no five-year survivors. In another report, three patients survived for 14, 33, and 93 months.[36] Only three small studies specifically outline the management of patients with primary carcinomas of the right colon invading the duodenum and pancreas.[72–74] Many other studies have looked at the overall approach to advanced colonic cancer at any site and suggest that in approximately 40% of cases with tumor adherence to duodenum or pancreas, fixation of the tumor to surrounding structures is caused by nonmalignant inflammatory adhesions rather than direct tumor invasion.[75,76] Other authors suggest that the figure may be higher, but clearly it is impossible to be certain at the time of operation; frozen section can be inaccurate and carries the risk of tumor spillage.

The unusual behavior of colonic tumors large enough to invade adjacent organs without coexistent metastatic disease probably explains prolonged survival in some patients after resection. Only 25% of these tumors have been reported as lymph-node positive.[72] Tumor size alone is not a risk factor for regional node involvement or for overall survival.[77] Low morbidity and mortality rates have been reported for these extended resections of colorectal cancers, albeit from specialist centers. Complete colonic tumor resection along with adjacent organs (pancreas, duodenum, or other) is associated with a mean survival of 40 months and a 5-year survival rate of 54%. These figures compare favorably to palliative bypass with a mean survival time of 9 months and to an incomplete resection, where patients survive a mean of 11 months.[77] Those without lymph node involvement and with only inflammatory adherence will have an even better prognosis. Information specifically related to pancreaticoduodenectomy for colonic cancer is scarce. In one study three out of four patients were alive with no evidence of disease at a mean follow-up of 23 months[74] and another study reported four patients free of disease at a median follow-up of 42 months after combined colonic and PD resection.[77]

2

Gastrectomy

Extension of pancreatectomy to include the stomach (other than a Whipple's resection) is seldom reported. In a series of 23 total gastrectomies for advanced pancreatic cancers 16 procedures were combined with total pancreatectomy, six with distal pancreatectomy and only one with a Whipple's resection.[45] Four of the 23 patients died in the early postoperative period, but among the survivors the median survival was 7.4 months with a 5-year survival of 13.6%; these figures were identical to those reported for standard pancreatic resections in the same series.

Portal Vein Resection

Centers that perform PD regularly report no increase in mortality rate with PV resection.[26,46,48–50,52,54,78] However, in patients with marked stenosis or obstruction of the PV with collaterals, resection of the PV provides no survival advantage.[52,60,46,55] In those with suspected PV invasion, the rate of curative resection even with portal vein resection may be as low as 15–30%.[46,78] The presence of tumor at other margins suggests that PV involvement is generally a sign of advanced carcinoma. PV/SMV resection should only be undertaken if it seems likely to permit a curative resection. Tumor involvement of the SMA represents locally advanced disease and curative resection will not be possible even with arterial resection.[47,60]

In an attempt to quantify PV involvement preoperatively from angiographic findings, Ishikawa and coworkers proposed a classification system.[49] If preoperative imaging suggested involvement of half or less of the circumference or less than 1.4 cm length of PV involvement, the 3-year survival was 59%. By contrast, if more than half the circumference was involved or more than 1.4 cm length of PV was involved, there were no survivors beyond 18 months. This classification is not yet widely used and the data on PV resection are difficult to interpret as most authors do not state their philosophy regarding this step or give an indication of the "curative" nature of their resection. It seems that in expert hands resection of the PV can be performed with no extra risk but with little or no survival benefit. In a comparison of 44 patients without venous resection compared to 31 with PV resection, there was no significant difference in survival.[47] Another study actually reported a worse prognosis for patients undergoing PV resection, even though there was no procedure-related mortality in this group. They attributed this outcome to a preponderance of large, node-positive, multicentric tumors in the PV resection group. In review of 841 patients undergoing PV resection, morbidity and mortality rates were not significantly increased, but the usefulness of the procedure was not established.[79] Overall, the 2-year survival after PV resection ranges from 15–37%.[51,54] Nakao and co-workers found that survival of 44 patients with histologically confirmed PV involvement after resection was less than 10% at 1 year compared to 39% among the 44 patients without vascular involvement who had also undergone resection.[52] Again, it seems that the addition of PV resection per se has no bearing on survival.[48] This lack of difference is multifactorial. First, it may be that the overall survival is so poor that small differences are difficult to detect. Second, the need for PV resection may simply reflect the tumor size and location rather than a biologically aggressive tumor.[26]

Lymphadenectomy

From a theoretical point of view, more radical removal of lymphatic tissue in cases of pancreatic cancer might be expected to improve long-term survival if the entire tumor is removed. Some retrospective studies from Japan have shown apparently better 5-year survival rates after extended lymphadenectomy[80–83] while other studies have reported no improvement in survival.[52,84] In a review of 29 papers reporting extended lymphadenectomy there does not appear to be an increase in mortality or morbidity rate,[85] but the data on long-term survival are conflicting.[79] About 40% of patients die from distant metastases within 12 months regardless of the operation and the incidence and site of relapse is the same whatever the initial surgical procedure undertaken

A Japanese retrospective review of 501 cases from 77 centers found that the extent of lymph node dissection did not affect prognosis for tumors of the head of the pancreas at any stage of the disease. They suggested that those undergoing a radical operation with radical lymph node dissection may survive longer than those undergoing excessive lymph node dissection. The European experience suggests that for patients with locally advanced disease but without nodal involvement, extended resection may have a small survival benefit. Those with node-positive disease have no benefit from radical resection.[86] Lymph node status plays a major role in determining survival. It is unlikely that patients will be understaged by a standard resection. In a review of the histology of 58 patients undergoing a radical resection, it was found that in no patient was there histologic evidence of involved nodes in the "extended" nodal area without there also being nodal disease in the "standard" nodal resection area. As a consequence, the radical procedure did not upstage a single patient.[87]

There have only been two prospective, randomized trials comparing standard against extended lymphatic clearance in association with PD.[27,87] Although both trials demonstrated that extended operations can be performed safely, neither study was able to show any benefit from extended lymphadenectomy in terms of long-term survival.

Quality of Life

A retrospective study from Japan[88] compared survival after 29 extended resections, of which 17 were curative, to that of patients undergoing palliative bypass for locally advanced cancer. Mean survival was longer after resective surgery compared to palliative bypass (8 months curative, 7 months noncurative, and 3 months after bypass). The quality of life was better after resection than palliative bypass. Another review of 12 patients undergoing extended PD resections reported a satisfactory performance status in 8 out of the 10 patients who survived the operation.[36]

Conclusion

Although we have described many variations on the standard pancreatic resection, it has not been our intention to suggest that surgeons immediately incorporate these procedures into their practice. We accept that in the infinitely variable world of surgical practice there will be times when it is necessary and appropriate to extend the standard operation to include vessels or adjacent organs. This decision has to be well thought through and made in the best interests of the individual patient. The data to support these procedures are sparse but some patients will surely benefit from extended resection. The aim of this chapter is to describe and teach new techniques that the cancer upper gastrointestinal surgeon can use and practice when he/she is faced with locally advanced pancreatic cancer and, therefore, to standardize these techniques to a higher level of organization, not yet reached in the surgical literature. Obvious examples will be those with less aggressive neoplasms such as neuroendocrine tumors or those in whom the apparent extension represents inflammatory adhesions and a curative resection would not otherwise have been undertaken. The cancer surgeon must feel, in the operative field, that the local clearance of the pancreatic tumor offers a superior disease-free survival and a better quality of life than a palliative procedure and is on an intellectual and oncologic point of view more satisfying. Ultimately the surgeon will be guided by his/her attitude to pancreatic cancer and by his/her expertise in performing these demanding and potentially risky procedures. The "art" of selecting the right operation for each patient that we treat is always a crucial part of the management algorithm and never more so than in the management of advanced pancreatic tumors.

Pancreaticoduodenectomy as a palliative procedure has been advocated largely because of the very low mortality rates reported by large centers.[89] Although we generally avoid obviously palliative resections, it may not be until quite late in the procedure or even after histologic confirmation that the palliative nature of the procedure is realized. We believe that all patients who are reasonably fit and have potentially resectable disease should be explored even those with large tumors in proximity to the portal vein.

2

References

1. Sohn TA, Lillemoe KD, Cameron JL, Huang JJ, Pitt HA, Yeo CJ. Surgical palliation of unresectable periampullary adenocarcinoma in the 1990s. *J Am Coll Surg.* 1999;188:658–666.
2. American Cancer Society. *Cancer Facts and Figures*. Oakland, CA: American Cancer Society; 1991.
3. Gudjonsson B. Carcinoma of the pancreas: Critical analysis of costs, results of resections and the need for standardized reporting. *J Am Coll Surg.* 1995;181:483–503.
4. Carter DC. Cancer of the pancreas. *Gut.* 1990;31:494–496.
5. Trede M. Treatment of pancreatic carcinoma: the surgeon's dilemma. *Br J Surg.* 1987;74:79–80.
6. Gudjonsson B. Treatment and survival in 13 560 patients with pancreatic cancer and incidence of the disease, in the West Midlands: an epidemiological study (letter). *Br J Surg.* 1996;83:874.
7. Takada T, Yasuda H, Amano H, Yoshida M, Uchida T. Simultaneous hepatic resection with pancreato-duodenectomy for metastatic pancreatic head carcinoma: does it improve survival? *Hepatogastroenterology.* 1997;44:567–573.
8. Makary MA, Warshaw AL, Centeno BA, Willet CG, Rattner DW, Fernandez-del Castillo C. Implications of peritoneal cytology for pancreatic cancer management. *Arch Surg.* 1998;133:361–365.
9. Bottger TC, Boddin J, Duber C, Heintz A, Kuchle R, Junginger T. Diagnosing and staging of pancreatic carcinoma-what is necessary? *Oncology.* 1998;55:122–129.
10. Warshaw AL. Implications of peritoneal cytology for staging of early pancreatic cancer. *Am J Surg.* 1991;161:26–30.
11. Lundstedt C, Stridbeck H, Andersson R, Tranberg KG, Andren-Sandberg A. Tumor seeding occurring after fine-needle biopsy of abdominal malignancies. *Acta Radiol.* 1991; 32:518–520.
12. Smith AC, Dowsett JF, Russel RCG, Hatfield ARW, Cotton PB. Randomized trial of endoscopic stenting versus surgical bypass in malignant low bile duct obstruction. *Lancet.* 1994;344:1655–1660.
13. Campbell JP, Wilson SR. Pancreatic neoplasms: How useful is evaluation with US? *Radiology.* 1988;167:341–344.
14. Lee YT. Tissue diagnosis for carcinoma and periampullary structures. *Cancer.* 1982;49:1035–1039.
15. Freeny PC, Marks WM, Ryan JAL, Traverso W. Pancreatic ductal adenocarcinoma: Diagnosis and staging with dynamic CT. *Radiology.* 1988;166:125–133.

16. Dooley WC, Cameron JL, Pitt HA, Lillemoe KD, Yue NC. Is preoperative angiography useful in patients with periampullary tumors? *Ann Surg*. 1990;211:649–654.
17. Warshaw AL, Gu ZY, Wittenberg J, Waltman AC. Preoperative staging and assessment of resectability of pancreatic cancer. *Arch Surg*. 1990;125:230–233.
18. Warshaw AL, Tepper JE, Shipley WU. Laparoscopy in the staging and planning of therapy for pancreatic cancer. *Am J Surg*. 1986;151:76–80.
19. Andren-Sandberg A, Wagner M, Tihanyi T, Lofgren P, Friess H. Technical aspects of left-sided pancreatic resection for cancer. *Dig Surg*. 1999;16:305–312.
20. Povoski SP, Karpeh MS, Jr., Conlon KC, Blumgart LH, Brennan MF. Association of preoperative biliary drainage with postoperative outcome following pancreaticoduodenectomy. *Ann Surg*. 1999;230:131–142.
21. Fleming WR, Williamson RC. Preservation of the pylorus in resection of the head of the pancreas. *J Hep Bil Pancr Surg*. 1994;4:355–366.
22. Watanapa P, Williamson RC. Resection of the pancreatic head with or without gastrectomy. *World J Surg*. 1995;19: 403–409.
23. Klempnauer J, Ridder GJ, Piso P, Pichlmayr R. Is liver resection in metastases of exocrine pancreatic carcinoma justified? *Chirurg*. 1996;67:366–370.
24. Ogata Y, Hishinuma S, Matsui J, Ozawa I, Takahashi S. Pylorus-preserving pancreaticoduodenectomy with combined resection of the portal vein and gastrointestinal reconstruction by Imanaga procedure for ductal cancer of the head of the pancreas. *J Hep Bil Pancr Surg*. 1994;4: 372–378.
25. Nagakawa T, Konishi I, Ueno K et al. The results and problems of extensive radical surgery for carcinoma of the head of the pancreas. *Jpn J Surg*. 1991;21:262–267.
26. Fuhrman GM, Leach SD, Staley CA et al. Rationale for en bloc vein resection in the treatment of pancreatic adenocarcinoma adherent to the superior mesenteric-portal vein confluence. Pancreatic Tumor Study Group. *Ann Surg*. 1996; 223:154–162.
27. Pedrazzoli S, DiCarlo V, Dionigi R et al. Standard versus extended lymphadenectomy associated with pancreatoduodenectomy in the surgical treatment of adenocarcinoma of the head of the pancreas: a multicenter, prospective, randomized study. Lymphadenectomy Study Group. *Ann Surg*. 1998;228:508–517.
28. Williamson RCN, Usatoff V. Pancreas. In: Kirk RM, ed. *General Surgical Operations*. 4th ed. London: Harcourt Brace; 2000.
29. Kasakura Y, Fujii M, Mochizuki F, Kochi M, Kaiga T. Is there a benefit of pancreaticosplenectomy with gastrectomy for advanced gastric cancer? *Am J Surg*. 2000;179:237–242.
30. Fabre JM, Houry S, Manderscheid JC, Huguier M, Baumel H. Surgery for left-sided pancreatic cancer. *Br J Surg*. 1996;83:1065–1070.
31. Aldridge MC, Williamson RC. Distal pancreatectomy with and without splenectomy. *Br J Surg*. 1991;78:976–979.
32. Schwarz RE, Harrison LE, Conlon KC, Klimstra DS, Brennan MF. The impact of splenectomy on outcomes after resection of pancreatic adenocarcinoma. *J Am Coll Surg*. 1999; 188:516–521.
33. Horvath KD, Chabot JA. An aggressive resectional approach to cystic neoplasms of the pancreas. *Am J Surg*. 1999;178: 269–274.
34. Andren-Sandberg A, Lindberg CG, Lundstedt C, Ihse I. Computed tomography and laparosocpy in the assessment of the patient with pancreatic cancer. *J Am Coll Surg*. 1998; 186:35–40.
35. Brennan MF, Moccia RD, Klimstra D. Management of adenocarcinoma of the body and tail of the pancreas. *Ann Surg*. 1996;223:506–511.
36. Civello IM, Frontera D, Viola G, Cina G, Sganga G, Crucitti F. Extensive resection in pancreatic cancer: review of the literature and personal experience. *Hepatogastroenterology*. 1998;45:1877–1883.
37. Johnson CD, Schwall G, Flechtenmacher J, Trede M. Resection for adenocarcinoma of the body and tail of the pancreas. *Br J Surg*. 1993;80:1177–1179.
38. Sarr MG, Behrns KE, van Heerden JA. Total pancreatectomy. An objective analysis of its use in pancreatic cancer. *Hepatogastroenterology*. 1993;40:418–421.
39. Launois B, Franci J, Bardaxoglou E et al. Total pancreatectomy for ductal adenocarcinoma of the pancreas with special reference to resection of the portal vein and multicentric cancer. *World J Surg*. 1993;17:122–126.
40. Kloppel G, Lohse T, Bosslet K, Ruckert K. Ductal adenocarcinoma of the head of the pancreas: incidence of tumor involvement beyond the Whipple resection line. Histological and immunocytochemical analysis of 37 total pancreatectomy specimens. *Pancreas*. 1987;2:170–175.
41. Pedrazzoli S, Beger HG, Obertop H et al. A surgical and pathological based classification of resective treatment of pancreatic cancer. Summary of an international workshop on surgical procedures in pancreatic cancer. *Dig Surg*. 1999; 16:337–345.
42. Swope TJ, Wade TP, Neuberger TJ, Virgo KS, Johnson FE. A reappraisal of total pancreatectomy for pancreatic cancer: results from U.S. Veterans Affairs hospitals, 1987–1991. *Am J Surg*. 1994;168:582–585.
43. Taschieri AM, Elli M, Cristaldi M, Montecamozzo G, Porretta T, Danelli PG. Total versus partial pancreatectomy in the surgical treatment of carcinoma of the pancreatic head. *Chir Ital*. 1994;46:44–50.
44. Ihse I, Anderson H, Andren S. Total pancreatectomy for cancer of the pancreas: is it appropriate? *World J Surg*. 1996;20:288–293.
45. Klempnauer J, Ridder GJ, Bektas H, Pichlmayr R. Extended resections of ductal pancreatic cancer—impact on operative risk and prognosis. *Oncology*. 1996;53:47–53.
46. Roder JD, Stein HJ, Siewert JR. Carcinoma of the periampullary region: who benefits from portal vein resection? *Am J Surg*. 1996;171:170–174.
47. Leach SD, Lee JE, Charnsangavej C et al. Survival following pancreaticoduodenectomy with resection of the superior mesenteric-portal vein confluence for adenocarcinoma of the pancreatic head. *Br J Surg*. 1998;85:611–617.
48. Harrison LE, Klimstra DS, Brennan MF. Isolated portal vein involvement in pancreatic adenocarcinoma. A contraindication for resection? *Ann Surg*. 1996;224:342–347.
49. Ishikawa O, Ohigashi H, Imaoka S et al. Preoperative indications for extended pancreatectomy for locally advanced pancreas cancer involving the portal vein. *Ann Surg*. 1992;215:231–236.
50. Takahashi S, Ogata Y, Tsuzuki T. Combined resection of the pancreas and portal vein for pancreatic cancer. *Br J Surg*. 1994;81:1190–1193.
51. Tashiro S, Uchino R, Hiraoka T et al. Surgical indication and significance of portal vein resection in biliary and pancreatic cancer. *Surgery*. 1991;109:481–487.

2

52. Nakao A, Harada A, Nonami T, Kaneko T, Inoue S, Takagi H. Clinical significance of portal invasion by pancreatic head carcinoma. *Surgery*. 1995;117:50–55.
53. Cameron JL, Crist DW, Sitzmann JV et al. Factors influencing survival after pancreaticoduodenectomy for pancreatic cancer. *Am J Surg*. 1991;161:120–124.
54. Launois B, Stasik C, Bardaxoglou E et al. Who benefits from portal vein resection during pancreaticoduodenectomy for pancreatic cancer? *World J Surg*. 1999;23:926–929.
55. Clavien PA, Rudiger HA. A simple technique of portal vein resection and reconstruction during pancreaticoduodenectomy. *J Am Coll Surg*. 1999;189:629–634.
56. Starzl TE, Iwatsuki S, Shaw BW, Jr. A growth factor in fine vascular anastamoses. *Surg Gynecol Obstet*. 1984;159: 164–165.
57. Evans DB, Lee JE, Leach SD, Fuhrman GM, Cusack JC, Jr., Rich TA. Vascular resection and intraoperative radiation therapy during pancreaticoduodenectomy: rationale and technique. *Adv Surg*. 1996;29:235–262.
58. Cusack JC, Fuhrman GM, Lee JE, Evans DB. Managing unsuspected tumor invasion of the superior mesenteric-portal venous confluence during pancreaticoduodenectomy. *Am J Surg*. 1994;168:352–354.
59. Konishi M, Kinoshita T, Nakagori T et al. Distal pancreatectomy with resection of the celiac axis and reconstruction of the hepatic artery for carcinoma of the body and tail of the pancreas. *J Hepatobiliary Pancreat Surg*. 2000;7:183–187.
60. Baulieux J, Adham M, Oussoultzoglou E et al. Is pancreatectomy with resection of the retro-pancreatic vessels for cancer justified? *Chirurgie*. 1998;123:438–444.
61. Berberat PO, Friess H, Uhl W, Buchler MW. The role of octreotide in the prevention of complications following pancreatic resection. *Digestion*. 1999;60:15–22.
62. Yeo CJ, Cameron JL, Lillemoe KD et al. Does prophylactic octreotide decrease the rates of pancreatic fistula and other complications after pancreaticoduodenectomy? Results of a prospective randomized placebo-controlled trial. *Ann Surg*. 2000;232:419–429.
63. Yeo CJ, Barry MK, Sauter PK et al. Erythromycin accelerates gastric emptying after pancreaticoduodenectomy. A prospective, randomized, placebo-controlled trial. *Ann Surg*. 1993;218:229–238.
64. de Rooij PD, Rogatko A, Brennan MF. Evaluation of palliative surgical procedures in unresectable pancreatic cancer. *Br J Surg*. 1991;78:1053–1058.
65. Ishikawa O. Surgical technique, curability and postoperative quality of life in an extended pancreatectomy for adenocarcinoma of the pancreas. *Hepatogastroenterology*. 1996;43:320–325.
66. Williamson RC, Bliouras N, Cooper MJ, Davies ER. Gastric emptying and enterogastric reflux after conservative and conventional pancreatoduodenectomy. *Surgery*. 1993; 114: 82–86.
67. Morel P, Mathey P, Corboud H, Huber O, Egeli RA, Rohner A. Pylorus preserving duodenopancreatectomy: Long-term complications and comparison with the Whipple procedure. *World J Surg*. 1990;14:642–647.
68. Fortner JG. Regional pancreatectomy for cancer of the pancreas: A new surgical approach. *Surgery*. 1973;73:307–320.
69. Fortner JG. Regional pancreatectomy for cancer of the pancreas, ampulla and other related sites. *Ann Surg*. 1984;199: 418–425.
70. Dalton RR, Sarr MG, van Heerden JA, Colby TV. Carcinoma of the body and tail of the pancreas: is curative resection justified? *Surgery*. 1992; 111:489–94.
71. Moossa AR. Pancreatic cancer. Approach to diagnosis, selection and surgery and choice of operation. *Cancer*. 1982;50:2689–2698.
72. Curley SA, Evans DB, Ames FC. Resection for cure of carcinoma of the colon directly invading the duodenum or pancreatic head. *J Am Coll Surg*. 1994;179:587–592.
73. Ellis H, Morgan MN, Wastell C. 'Curative' surgery in carcinoma of the colon involving duodenum. A report of 6 cases. *Br J Surg*. 1972;59:932–935.
74. Koea JB, Conlon K, Paty PB, Guillem JG, Cohen AM. Pancreatic or duodenal resection or both for advanced carcinoma of the right colon: is it justified? *Dis Colon Rectum*. 2000;43:460–465.
75. Davies GC, Ellis H. Radical surgery in locally advanced cancer of the large bowel. *Clin Oncol*. 1975;1:21–26.
76. Polk HCJ. Extended resection for selected adenocarcinomas of the larger bowel. *Ann Surg*. 1972;175:892–899.
77. Curley SA, Carlson GW, Shumate CR, Wishnow KI, Ames FC. Extended resection for locally advanced colorectal carcinoma. *Am J Surg*. 1992;163:553–559.
78. Allema JH, Reinders ME, van Gulik TM et al. Portal vein resection in patients undergoing pancreatoduodenectomy for carcinoma of the pancreatic head. *Br J Surg*. 1994;81: 1642–1646.
79. Pedrazzoli S, Pasquali C, Sperti C. General aspects of surgical treatment of pancreatic cancer. *Dig Surg*. 1999;16: 265–275.
80. Ishikawa O, Ohhigashi H, Sasaki Y et al. Practical usefulness of lymphatic and connective tissue clearance for the carcinoma of the pancreas head. *Ann Surg*. 1988;208:215–220.
81. Manabe T, Ohshio G, Baba N et al. Radical pancreatectomy for ductal cell carcinoma of the head of the pancreas. *Cancer*. 1989;64:1132–1137.
82. Naganuma T, Isaji S, Kawarada Y. Staging and extended resection for pancreatic cancer. *Pancreas*. 1998;16: 355–362.
83. Satake K, Nishiwaki H, Yokomatsu H et al. Surgical curability and prognosis for standard versus extended resection for T1 carcinoma of the pancreas. *Surg Gynecol Obstet*. 1992;175:259–265.
84. Mukaiya M, Hirata K, Satoh T et al. Lack of survival benefit of extended lymph node dissection for ductal adenocarcinoma of the head of the pancreas: retrospective multi-institutional analysis in Japan. *World J Surg*. 1998;22: 248–252.
85. Iacono C, Bortolasi L, Facci E et al. Does extended pancreaticoduodenectomy increase operative morbidity and mortality vs. standard pancreaticoduodenectomy? *J Gastrointest Surg*. 1997;1:446–453.
86. Gall FP, Kessler H, Hermanek P. Surgical treatment of ductal pancreatic carcinoma. *Eur J Surg Oncol*. 1991;17:173–181.
87. Yeo CJ, Cameron JL, Sohn TA et al. Pancreaticoduodenectomy with or without extended retroperitoneal lymphadenectomy for periampullary adenocarcinoma: comparison of morbidity and mortality and short-term outcome. *Ann Surg*. 1999;229:613–622.
88. Miyata M, Nakao K, Takao T et al. An appraisal of pancreatectomy for advanced cancer of the pancreas based on survival rate and postoperative physical performance. *J Surg Oncol*. 1990;45:33–39.
89. Lillemoe KD, Cameron JL, Yeo CJ et al. Pancreaticoduodenectomy. Does it have a role in the palliation of pancreatic cancer? *Ann Surg*. 1996;223:718–725.

7 Liver and Bile Duct

William C. Meyers and Andres E. Castellanos

2

Abbreviations

CT: computed tomography
GIA: gastrointestinal anastomosis
IVC: inferior vena cava
SMA: superior mesenteric artery

Extended multivisceral resections involving the liver contribute to the armamentarium of an experienced liver surgeon.[1] From to time-to-time the experienced liver surgeon is faced with a large tumor that requires an aggressive approach for complete resection.[2] Each particular tumor that requires this type of resection is different with respect to the precise anatomy necessary to consider.[3] This chapter presents four such radical resections which we have encountered in our Department of Surgery. We hope that depicting these resections in some detail might help assist other experienced liver surgeons in thinking through aggressive approaches to the resection of similar tumors in other patients. In other words we do not recommend that anyone necessarily follow the precise details of any of the descriptions below. Instead, we are providing only some organized approaches for particular cases.

Preoperative Evaluation

Initial evaluation of patients with large hepatic tumors should be aimed at determining the extent of invasion into adjacent structures and organs. In our institution we prefer the use of a spiral CT scan with i.v. contrast. We are usually able to determine vascular extension without further need for extra testing. In selected cases we complement this with a staging laparotomy and the use of intraoperative ultrasound.

We do not consider vascular invasion as a criterion for unresectability[4]; but it may determine the planned procedure: extensive resection versus transplantation. The evidence of multicentric disease that precludes an en bloc dissection is used as a contraindication for surgery.

Preoperative testing is particular to each institution but we recommend obtaining a baseline hemoglobin, liver function test, and coagulation profile. The evaluation of hepatic function is critical in patients with underlying cirrhosis. Severe liver disease (Child-Pugh's class C) is considered a contraindication for major partial hepatic resection. We acknowledge that without the possibility of liver transplantation some of these resections will be impossible to perform and this may be a limiting factor in some institutions.

Special attention should be taken to correct any underlying coagulopathy. Blood, fresh frozen plasma and platelets should be available at the time of surgery. Extensive pulmonary and cardiac evaluation may be required at times and a good review of systems and past medical history are fundamental in making this determination.

Surgical Technique

Resection of Hepatic Tumor Involving the Vena Cava

This is a challenging problem that we have encountered with certain frequency. Even though their numbers may be small as a general group, in a very busy liver practice it may be encountered once or twice a year. This section describes the technique used in a young patient with a large hepatocellular tumor, which was invading the liver substance and the vena cava. We can't emphasize enough the importance of good preoperative evaluation.

The patient is placed in a supine position. A right subcostal incision extending 2.5–3.0 cm above the xiphoid is performed. The incision can be extended to the left subcostal area if necessary. One of the most common mistakes made is limiting the exposure, which is why we advocate a generous incision. We very rarely use a thoracic extension, but this is a consideration for reoperative surgery or removal of tumors that extend above the diaphragm (Fig. 7.**1**).

Once the incision is made, we recommend a meticulous exploration to rule out extrahepatic disease or other concomitant pathology.

We usually remove the gallbladder as an initial maneuver; this facilitates the approach to the portal hilum and prevents the possibility of a second operation for gallbladder related problems in a scarred right upper quadrant.

The liver is subsequently mobilized. This begins with the division of the falciform ligament. The right and left triangular ligaments are divided as well, detaching the liver segments from the diaphragm. These maneuvers

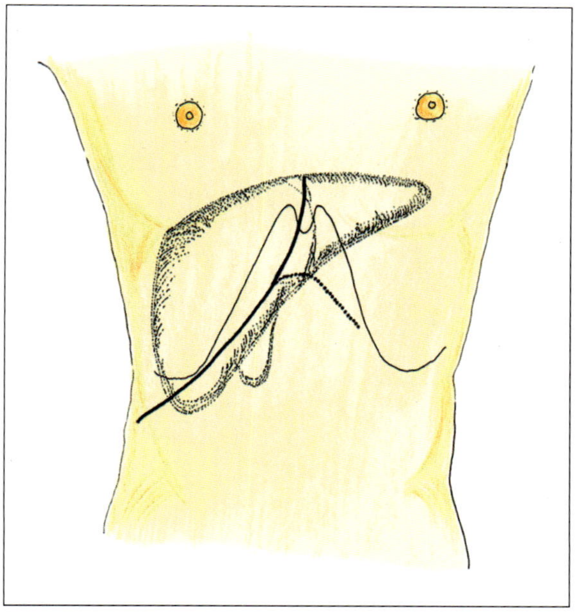

Fig. 7.1 Initial sub-costal incision for extended liver resection. The xiphoid extension may be optional.

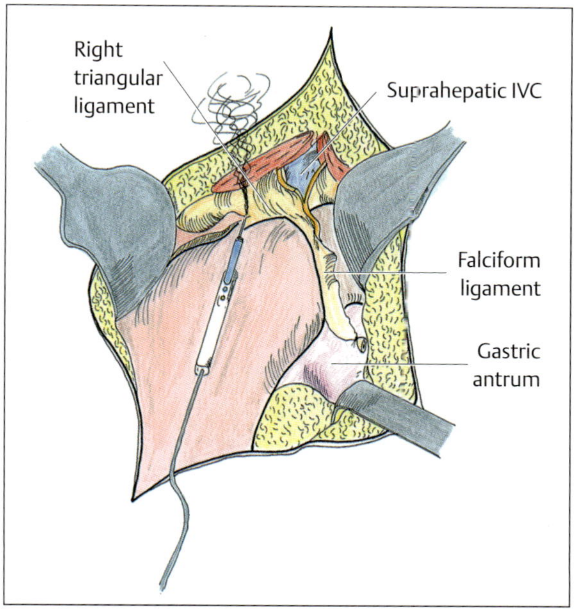

Fig. 7.2 The liver is mobilized dividing the triangular ligament and lateral attachment.

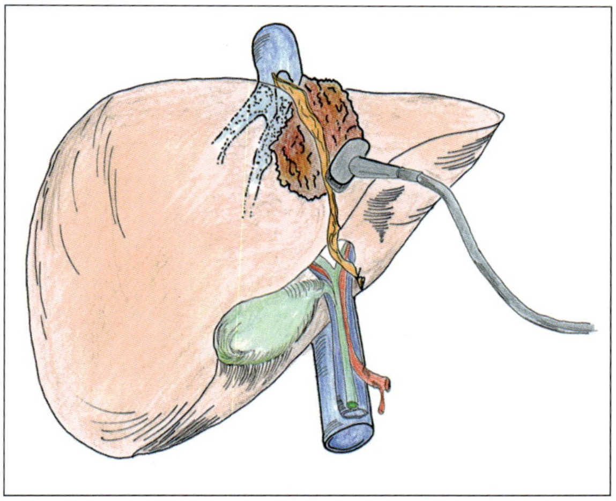

Fig. 7.3 Intraoperative ultrasonography is performed to localize the tumor and its relationship with the major structures.

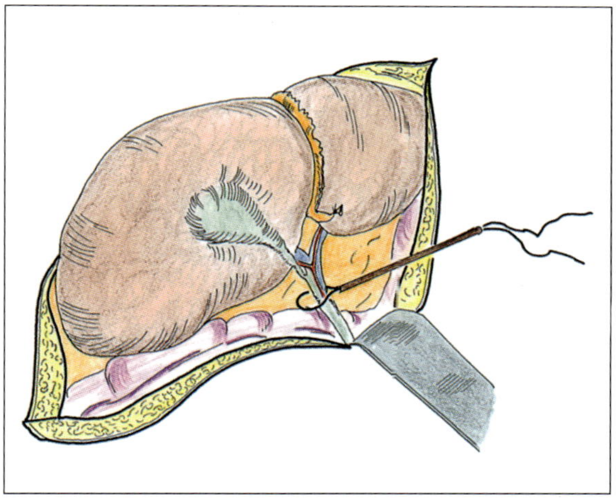

Fig. 7.4 The portal triad is secured using a Rummel tourniquet.

allow exposure to the suprahepatic vena cava, facilitating further vascular control when indicated. Care should be taken when incising the ligaments near the suprahepatic cava; the hepatic veins and diaphragmatic veins may be encountered superficially within these ligaments. Special attention should be directed to the examination of the gastrohepatic ligament when mobilizing the left lateral segment. Very often a large left hepatic artery originating from the left gastric artery can be found (Fig. 7.2).

Once the liver is fully mobilized we evaluate the liver using intraoperative ultrasound. It is very important to determine the exact location of the tumor and its relation to the vascular structures. Tumors invading the IVC often arise from the posterior segments. Intraoperative ultrasound is more sensitive than any preoperative evaluation to determine the extent of these relationships and subsequent degree of invasion (Fig. 7.3).

We proceed to obtain control of the portal triad. This is a simple maneuver that should be performed without difficulty. The foramen of Winslow is identified and by placing a finger in the foramen and out through the gastrohepatic omentum, the portal triad is encircled. We prefer to use an umbilical tape to secure the portal triad. This procedure provides access for the subsequent Pringle maneuver when indicated. Traction can be applied using a Rummel tourniquet (Fig. 7.4).

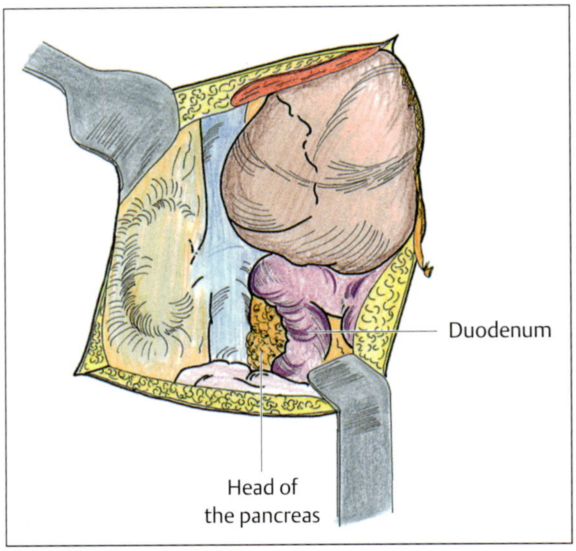

Fig. 7.5 A Kocher maneuver is performed to facilitate control of the IVC.

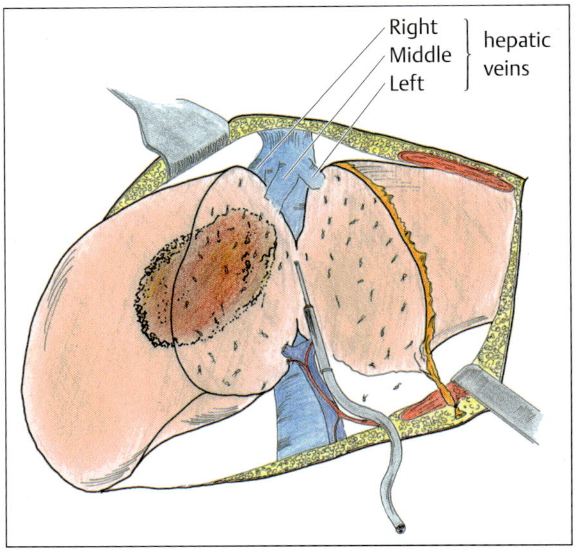

Fig. 7.6 The liver is divided using the ultrasonic dissector; at least 1 cm of margin is preserved around the tumor.

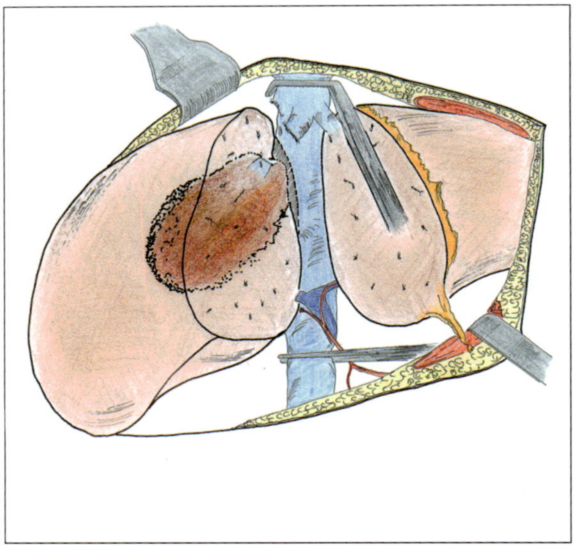

Fig. 7.7 The IVC attached to the tumor is removed en bloc.

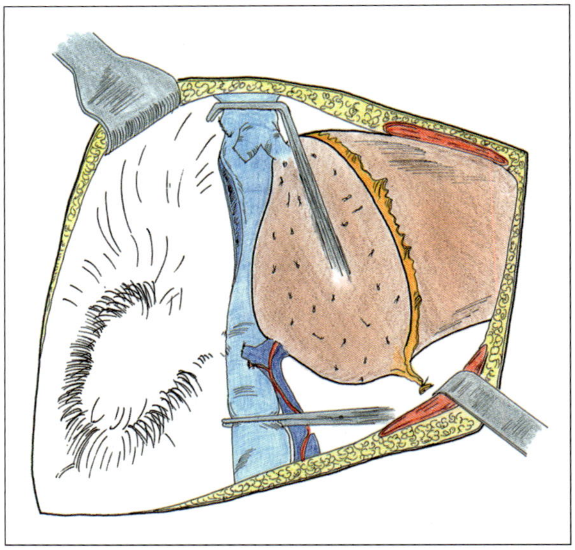

Fig. 7.8 Surgical field after specimen is removed.

In order to facilitate exposure and subsequent control of the infrahepatic vena cava a Kocher maneuver is performed. The IVC is exposed and suprarenal control is obtained (Fig. 7.**5**).

Once we have complete vascular control we are ready to start our hepatic dissection. This is going to be determined by the size of the tumor and its anatomic location within the different segments of the liver. We try to preserve as much healthy parenchyma as possible. We prefer to use the Cavitronic Ultra Sonographic Aspirator (CUSA) for our dissection, but finger fracture, clamp crushing, and the harmonic scalpel have been used. The intermittent Pringle maneuver can be used to limit bleeding and control bleeding vessels within the liver parenchyma. We limit portal occlusion to 15 to 20 minutes reserving its use only if necessary. This dissection can be meticulous and requires considerable practice. We try to preserve at least a 1 cm margin around the tumor (Fig. 7.**6**). We reserve the dissection of the tumor involving the IVC for the end. Once the entire tumor is dissected from the liver and it is only attached to the IVC, after performing the Pringle with the previously placed tourniquet, we proceed to perform proximal and distal clamping of the IVC. At this point the IVC is opened and the part attached to the tumor is resected. Any residual thrombus is removed as well (Fig. 7.**7**). The specimen is passed off the field and sent for pathologic examination. The surgical field is inspected (Fig. 7.**8**).

Depending on the size of the defect in the IVC, this can be primarily closed with continuous running 3–0 Prolene suture or equivalent suture. Attention should be taken not to narrow the lumen of the inferior vena cava but some degree of narrowing is acceptable (Fig. 7.**9**). Large defects can be repaired with a femoral or saphenous vein patch or synthetic material. Once the patch is sutured in place with nonabsorbable suture the proximal and distal control of the IVC is released.

Hemostasis of the remaining liver parenchyma is assured and any bleeding vessels are ligated. Cryoprecipitate glue or hemostatic agents may be used to reinforce hemostasis. A careful search for bile leakage is also accomplished. Drains are left in place and the incision is closed in layers (Fig. 7.**10**). We have seen some postoperative biliary leakage from the cut surface even after this was not detected at the operation. Severe leakage is usually treated expectantly with drains left in place as long as necessary.

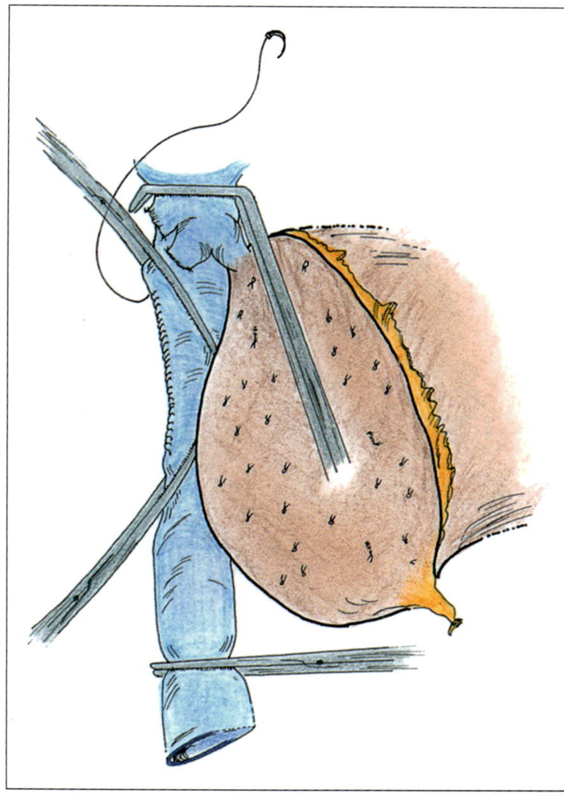

Fig. 7.**9** The IVC can be primarily closed with Prolene suture. A large defect can be repaired with a synthetic or venous patch.

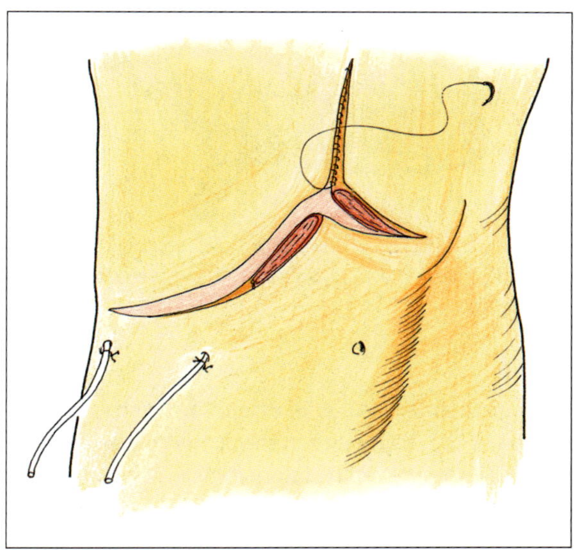

Fig. 7.**10** The incision is closed after proper drains have been placed.

☐ Resection for Tumors with Extensive Vascular Involvement using Autotransplantation

We describe below the resection of a large peripheral cholangiocarcinoma originating from the right hepatic duct but involving portal structures, inferior vena cava, and key structures of the left lateral segment. The patient mentioned was suffering from severe abdominal pain. Even though the cell type surprised us, nonetheless the relatively well differentiated tumor, as well as her young age seemed to warrant an aggressive approach. We currently perform similar autotransplantations safely.

The approach we choose for this resection is to perform the dissection on a back table after the liver has been completely removed. This technique requires a venovenous bypass while the liver is explanted or extracorporeal.

Similar to the previously described procedure the patient is placed in a supine position and a generous right subcostal incision extended above the xiphoid and into the left subcostal space is performed (Fig. 7.**1**). The liver is completely mobilized as is done for an extensive hepatic resection (Fig. 7.**11**).

The left axillary and left femoral region are also prepared and the left axillary vein and left femoral vein are exposed and cannulated in preparation for the venovenous bypass (Fig. 7.**12**).

The porta hepatis is dissected and the common bile duct is identified and divided with a 2.0 cm long stump (Fig. 7.**13**). The hepatic artery is dissected from the bifurcation to the take off of the gastroduodenal artery. Attention is paid to identify replaced right or left hepatic arteries. A generous segment of the portal vein is dissected as well. The supra- and infrahepatic vena cava are dissected. The latter is isolated between the adrenal and the renal vein (Fig. 7.**14**).

Once this dissection is completed, the liver resection may begin. The portal vein is clamped and divided near its bifurcation (Fig. 7.**15a**). The suprahepatic and the infrahepatic IVC is clamped (Fig. 7.**15b**). When clamping

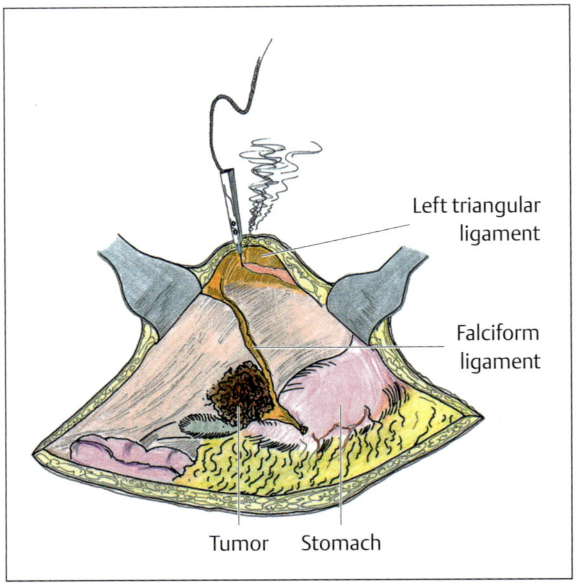

Fig. 7.**11** The liver is mobilized dividing the falciform and triangular ligaments.

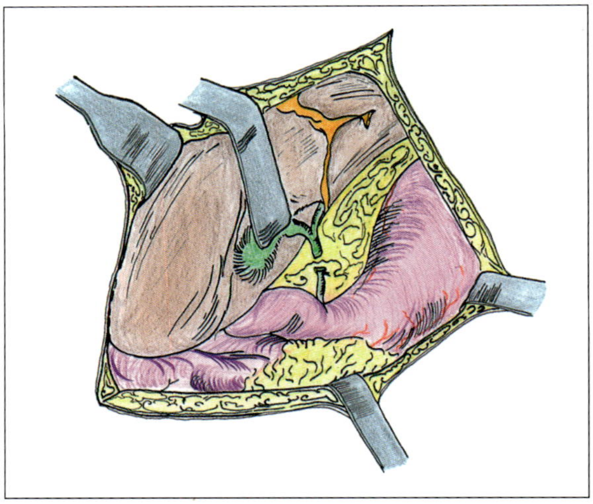

Fig. 7.**13** The portal triad is dissected and the common bile duct divided.

the suprahepatic IVC, it is essential to incorporate a portion of the diaphragm in the clamp to prevent slippage. The segment of the inferior vena cava attached to the tumor is resected en bloc with the liver (Fig. 7.**15c**). The specimen is passed to the back table, where the liver is irrigated with cold preserving solution and placed on ice. The operative field is inspected (Fig. 7.**15d**).

After the liver is removed a cannula is placed in the portal vein. The vascular clamp is removed and the cannula is introduced and secured with a Rummel tourniquet. The cannula is connected to the venovenous bypass system (Fig. 7.**16**).

On the back table, ex situ tumor resection is performed. This minimizes blood loss and allows a more meticulous dissection. Remember that this maneuver

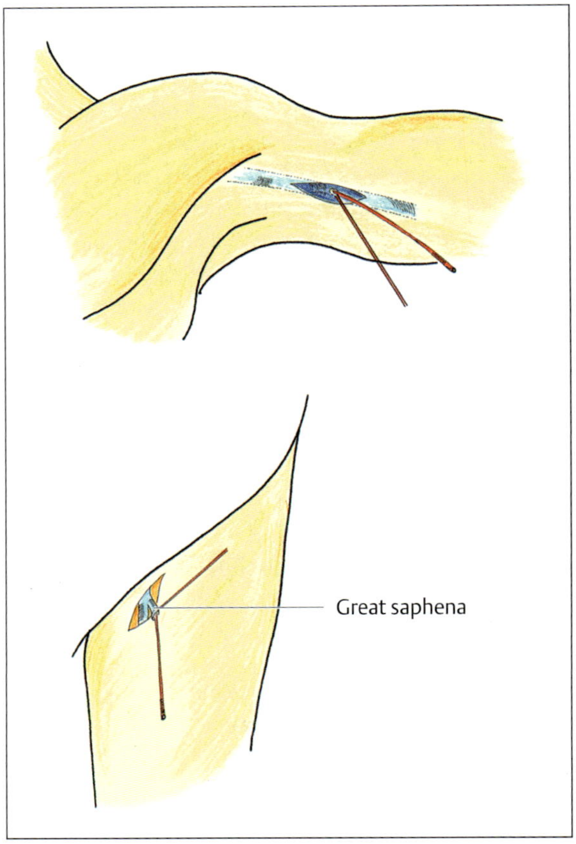

Fig. 7.**12** The axillary and femoral veins are cannulated in preparation for the venovenous bypass.

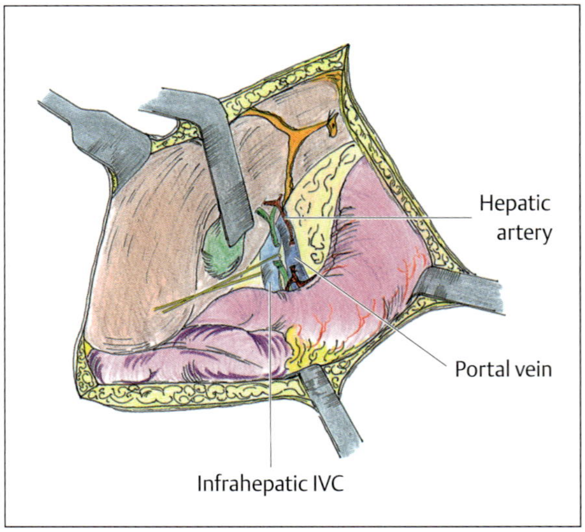

Fig. 7.**14** The portal vein and the vena cava are dissected.

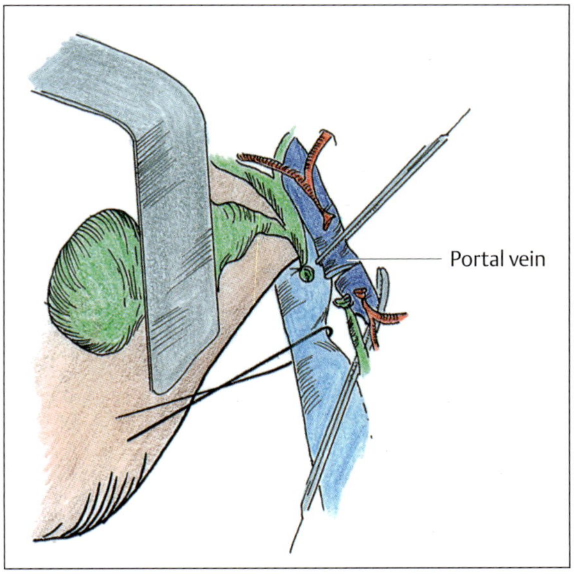

Fig. 7.**15a** The portal vein is clamped and divided.

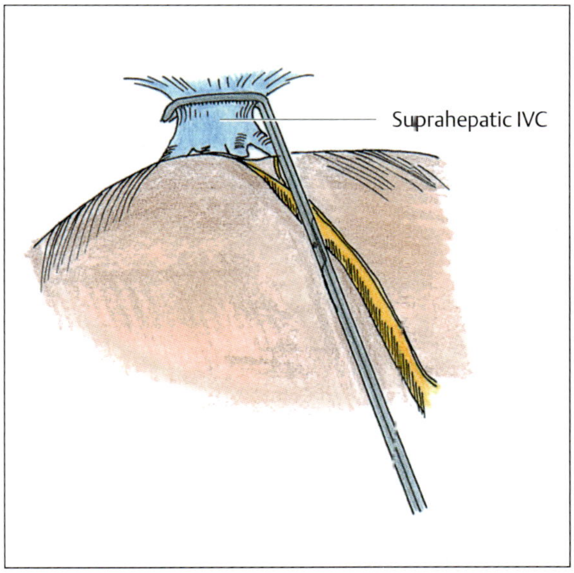

Fig. 7.**15b** The suprahepatic and infrahepatic vena cava is clamped.

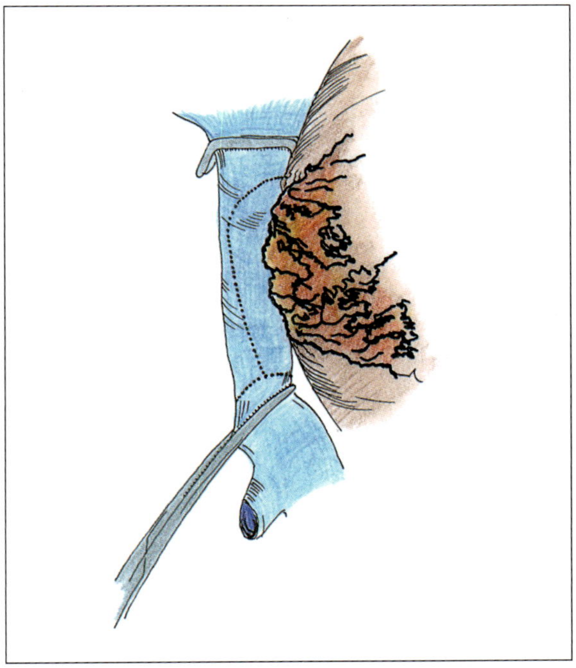

Fig. 7.**15c** The invaded segment of the IVC is removed en bloc with the liver.

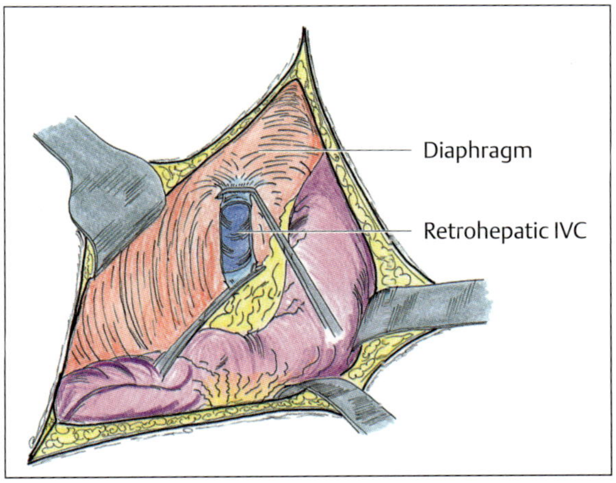

Fig. 7.**15d** Operative field after liver removal.

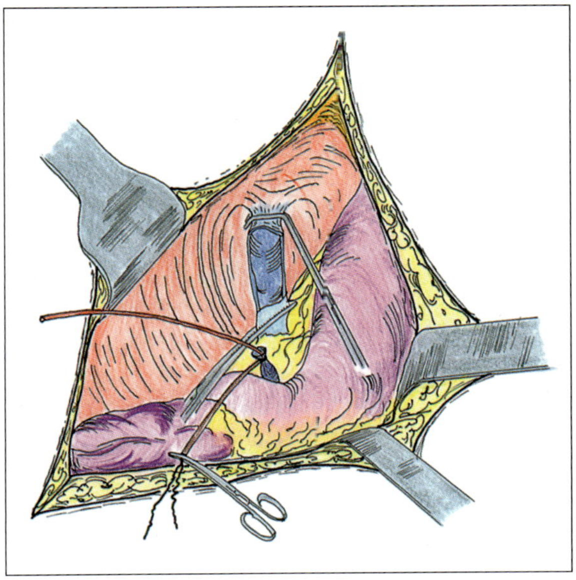

Fig. 7.**16** A cannula is inserted in the portal vein and the patient is placed in venovenous bypass until the back table dissection is completed.

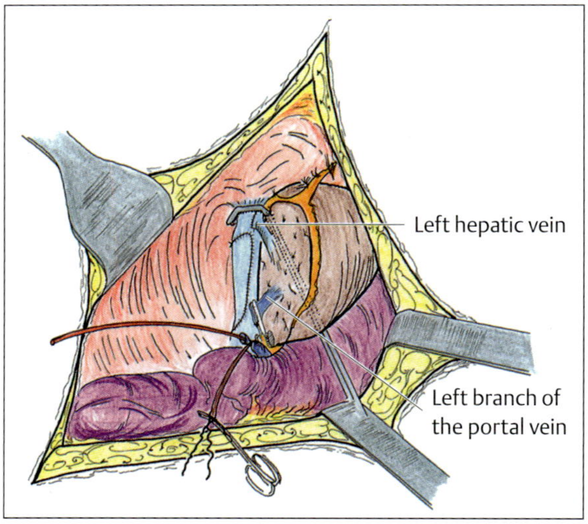

Fig. 7.**17** The specimen is reconnected. The IVC may require some type of patch graft to prevent narrowing of the lumen. The suprahepatic and remnant of the IVC are connected to this patch.

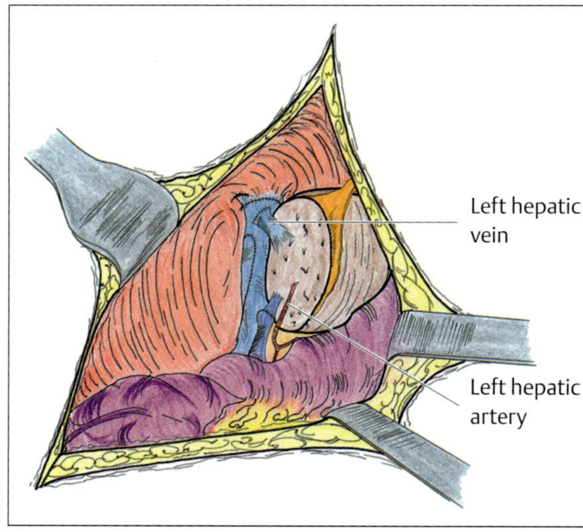

Fig. 7.**18** The portal vein and hepatic artery are reanastomosed.

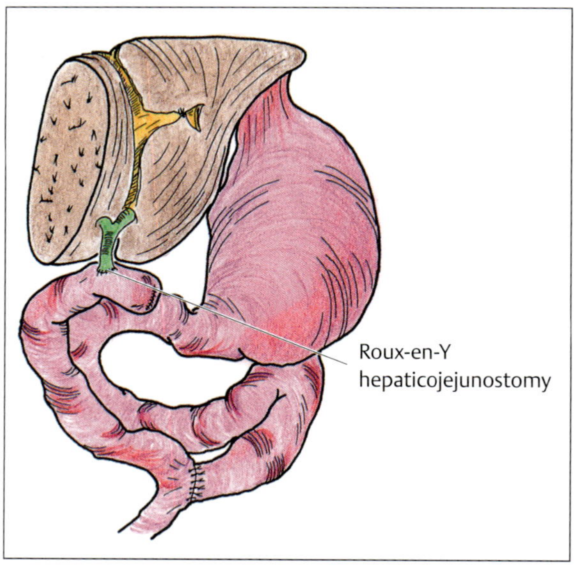

Fig. 7.**19** The biliary anastomosis is performed using a Roux-en-Y hepaticojejunostomy.

may compromise the length of the vascular pedicles and effort should be made to preserve them as much as possible. In this particular case we were able to preserve the left lateral lobe with an adequate vascular pedicle and bile duct. Frequently, the inferior vena cava requires some type of patch graft in order to correct the large defect and prevent narrowing of the lumen; this is also performed at the back table. The femoral vein, saphenous vein, or internal jugular can be used to assist the repair.

Once the dissection is completed the specimen is ready to be reconnected. The IVC is reanastomosed to the remnant of the supra and infrahepatic IVC, respectively, using nonabsorbable vascular suture (Fig. 7.**17**). The portal vein anastomosis is performed with 5–0 Prolene sutures. Once completed the portal cannula is removed. The hepatic artery is reanastomosed using 6–0 Prolene sutures. The clamps are released and hemostasis achieved (Fig. 7.**18**).

The biliary anastomosis can be performed using different methods. It can be performed by direct choledochocholedochostomy using interrupted 4–0 Prolene and placement of an intraluminal stent. It can also be repaired with the use of a T-tube. We prefer to perform a Roux-en-Y hepaticojejunostomy with a 45 cm Roux-en-Y segment. This technique has less morbidity in terms of biliary stenosis (Fig. 7.**19**).

Two drains are placed in the surgical area and the abdominal incision is closed in layers. The femoral and axillary cannulas are removed and the venotomies repaired with 6–0 Prolene sutures. The incisions are closed with absorbable suture.

Extended Hepatic Resection for Tumor Involving the Stomach

Tumors arising from the left hepatic lobe can invade the gastrohepatic ligament and the distal stomach requiring an en bloc resection of the stomach and left lateral segment. The following resection was performed on a patient with a massive fibrolamellar cholangiocarcinoma. He had undergone preoperative chemotherapy with impressive shrinking of his tumor basically separating some of the tumor from the important hilar structures. Nonetheless, most of the stomach was involved.

The procedure is best performed through a bilateral subcostal incision, as previously described (Fig. 7.**1**);

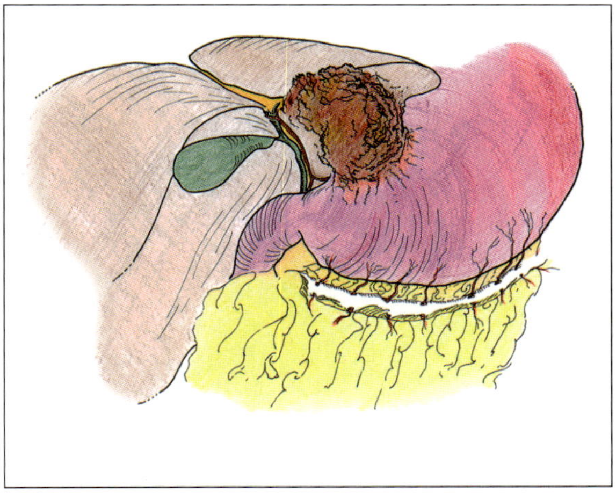

Fig. 7.20 Once the tumor is found to be resectable the dissection starts along the greater curvature where the gastroepiploic arcade and short vessel are ligated.

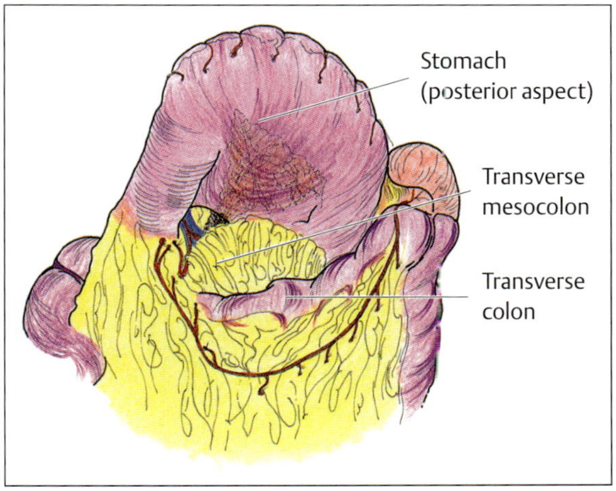

Fig. 7.21 The right gastroepiploic artery is ligated and divided.

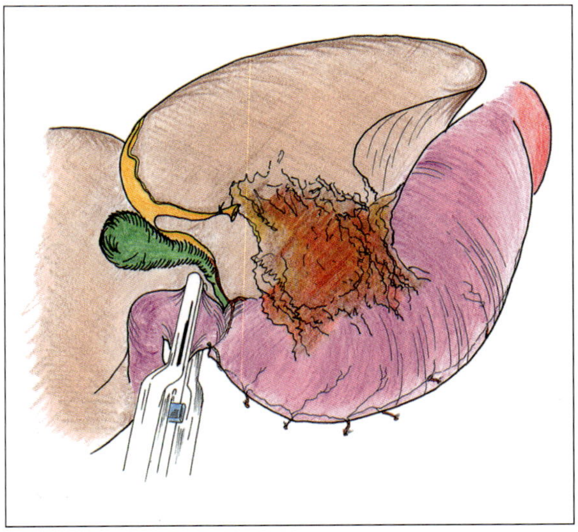

Fig. 7.22 The duodenum is divided using the linear stapler.

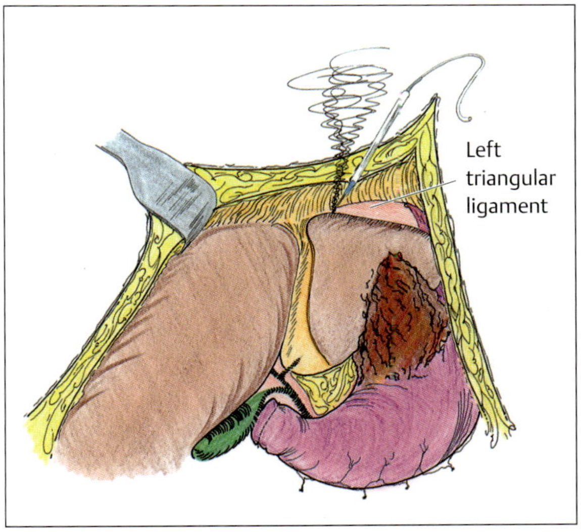

Fig. 7.23 The liver is mobilized dividing the left triangular ligament.

this allows excellent exposure of the liver and the stomach. The abdominal cavity is explored and the tumor with its relationships to the adjacent structures is determined.

Once the tumor is found to be resectable, the dissection starts along the greater curvature, where the gastroepiploic arcade and short gastric vessels are ligated. Any adhesions or peritoneal attachments to the pancreas and peritoneum are divided to mobilize the entire stomach (Fig. 7.**20**).

As the dissection proceeds toward the duodenum, the right gastroepiploic artery arises from the gastroduodenal artery in proximity to the anterosuperior pancreaticoduodenal artery branches; this requires careful dissection. The right gastroepiploic artery is ligated and divided including a small branch of the right gastric artery serving the pylorus (Fig. 7.**21**). The dissection is continued to include at least 2 cm of the duodenum proximally. Here the duodenum is divided using a linear stapler. Dissection continues along the lesser curvature in order to mobilize the stomach (Fig. 7.**22**).

The left gastric artery is ligated and divided with 2–0 silk suture ligatures. This dissection can be limited based on tumor location.

The liver is then fully mobilized dividing the avascular ligaments. The falciform and the right and left triangular ligaments are divided (Fig. 7.**23**). Intraoperative ultrasound is used to determine the relationship of the tumor to the middle and left hepatic veins. This will determine the need for a formal left hepatic lobectomy or a left lateral segmentectomy. If a formal left hepatic lobectomy is required, the left branches of the portal vein and hepatic artery are divided. We do not dissect the portal triad if it is not necessary. In a left

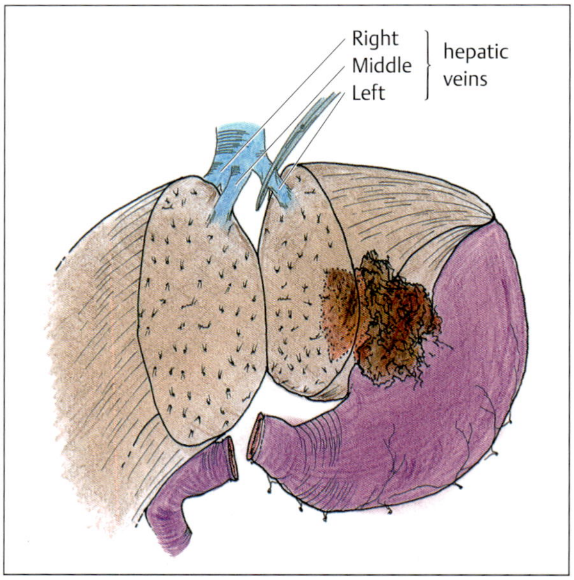

Fig. 7.**24** The hepatic parenchyma including the tumor is divided.

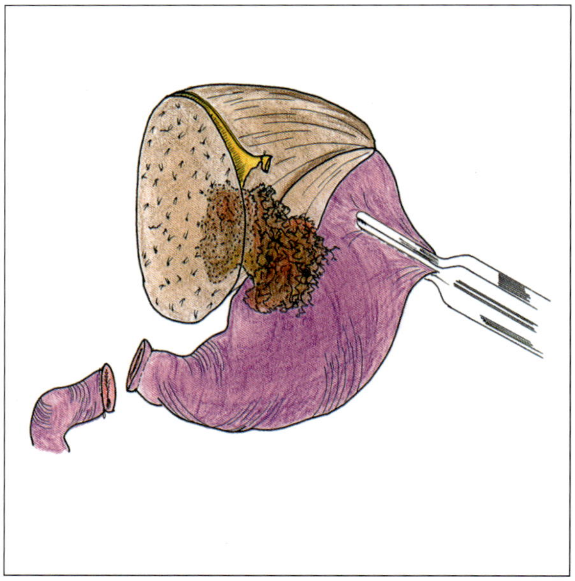

Fig. 7.**25** The stomach is divided using linear staples.

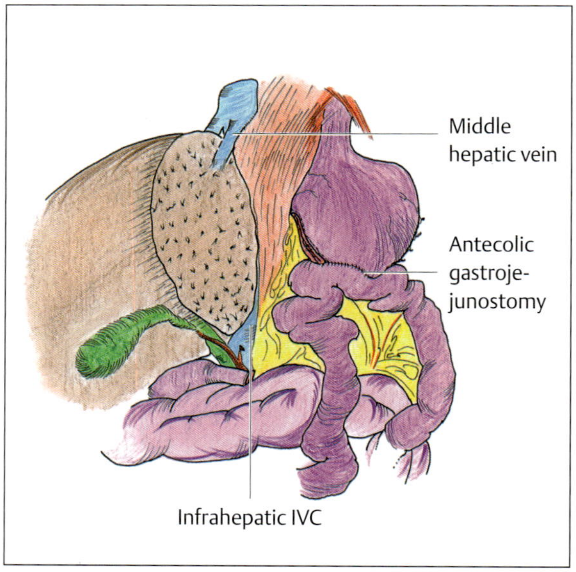

Fig. 7.**26** A gastrojejunostomy is performed to reestablish gastrointestinal continuity.

lateral segmentectomy this dissection is not indicated and only predisposes the patient to unnecessary risk. Dissection of the hepatic parenchyma is performed with the ultrasonic aspirator. The middle and left hepatic veins may be encountered and if necessary they can be suture ligated. The left and middle hepatic veins usually join for a very short distance prior to the junction with the suprahepatic vena cava (Fig. 7.**24**). Hemostasis of the remaining liver segment is reinforced to secure a dry field.

Once the liver is dissected, attention is moved to the stomach. In most cases we can preserve part of the stomach and perform a subtotal gastrectomy, preserving most of the gastric antrum and greater curvature. The stomach is divided using linear staplers; the distal stomach remains attached to the left lateral segment (Fig. 7.**25**). The specimen including the left hepatic lobe and the proximal stomach are passed off the field. A loop of proximal jejunum is brought anterior to the colon and an anastomosis between the proximal stomach and the jejunum is created (Fig. 7.**26**). We prefer a hand-sewn, double layer, interrupted, 3–0 silk suture technique for the anastomosis but stapled anastomoses are also acceptable. Regardless of the technique the most important thing is a tension free anastomosis.

Drains are placed around the liver parenchyma and in the gastrojejunostomy area. The abdomen is closed in standard fashion.

□ Hepatico-Bilio-Pancreaticoduodenectomy Combined with Liver Transplantation

Large hepatic tumors can invade the portal triad and the duodenum, especially sarcomas.

This requires an en bloc resection of the liver, duodenum, and pancreas combined with a liver transplant. This is a very challenging procedure that requires optimal preoperative evaluation.

The following procedure was performed for a 40-year-old woman with a large leiomyosarcoma of the duodenum involving most of the liver including the portal structures and vena cava (Fig. 7.**27**). The tumor also invaded the ampulla and head of the pancreas as well. There is no good way to resect this tumor without performing an aggressive approach.

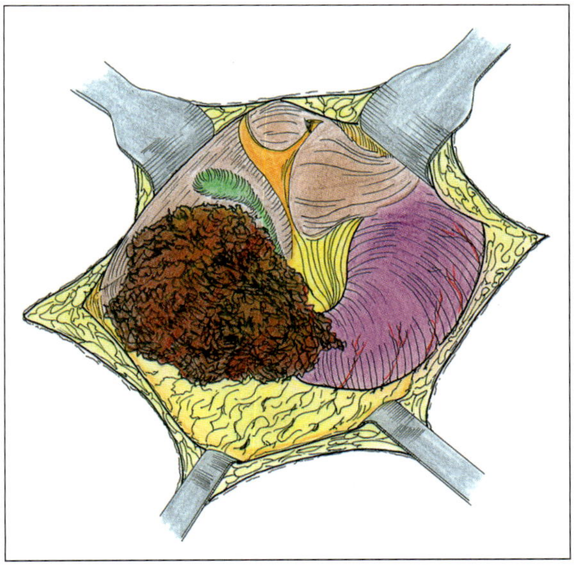

Fig. 7.**27** The abdominal cavity is initially explored and resectability is determined.

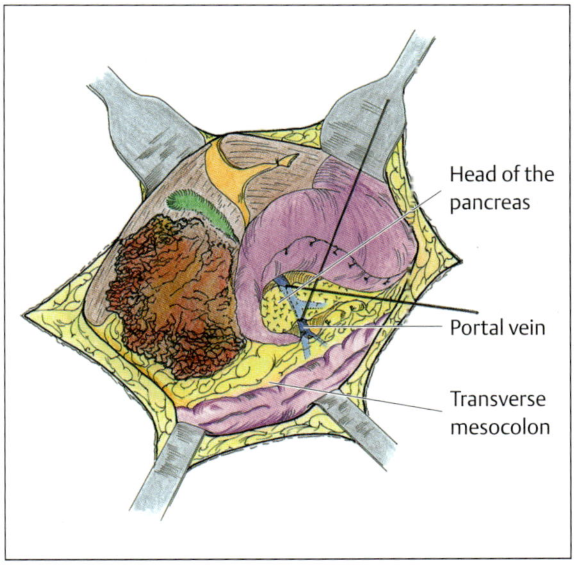

Fig. 7.**28** The space between the portal vein and the pancreas is developed.

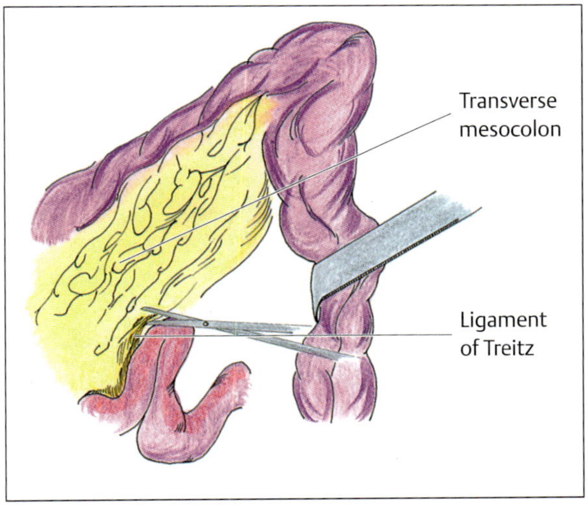

Fig. 7.**29** The ligament of Treitz is divided in its avascular segment.

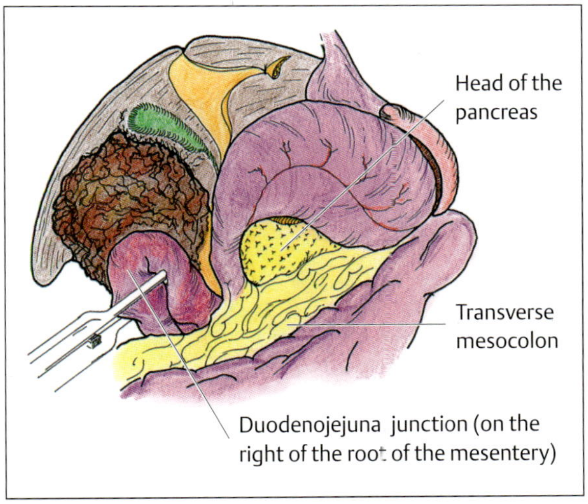

Fig. 7.**30** The proximal jejunum is divided. Dissection continues proximally until the short duodenal mesentery is divided.

The patient is placed in a supine position and the abdomen is approached through a bilateral subcostal incision. A xiphoid extension can be used if necessary. The abdomen is explored to rule out other pathologies and confirm the extent of tumor invasion and its relationship to adjacent structures.

As an initial step the duodenum is mobilized with the Kocher maneuver. The lesser sac is exposed by dividing the gastrocolic ligament. A plane is created between the pancreas and the portal vein. At this point, the portal vein originates behind the pancreas at the confluence of the splenic and superior mesenteric vein. This is normally an avascular plane and adherence here should raise concern of tumor involvement at this distinct location. After opening the gastrohepatic omentum, the surgeon should be able to pass a finger from superior to inferior along this plane. This should open in the inferior border of the pancreas just above the superior mesenteric vein (Fig. 7.**28**).

The ligament of Treitz is mobilized by dividing the avascular plane between the aorta and the third portion of the duodenum from the right side of the abdomen and then dividing the attachment of the fourth portion of the duodenum to the ligament of Treitz (Fig. 7.**29**). The duodenojejunal junction can be mobilized into the right upper quadrant, underneath the root of the mesentery. At this level the bowel is divided with a GIA stapler (Fig. 7.**30**). The short duodenal mesentery is divided between clamps and tied with 3-0 silk ligature.

The pancreas is divided at this level. We prefer to use a GIA stapler. We found this to be more hemostatic

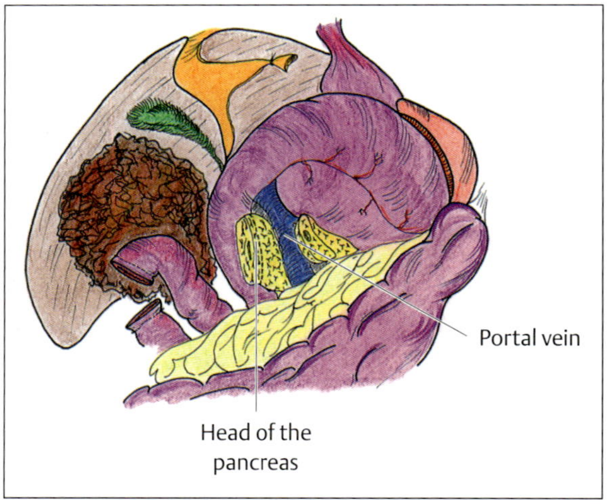

Fig. 7.**31** The pancreas is divided using a GIA stapler. This can also be done sharply using the knife.

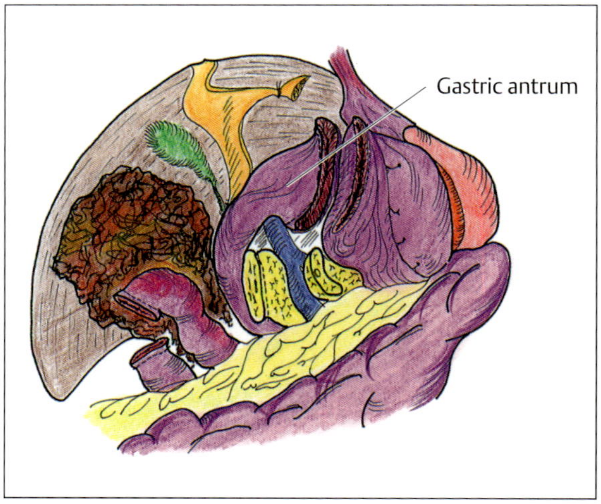

Fig. 7.**32** The distal stomach is divided at the upper border of the antrum.

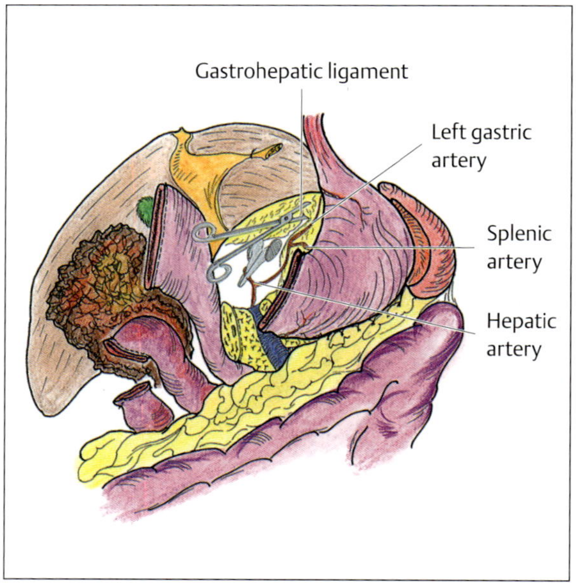

Fig. 7.**33** The hepatic artery is clamped and dissection continues along the lesser curvature.

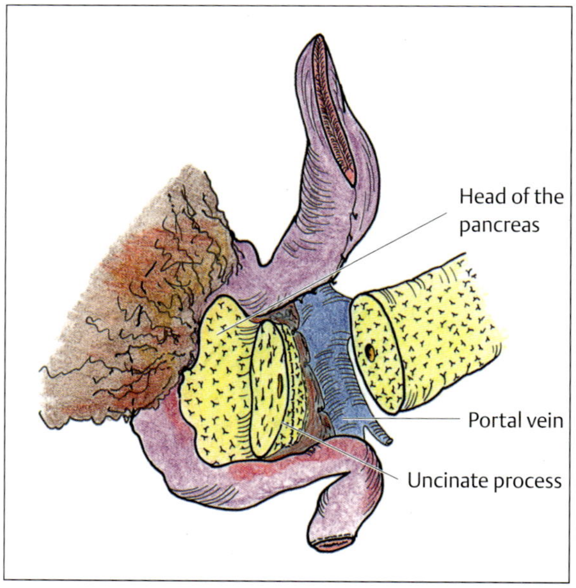

Fig. 7.**34** The uncinate process is dissected off the retroperitoneum.

(Fig. 7.**31**). It can also be sharply divided and the hemostasis is secured with fine (4–0) Vicryl sutures. Any bleeding point should be controlled at this time with a 3–0 silk suture. This exposes the portal vein proximal to the site of the tumor.

We proceed to divide the distal stomach at the upper border of the antrum. This is accomplished with a 90-mm linear stapler (Fig. 7.**32**). The upper border of the duodenum is mobilized by blunt dissection. The hepatic artery is identified at this level and divided between clamps and secured with 2–0 silk suture. The gastrohepatic ligament along the lesser curvature is also divided (Fig. 7.**33**). The left gastric artery is carefully preserved.

If the pylorus is spared from tumor invasion, its preservation can be attempted. We have found that, in this type of tumor, it is often impossible and very time consuming.

The pancreatic head and uncinate process are mobilized off the portal vein and SMA. Small vessels draining into the portal vein should be clipped and divided.

The uncinate process is dissected off the retroperitoneum. The head of the pancreas and duodenum remain attached to the tumor (Fig. 7.**34**).

We proceed to mobilize the liver, as previously described, by dividing the falciform ligament and the left and right triangular ligaments. The suprahepatic IVC is exposed (Fig. 7.**35**).

The infrahepatic IVC is also dissected between the adrenal and the renal veins. At this point the portal vein, the suprahepatic vena cava, and the infrahepatic IVC are clamped and divided. This allows the liver with

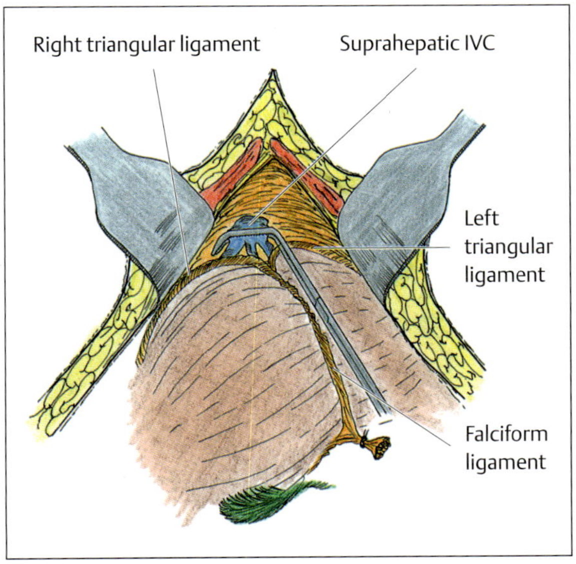

Fig. 7.**35** The liver is mobilized and the suprahepatic vena cava is exposed.

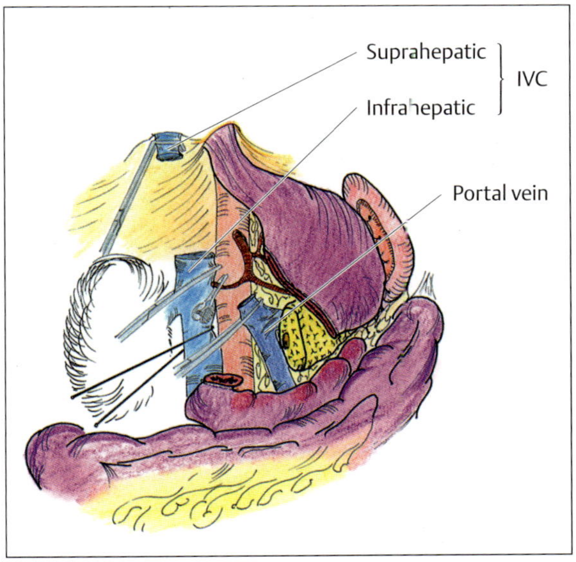

Fig. 7.**36** The portal vein, the supra- and infrahepatic cava vein are divided and the specimen is passed off the field en bloc.

the tumor attached to the previously mobilized pancreas and duodenum to be removed en bloc (Fig. 7.**36**).

At this point, the patient can be placed on a venovenous bypass, as previously described, or the anastomosis with the new liver can be directly performed. This will be based on the expertise of the surgeon.

The liver, which has been prepared at the back table, is placed into the patients' abdomen with cold slush packing. The suprahepatic vena cava is anastomosed first with 3–0 Prolene suture (Fig. 7.**37**). The infrahepatic vena cava is anastomosed after the liver is retracted superiorly, using 3–0 Prolene suture as well. The donor portal vein is flushed with 5% albumin in Ringer's solution to remove the high potassium and then the anastomosis between the new liver and the receiver's portal vein stump is completed with 5–0 Prolene sutures.

The hepatic artery is anastomosed to the patient's common hepatic artery stump or directly to the aorta.

Once all the vascular anastomoses are completed, the clamps are removed and the reperfusion of the new liver is initiated. Hemostasis is secured.

The final step is to complete the pancreatic, biliary, and gastric anastomosis.

A loop of proximal jejunum is brought antecolic into the right upper quadrant. The pancreaticojejunostomy is created first. The anastomosis is accomplished with an outer layer of suture between the serosa of the small bowel and the capsule of the pancreas and an inner layer mucosa to mucosa; we prefer to use 4–0 PDS for this anastomosis. No stent is used for the pancreatic anastomosis (Fig. 7.**38**).

The biliary anastomosis is done end-to-side between the jejunum and the donor common bile duct. This is a single layer anastomosis of 4–0 PDS suture. Absorbable suture allows us to place the knots inside the bile duct for technical ease. No stents are required (Fig. 7.**39**).

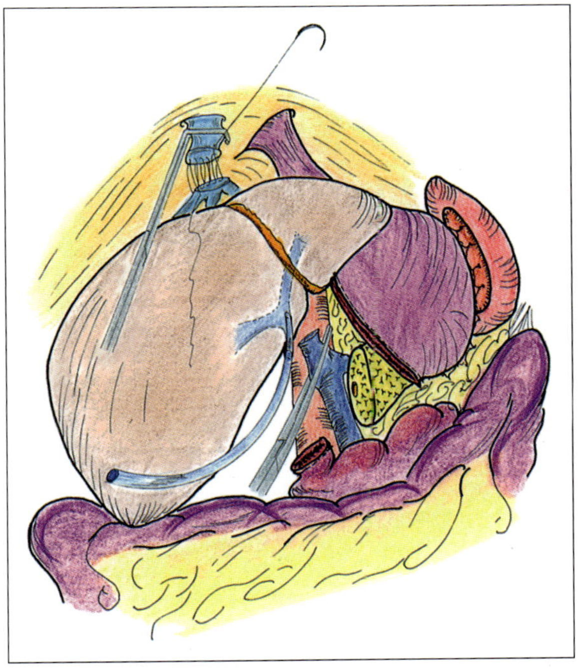

Fig. 7.**37** The liver transplant is reanastomosed. The suprahepatic vena cava is reanastomosed first.

The gastrojejunostomy is created 45 cm distal to the biliary anastomosis. This can be done hand-sewn or with the staple device (Fig. 7.**40**).

Multiple closed suction drains are placed around the pancreatic and biliary anastomosis. The abdomen is closed in standard fashion.

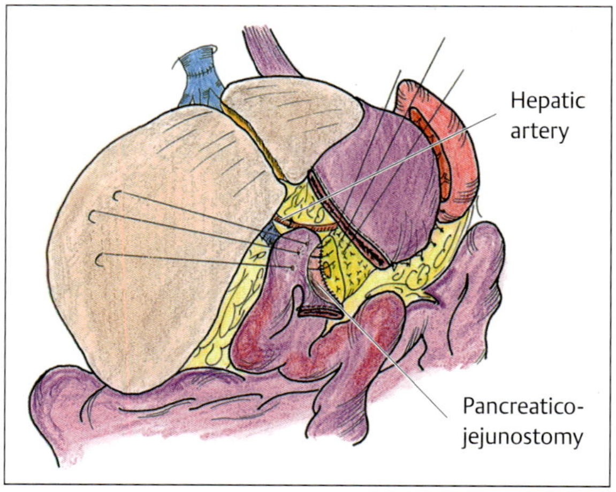

Fig. 7.**38** The pancreaticojejunostomy is created.

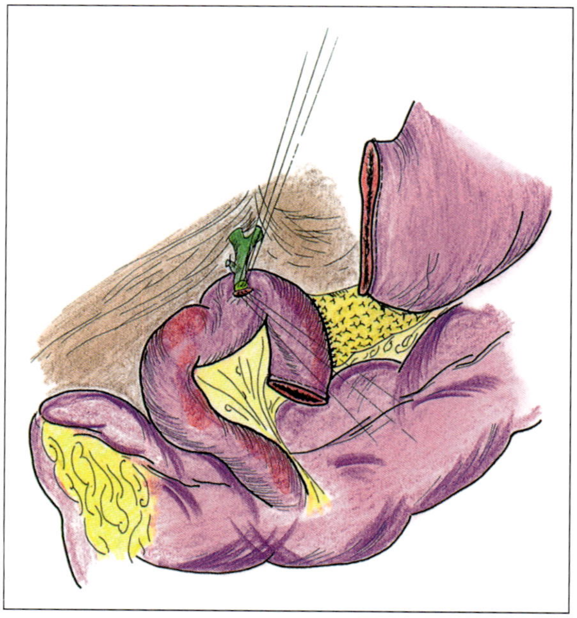

Fig. 7.**39** End-to-side biliary anastomosis.

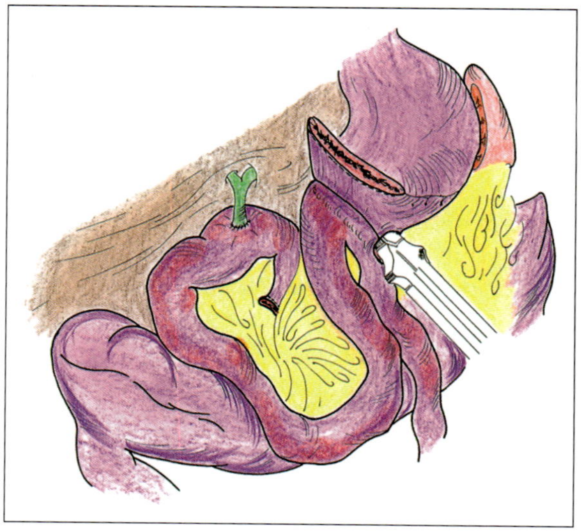

Fig. 7.**40** Stapled gastrojejunostomy. This can be performed handsewn.

Postoperative Care

After major hepatic resection or transplantation the patients should be admitted to the intensive care unit. Careful monitoring of hemodynamics and fluid balance is mandatory.

Hemoglobin, liver function test, and coagulation times are followed very closely after the initial surgery. Initial elevation of the liver function test is not uncommon, but this usually is transient and it should normalize within the first week. Up to 80 to 90% of the liver can be removed without consequences, except in patients with preexistent liver disease. This group of patients can have an increased risk for developing liver failure after resection.

Hypoglycemia and hypoproteinemia can occur in the immediate postoperative period, and this should be treated supportively. We recommend avoiding H2 blockers; they interfere with liver regeneration. Regeneration is almost complete within 3 weeks except in elderly patients where the liver grows back more slowly.

Drains are left in place as long as they are necessary. They can generally be removed within the first postoperative week. It is common to have bile-stained fluid after the initial resection. However, major bile leakage may not be evident until the patient resumes diet. Conservative management is appropriate because most of these leaks will resolve spontaneously.

Conclusion

In the preceding sections we have presented new approaches for extended liver resections involving adjacent organs. One should recognize that these resections might be controversial. In our experience, the aggressive approach turned out to be favorable for the patient. Experience in hepatobiliary surgery and transplantation techniques is one of the elements for success of these procedures.[5] Each patient should be individualized and the procedures adapted to each particular case. We believe that, with the current improvement in adjuvant therapies, these procedures will play a larger role in the care of advanced hepatic or biliary cancer invading adjacent organs.

References

1. Sabiston DC. *Atlas of General Surgery*. Philadelphia: Saunders; 1994.
2. Meyers WC, Chari RS, Schaffer BK, Shah SA. Staging, resection and ablation of liver tumors. In: Sabiston DC, ed. Sabiston Textbook of Surgery. Philadelphia: Saunders; 2001:1035–1043.
3. Meyers WC, Jackson DM, DeCaesteker JE, Castellanos AE. Anatomy of the biliary tree and gallbladder. In: *Gastrointestinal Disease: an Endoscopic Approach*. Thorofare, NJ: Slack Inc; 2002: 993–1008.
4. Chari RS, Foley DP, Meyers WC. Primary hepatic neoplasm. In: *Surgical Oncology. Contemporary Principles Practice*. New York, NY: McGraw-Hill; 2001: 659–671.
5. Hess W, Berci G. Textbook of Bilio-Pancreatic Diseases. Padova, Italy: Piccin; 1997: vol 3.

Lower Gastro-intestinal Tract

3

8 Right Colon

Feza H. Remzi and Mustafa Oncel

During 2000, 130 200 new cases of colon and rectal cancer were reported in the United States.[1] It is the third most common malignancy and the second leading cause of cancer death in both women and men. The average person has about 6% chance of developing colorectal cancer in his or her lifetime.[2] The cecum and right colon are the most common locations for colorectal cancer after the rectum and sigmoid.[3] Surgery is the primary modality of treatment in 92% of patients with colon cancer.[4] Although surgery may be performed for palliative control of symptoms in advanced cases, in most circumstances it is performed for curative intent.[5]

Advanced Colon Cancer

A small but significant number of patients for whom a curative operation was planned have big bulky tumors that extend beyond the intestinal wall and adhere to adjacent tissues or organs. When colon cancer has grossly invaded or has densely adhered to an adjacent organ in the absence of distant metastasis, it is called advanced colon cancer, which represents approximately 10% of all colorectal cancers.[6–10] Advanced colon cancers can present with lymph node metastasis (Dukes C2 or Astler–Coller T4N1–2) or without lymph node metastasis (Dukes C1 or Astler–Coller TN0). Almost half of these tumors are node-positive. Many locally advanced cancers, even if they are large in size or attached to other organs, are potentially curable with surgery, especially if the regional lymph nodes are free of metastases, which is surprisingly frequent.[7]

In 1959, Butcher and Spjut reported a variant of a very large, bulky colon cancer, which did not tend to metastasize to lymph nodes even though it invaded adjacent organs.[11] Spratt et al. analyzed 1137 consecutive colorectal patients and found that of the largest resected colorectal carcinomas (more than 13 cm in diameter), 66.7% had no metastases in resected lymph nodes.[12] Although these tumors tend to penetrate the intestinal wall, grow to a large size, and occupy the adjacent tissues or organs, they remain localized for long periods without spreading to regional lymph nodes and appear to be curable by aggressive resection. This biologic behavior is unlike that of most other epithelial tumors in which locoregional invasion is usually associated with contiguous regional or distant metastases, as is particularly true of other gastrointestinal adenocarcinomas.[7]

The sigmoid colon and rectum are the most common locations for locally advanced colon cancer.[8] Thus, extracolonic extension more often occurs in sigmoid colon and rectum where pelvic structures and organs may be involved.[13] Locally advanced carcinoma of the right colon and proximal transverse colon adhere to adjacent organs in as many as 11 to 28% of cases.[10,14] Right-sided carcinomas of the colon can invade the small bowel, abdominal wall, the right kidney, ureter and bladder, genital organs (uterus, fallopian tubes, and ovary), duodenum, pancreas, and liver. Extensive surgical procedures have been performed to completely resect locally advanced primary colon cancers, and multivisceral en bloc resection of these tumors has resulted in cure in many patients.[15,16]

En Bloc Resection

Resections for colon cancers are categorized as follows: R0, all gross disease resected by en bloc resection with margins histologically free of disease; R1, all gross disease resected by en bloc resection with margins histologically positive for disease; R2, residual gross disease remains unresected.[5]

Curative surgery must always follow the oncologic criteria of an en bloc resection established for the treatment of colorectal cancer. Unless en bloc resection is surgically and pathologically confirmed in a patient (R0 resection), the resection cannot be considered curative.[5] True tumor infiltration is generally confirmed pathohistologically in 43 to 70% of patients, whereas the remaining tend to have only inflammatory changes that mimic tumor invasion.[17–20] In a recent study, the true infiltration rate was observed in only 116 (34%) of 341 patients.[18] These findings may lead some to suggest that the colon may be separated from a structure that has been adhered to the colon cancer, since these infiltrations are not always associated with malign invasions, but when this concept was followed, the local recurrence rate was 26% and the 5-year survival rate was only 30% in 35 patients, probably because dissection caused dissemination of tumor cells. [18,21] Other studies have revealed similar results. In a group of 43 patients with adjacent organ involvements, local recurrence rates were exceedingly high when adherent organs were separated from the tumor (77 vs. 36%).[22] Conversely, the 5-year survival was significantly higher when an en bloc technique was performed (61 vs. 23%).[22] In two studies, early recurrence was reported in 70–100% of the patients treated with non en bloc resections.[22,23] Hunter et al. reported that en bloc resection of colorectal cancers that are adherent to other organs resulted in local recurrence and 5-year survival rates that were comparable with the stage-matched nonadherent colorectal cancers.[6] En bloc resection is now considered mandatory for curative colon cancer surgery because it reduces recurrence and maximizes the 5-year survival rates. An en bloc resection is warranted even for patients with regional lymph node metastases (the most important prognostic factor after potentially curative resection for colorectal carcinoma and adjacent organ involvement).[5,23]

3

Therefore, any attempt to separate the colon cancer from the adherent organs should be discouraged because it could lead to the dissemination of cancer cells into the abdomen, which increases the risk of recurrence. Similarly, finger-fracture separation of densely adherent viscera should be avoided because it can preclude cure.[24,25] With regard to the surgical approach for adherent carcinomatous masses, en bloc resection is an absolute necessity, because any effort to separate the carcinoma from neighboring organs will tear or transect the tumor and increase the attendant risk of intraoperative dissemination resulting in a significant and unacceptable worsening of the prognosis.[10,14,23]

Preventing Inadvertent Perforations

Inadvertent perforations during resection are not uncommon. The rectum is the most common location for accidental perforation, but it can occur during the resection of right colon tumors. Yu found that although tumor cells readily implant on traumatized serosa, the intact intestinal mucosa is quite resistant.[26] Bowel wall injury exposes the intraluminal bowel contents with its desquamated cancer cells to the traumatized fresh planes opened by surgical dissection. Gall et al. revealed that in 44 patients with positive tumor infiltration and multivisceral en bloc resection without tear or rupture of the tumor, the 5-year survival rate was 49%, which decreased significantly to 17% when the surgeon inadvertently tore or cut into tumor tissue during dissection.[17] Slanetz Jr reported a reduction in 5-year survival and an increase in local recurrence rates after inadvertent perforations during colon cancer surgery.[27] Therefore, during the surgical dissection of the tumor, the surgeon must be careful not to inadvertently perforate the tumor.

Extent of the Resection

The extent of the resection is one of the most important factors affecting cancer recurrence. Little controversy exists about the dissection margins in colon cancer. The ideal extent of bowel resection is defined by removing the blood supply and lymphatics at the level of the origin of the primary feeding arterial vessel.[5] When the primary tumor is equidistant from two feeding vessels, both vessels should be excised at their origin.[5]

The margin distal to the primary tumor is determined by the adequacy of the blood supply to the distal colon for anastomosis after appropriate vascular ligation, the downward lymphatic spread, and the intramural spread of the carcinoma.[28] Intramural spread of the tumor occurs through the submucosal and intramural lymphatics or perirectal fat.[29] Distal intramural spread rarely exceeds 4 cm even in the most unfavorable cases.[29] Recent studies have revealed that only 2.5% of patients will have tumors that have spread more than 2 cm, and these are generally anaplastic or poorly differentiated node-positive cancers.[2] Although there is some debate, 5 to 10 cm of normal bowel on either side of the primary colon tumor appears to be a minimum length to prevent anastomotic recurrence.[5,30,31] The length of resected ileum does not appear to affect local recurrence. Therefore, the shortest length of ileum needed to perform the surgical procedure should be excised to prevent malabsorption syndromes.[5] With regard to histologic assessments of distal margin, all margins must be microhistopathologically evaluated with a review of permanently fixed or frozen tissue sections.

Lymph node resection carries with it prognostic and therapeutic implications.[5] Tumor invasion to the lymph nodes directly affects survival rates in patients with advanced colon cancer. In a study of 58 patients with advanced colon cancers, Eisenberg et al. found that the mean survival and 5-year disease-free survival rates were 100.7 months and 76% for lymph-node negative patients respectively whereas they were 16.2 months and 0% for lymph-node positive patients respectively.[25]

An appropriate lymph node resection should extend to the level of the origin of the primary feeding vessel. As with the primary tumor, the lymph nodes should be removed en bloc. Lymph nodes at the origin of feeding vessels (apical nodes) should be removed when feasible and tagged for pathologic evaluation. Lymph nodes suspected of being positive for disease outside the field of resection need to be sampled or biopsied. If biopsy results of the suspected lymph nodes are positive for disease and the lymph nodes are resected with the apical nodes or the biopsy results are negative, the resection is considered to be a curative resection (R0 resection).[5] Otherwise the procedure is an incomplete resection for cure (R1 or R2 resections).[5] The apical node may also have prognostic significance in addition to the number of lymph nodes positive for disease in the specimen.[32] To achieve a high degree of accuracy (>90%), a minimum of 12 lymph nodes negative for disease must be examined to confirm that the disease does not involve the nodes.[33] Several retrospective studies have yielded conflicting results on the value of extended lymphadenectomy.[5,34,35]

No-Touch Technique

It has long been suspected that cancers may be disseminated through the bloodstream by the trauma of surgical removal. Viable tumor cells have been found in peripheral venous blood of patients whose colorectal cancer was intraoperatively manipulated.[36,37]

In 1952 Barnes described a special technique for resecting the right colon cancer in which the vascular pedicles are ligated and the bowel is divided before the cancer-bearing segment is handled.[38] Turnbull et al. demonstrated a difference in 5-year survival in a retrospective analysis.[39] In the only prospective randomized trial no statistical difference was observed in 5-year survival with the use of the no-touch technique in 236 patients (31.1% disease-related death in the conventional arm, 24.7% disease-related deaths in the no-touch technique); but the time to appearance of liver metastases was lower and the number of liver metastases was higher in the conventional arm.[40] The value of the no-touch technique has been debated.

Because malignant cells have been found within the lumen of the colon after operative manipulation, it is possible that viable tumor cells implant in the anastomotic line and cause recurrence in the suture line.[37] Therefore, at least one study recommended occluding the proximal and distal parts of primary tumor by ligating the colon externally with cotton tapes before manipulating the tumor.[37] No studies have been performed to evaluate the outcome of this technique.

Multivisceral Resection in Locally Advanced Right Colon Cancer

Colorectal cancer invades adjacent organs in 5.5–16.7% of all colorectal malignancies.[6–10,13,41,42] Because a high percentage of very large T4 tumors have not yet metastasized to the regional lymph nodes, a multivisceral resection offers radical removal of the local disease and results in cure.[19] Multivisceral resection of colon cancer is defined as en bloc removal of any organ or structure to which the primary tumor is adherent. Removal of unattached organs (e.g., liver resections for hepatic metastases, cholecystectomy for symptomatic gallbladder disease, splenic resection for iatrogenic injury, and resection of synchronous tumors) is not considered multivisceral resection.[18] The aim of multivisceral resection is an en bloc removal of the primary tumor and adherent organs or structures (R0 resection) without leaving any microscopic (R1 resection) or macroscopic (R2 resection) disease, in which survival and recurrence rates are unacceptable.

The invasion of colon cancer to other organs is rarely recognized before surgery. Most patients with colonic cancers who required extended resections have gastrointestinal tract symptoms such as anemia, weight loss, abdominal pain, nausea and vomiting, or diarrhea, but there is no correlation between any symptom or combination of symptoms and the presence of pathologic invasion of contiguous structures.[8,14,43,44] Pneumaturia and vaginal bleeding are pathognomonic, but they are extremely rare.[45] Polk emphasized that many right-sided carcinomas with contiguous organ involvement are palpable preoperatively, and that when a tumor is palpable and immobile, adjacent structures are most likely involved.[9,44]

The final decision for multivisceral resection is made at the time of laparotomy. However, the surgeon cannot distinguish between malignant and inflammatory adhesions. The adherence represents true malignant invasions of the contiguous organ in 36 to 70% percent of cases.[15,18,21,46,47] Intraoperative assessment should rarely be used to exclude a patient from multivisceral resection with curative intent because the postoperative pathohistologic examination reveals disease-free margins in many specimens in which the surgeon considered tumor resection to be incomplete.[18] Lehnert et al. encouraged surgeons not to decide intraoperatively to give up a resection because the inflammatory or malignant character of the adhesions during the laparotomy is not reliable and has a high negative predictive value.[18] They suggested that surgeons should make every effort to completely resect the invasive tumors with the adherent tissues.[18] In another series, re-exploration was performed in 52 consecutive patients who had originally been classified as having unresectable disease. An extended resection was performed in 32 of them, with a 5-year survival rate of 36%.[48] Thus, the surgeon should perform an en bloc, complete resection of the tumor with adjacent tissues unless it is obviously not possible to achieve a R0 resection.

Determining the nature of a dense adherence between a tumor and closely apposed organ is difficult. Attempts to biopsy tissues between colon cancer and an adherent organ may give false-negative results due to sampling error and more importantly can lead to tumor spillage. Thus, intraoperative frozen section should be avoided to determine the extent of resection in order not to cause tumor contamination.[18] When the surgeon suspects that the adherent tissue is microscopically invaded, en bloc resection is the best choice, because the differentiation of benign from malignant adhesions is inaccurate and because intraoperative biopsy risks tumor dissemination.[24] The nature of the adherence between the primary tumor and adjacent viscera should be determined only upon histologic assessment of the extended resection specimen.[9]

Before undertaking a major procedure such as multivisceral resection, the following issues should be kept in mind: the patient's condition, stage of the tumor, experience of the surgical team, operative factors, and postoperative outcome.[13] High-risk, unstable, elderly, and malnourished patients may not be good candidates for multivisceral resections. Although contentious, a recent study revealed that elderly patients, who had multivisceral resection procedures survived for a significantly shorter time than the younger patients.[18] The surgeon should remember that emergency operations are associated with worse outcomes when compared with elective multivisceral resections.[18] During laparotomy, peritoneal or liver metastasis must be ruled out before attempting a resection because patients with metastases would not benefit from multivisceral resections.[49]

3

Multiorgan resection for locally advanced colon cancers is not a standardized procedure. The following sections will attempt a standardization. In addition, the decision to perform multivisceral resection is usually made at the time of surgery because the need for multivisceral resection is rarely recognized before surgery for colon cancer. Therefore, good judgment is required as premature or irreversible steps that mandate an extended, but clearly palliative resection are best avoided. In this situation, it is important to evaluate the accuracy with which curative or palliative outcome of the treatment can be predicted during surgery. Long-term results are poor if en bloc resection of the primary tumor with any organ or structure to which it is adherent is not achieved.[50] It has been shown that mean survival is only 14 months in resections with histologically positive margins for disease, which is an extremely short amount of time.[8,50] Therefore, when dealing with a colorectal cancer that is adherent to adjacent organs, the surgeon must determine the resectability of the tumor. If the surgeon determines that the tumor is resectable, efforts must be made to perform an appropriate resection.[13]

Variations in surgical technique are the most important determinants of cancer recurrence and survival. Experience is needed to determine which surrounding organs are affected. If the surgeon is not familiar with the procedure, the abdominal wall should be closed and the patient referred to a specialized center.[13] A surgeon with limited experience may consider the tumor to be unresectable and prefer a palliative bypass as the only alternative for the patient, which would reduce his or her chance for cure.[13]

Specific Organ Involvements

The **small bowel** is the most common location of invasion; it is the affected organ in 15 to 25% of all cases with right colon cancer.[6,18,50] Generally, segmental resection with an adequate tumor-free margin and anastomosis is the choice of treatment. The **abdominal** wall is also a frequent location for tumor invasion.[6,50] The tumor infiltration rate of abdominal wall invasion is generally lower than that of other adherent organs.[18] Therefore, a small portion of peritoneum generally must be removed to obtain tumor-free margins. If the tumor invades a wide area such as the skin and underlying structures, a rare occurrence, a large en bloc removal of abdominal wall is needed.[51] If the surgeon has doubts about the subsequent abdominal closure that should never influence him or her to be less than thorough in the debridement or to accept less than adequate tumor resection, patient survival must always be the paramount consideration.[52] Mesh repair can be used in these patients. In patients who have a primary fascial closure without a mesh, the wound can be left open and closed in a delayed primary fashion.[52,53]

Larger tumors may also invade **urinary tract organs** including the kidney, ureter, and bladder. In this case, the affected organ must be resected to achieve cure.[13,14,18] Complete tumor resection with en bloc partial or total nephrectomy can be performed.[53] Occasionally, in bulky tumors, the ureter may appear to have been invaded by tumor. In this situation, the surgeon must assess if it is in contact with the tumor or encircled by it. In the former case, a careful dissection usually shows that it is not involved and can be separated. In the latter case, a resection is imperative. If a small portion of the ureter is invaded, an anastomosis can be safely done over a ureteral catheter after a partial ureteral removal (Fig. 8.**1**). If a long portion of ureter is removed or the resection site is near to the bladder, the reconstruction can be made with an ureteroneocystostomy.[54] Another technique for the reconstruction of missing ureter includes a defunctionalized segment of ileum anastomosed proximally to the proximal segment of ureter and distally to the bladder.[55] Bladder invasion can be managed by removing the involved portion of the bladder with a 2-cm tumor-free margin.[14,54]

Right colon tumors rarely invade the **genital organs**, uterus, fallopian tubes, and ovaries.[18] Although there are no current data to support routine prophylactic oophorectomy, en bloc or complete resection of the ovary is recommended if the tumor has obviously and directly invaded the ovary or if the ovary has a grossly abnormal appearance.[5] The incidence of synchronous ovarian metastases varies from 2 to 8%.[54] Because of the higher prevalence of ovarian cancer among women with colorectal cancer, oophorectomy may be per-

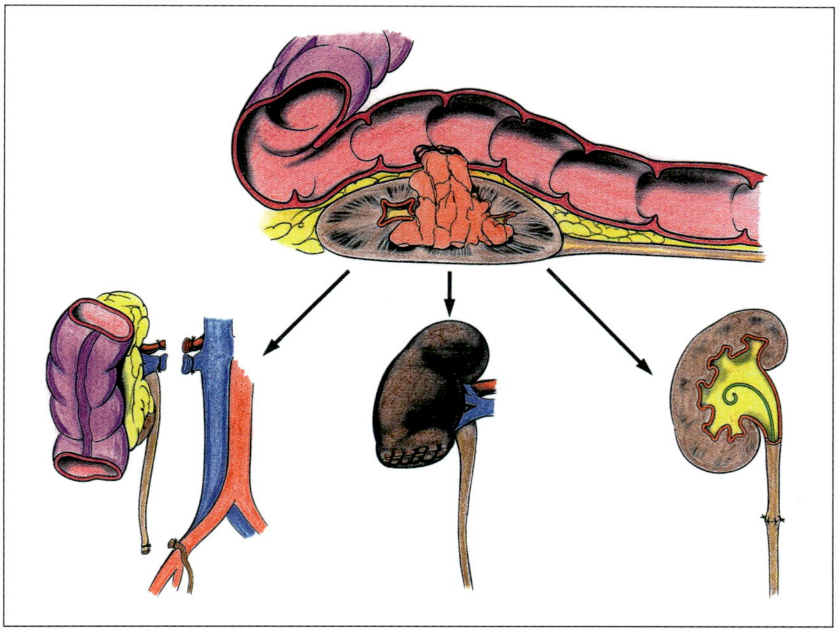

Fig. 8.1 When the kidney is invaded with a large tumor, complete tumor resection with en bloc partial or total nephrectomy can be performed. If the ureter is invaded, a partial removal is required and then an anastomosis can be safely done over a ureteral catheter in most cases.

3

formed in postmenopausal patients or in premenopausal patients who do not have a desire to conceive.[54] During the resection of these structures, the surgeon should strive for a tumor-free margin, which is the most important factor affecting survival and recurrence of the tumor.

Although a right-sided colon cancer does not frequently involve the **duodenum** and **pancreas**, this condition represents a challenge for the operating surgeon because an extended radical resection might be needed.[8,44,56] Studies reporting combined resection for the treatment of locally advanced cancer mention that the duodenum and pancreas are involved in 0 to 11% of cases.[10,14,17,22,23,57] Duodenal invasion can be managed with lateral duodenal resection with at least 1-cm tumor-free margin where the infiltration is limited to the duodenum (Fig. 8.**2**). This management avoids the need for a major procedure such as pancreaticoduodenectomy.[8,44,58,59] If the defect on the duodenum is small, it can be repaired with primary suturing, if it is large, however, the reconstruction should be made with duodenojejunostomy (Fig. 8.**3**).[8,43] Roux-en-Y duodenojejunostomy may be used as an alternative to duodenojejunostomy, and wider invasions may require pancreaticoduodenectomy. In some cases, involvement of the pancreas and duodenum is associated with widely metastatic disease and, in these instances, symptomatic patients can be palliated with endoscopic stenting, and operative biliary and/or gastric bypass.[60] Less frequently, patients with isolated metastatic or locally advanced tumors may be treated with pancreaticoduodenectomy for tumor clearance.[17,60] According to Koea et al., if the tumor invades superior mesenteric vessels, it is then unresectable for cure (Fig. 8.**4**).[44] However, Yoshimi et al. presented a patient with a successful mesenteric vein resection and end-to-end anastomosis.[61]

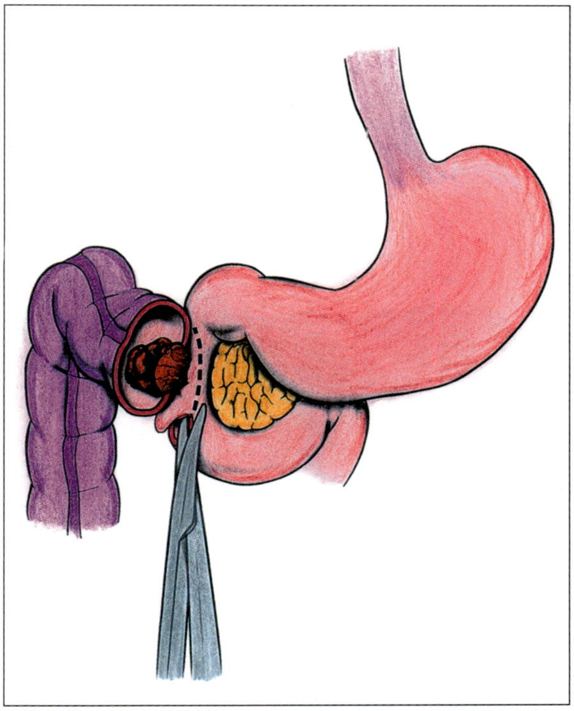

Fig. 8.2 Duodenal invasion can be managed with lateral duodenal resection with at least 1 cm tumor-free margin.

The guiding principle when the root of the mesentery is invaded by a colon cancer depends on the operative circumstances, the vascular experience of the surgeon, the general state and age of the patient, and the

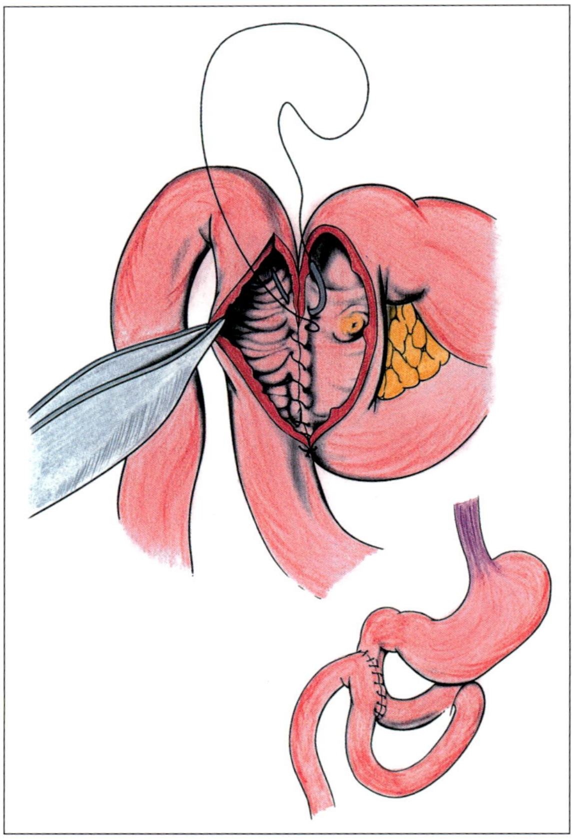

Fig. 8.3 Duodenojejunostomy is generally preferred for the reconstruction if the defect on the duodenum is large.

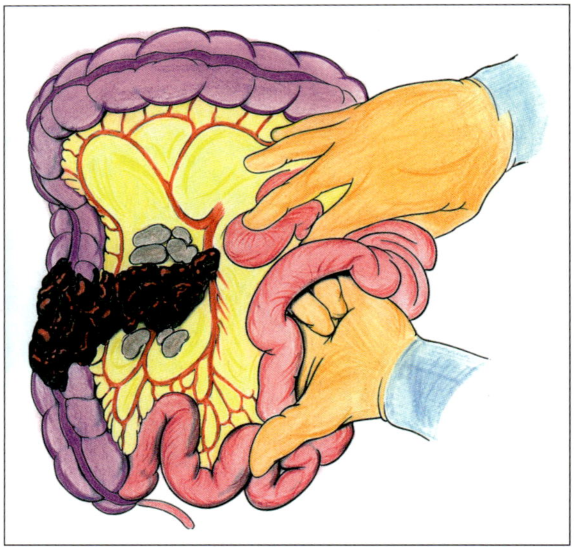

Fig. 8.4 If the superior mesenteric vessels are invaded, the tumor is generally considered as unresectable for cure.

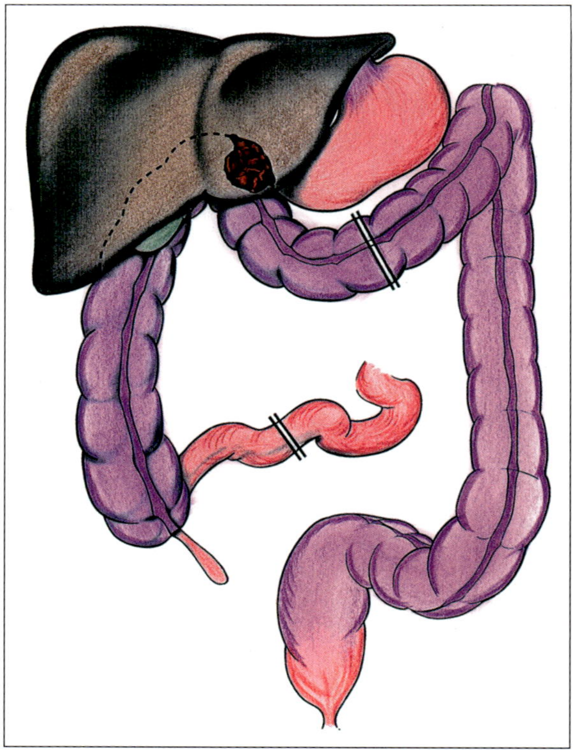

Fig. 8.5 Direct invasion of the liver is a very rare event occurring only after duodenal or pancreatic involvement.

logistical support allowing a major vascular resection and reconstruction.

The resection of the superior mesenteric vein (SMV) or portal vein is mainly reported with regard to a cancer of the head of the pancreas. The resection and reconstruction of the SMV for colon cancer can be approached in this analogy. It is known that SMV resection (for adenocarcinoma of the pancreas) increases operative time, number of transfusions, ICU stay, and total length of hospital stay but does not affect the postoperative morbidity or mortality and improves the surgical prognosis when the SMV is invaded.[62,63]

The resection and bypass of the superior mesenteric artery (SMA) is well described for visceral aneurysms or chronic intestinal ischemia. The technique gives good results. It is also occasionally reported for carcinoma of the pancreas.[64] SMA and/or SMV resection for colonic carcinomatous invasion is probably exceptional but technically feasible. However, this possibility should be foreseen before the operation because the saphena (for SMA replacement) or an internal jugular vein (for SMV replacement, for example) must be included in the operative field. After SM vessels resection, the sequence of reconstruction is to reestablish the SMV before the SMA.

Although the literature agrees that localized colon cancer that has invaded the pancreas and duodenum can safely be managed with extended resection and pancreaticoduodenectomy, publication bias may have resulted in the presentation of only successful cases.[44]

Direct invasion of the liver is a very rare event occurring only after duodenal or pancreatic involvement (Fig. 8.5).[17,23,56,65] Nonanatomic resection with a few centimeters' normal liver tissue, segmental resection, or lobectomy can be performed according to the size and location of the invasion (Fig. 8.6).[13,53,65]

Technical Details of Multivisceral Right Colon Resection

The patient is placed in the supine position on the operating table unless a left-sided invasion or synchronous tumor is present, or a colonoscopic examination under anesthesia is planned. After the induction of anesthesia, a nasogastric tube is inserted to decompress the stomach and it generally remains in place for 24 -hours or until bowel movements begin. A urinary catheter is inserted, which remains in place until the patient is mobile enough to urinate. An appropriately sized wound protector minimizes contamination of the wound as well as the chance of tumor cells' implanting if there are viable cells shed from the serosal surface during the procedure. A midline incision is made in the upper abdomen. Some form of self-retaining retractor is generally used to aid the procedure.[54]

Before performing the procedure, the surgeon explores the abdominal cavity to evaluate the extent of the disease. The tumor is examined only to confirm its resectability, and any additional manipulation—including palpation of the tumor—is avoided. The liver, regional lymph nodes, stomach, small bowel, and the remainder of the colon are examined. The pelvic cavity and gynecologic organs are examined to evaluate whether there is peritoneal seeding or whether there are implants on the ovaries.[54] Then the small bowel is reflected to the patient's left side and the root of the mesentery and the transverse mesocolon are examined to determine whether the tumor has invaded these structures or metastasized. The small bowel is reflected cephalad and to the patient's right side to expose the third portion of the duodenum. After dividing the peritoneum over the duodenum, a finger is passed under the superior mesenteric artery from left to the right, over the third and second portions of the duodenum (Fig. 8.**7**). A little hole in the mesentery may make the examination and palpation of the superior mesenteric vessels easier (Fig. 8.**8**). This maneuver will determine the local resectability of the tumor.[54] If there is a large tumor surrounding the superior mesenteric vessels and the aorta or inferior vena cava, a palliative operation should be considered (Fig. 8.**9**).[54]

Once resectability has been determined, the right colic artery is identified in the base of the transverse mesocolon. The hepatic flexure branch is divided just distal to where it is originated from the middle colic artery. Division of the main trunk of the middle colic artery is not recommended, because it is unnecessary for right-sided colon cancers and can cause the ischemia of the distal transverse colon. The mesentery of the ileum is divided between the ileocolic artery and the most distal ileal branch. The lesser sac is entered through the gastrocolic omentum. The right side of the gastrocolic omentum is divided and the gastroepiploic

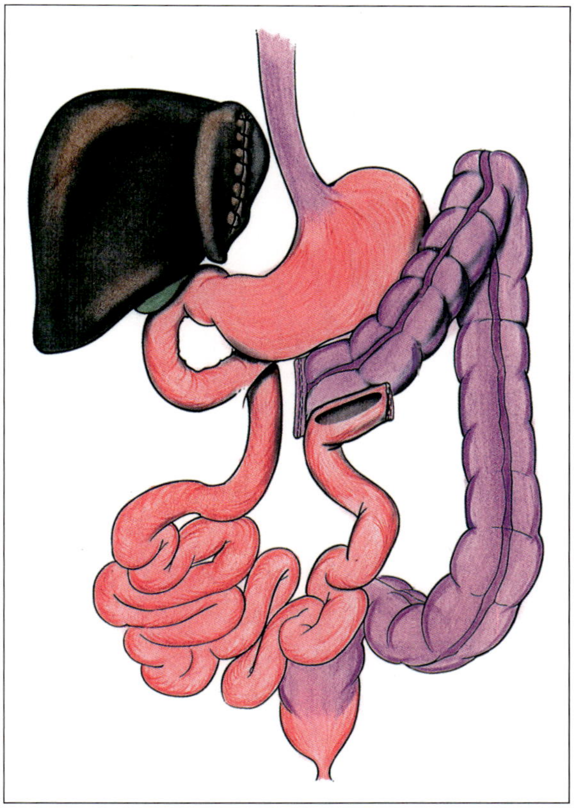

Fig. 8.**6** Lobectomy may be preferred for large invasions.

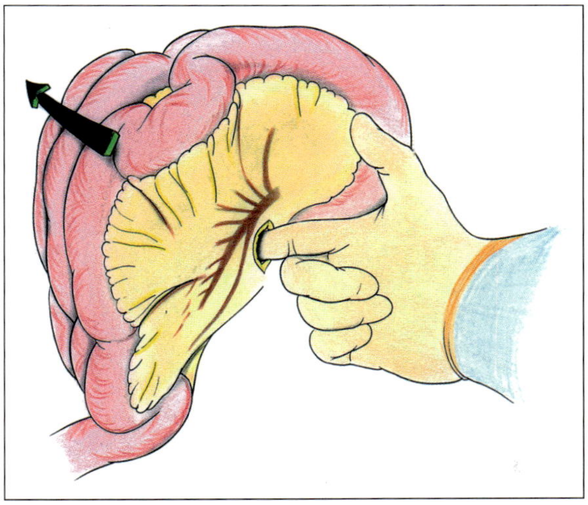

Fig. 8.**7** The examination and palpation of the superior mesenteric vessels. This is the initiation of the no-touch technique.

arcade is preserved until the hepatic mesocolon is mobilized and the stomach is separated from the mesocolon. The bowel is transected in its midportion, and the omentum is incised to the level of the anastomosis. The bowel is completely detached from its central connections. The peritoneum is divided from the base of the mesentery along the paracolic gutter to the hepatic flexure.[54]

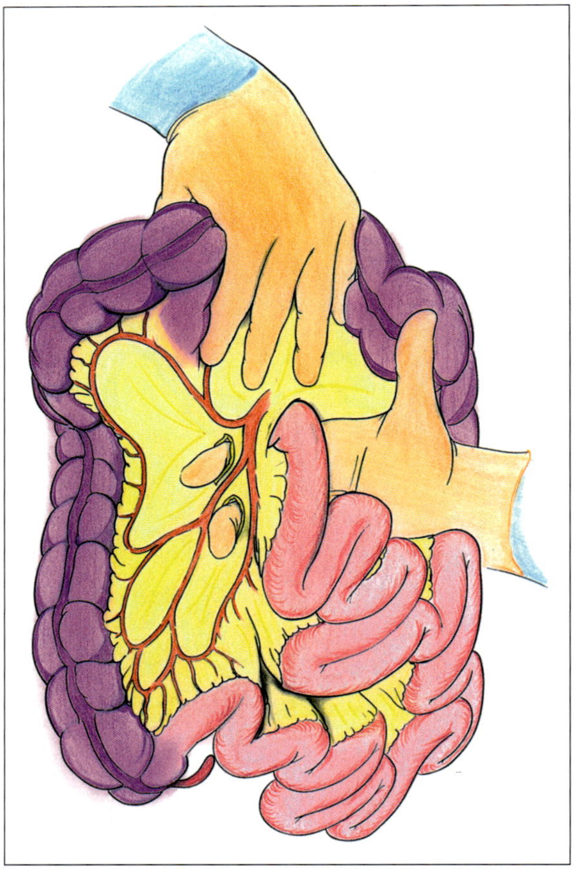

Fig. 8.8 The root of the mesentery and the base of the transverse colon are examined to determine whether the tumor has invaded these structures.

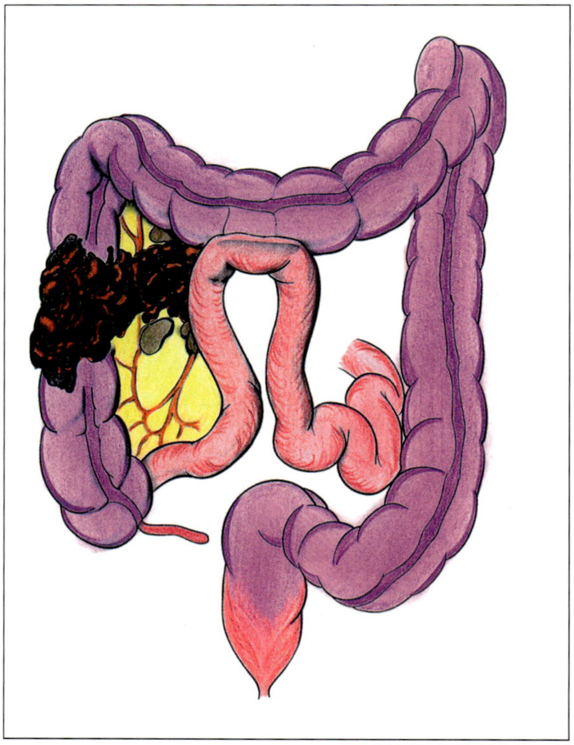

Fig. 8.9 Ileotransversostomy for an unresectable right colon cancer.

At any stage of the resection, when a structure that the tumor is attached to is identified, an en bloc resection with tumor-free margins is performed. After reconstruction of the attached organ, an end-to-end, end-to-side, or side-to-side anastomosis of terminal ileum and transverse colon is performed with either handsewn sutures or circular stapling instruments.

Outcome of Multivisceral Resections

The perioperative mortality and morbidity of multivisceral resections are similar to or slightly higher than that of conventional colectomies. Approximately 25 to 31 % of the patients develop complications which include anastomotic leak, wound infection, peritonitis, ileus, bleeding, fistula, abscess, and nonsurgical complications.[10,15,18,23–25] The high rate of morbidity may be related to increased blood loss and bacterial contamination of the operative field.[7] The operative time is also longer in these cases, and the procedure sometimes requires more than one anastomosis, which may increase the complication rates. Postoperative morbidity can be reduced using procedures such as omental pedicle flap or myocutaneous flaps that bring vascularized tissue to the resection or anastomosis region.[7]

Early postoperative mortality rates were roughly 10% in initial papers and as high as 22% in one series.[15,17,23,49,66,67] But recent series have demonstrated lower perioperative mortality rates ranging between 0 and 8%.[14,18–20,25,44] A recent study revealed that the early postoperative mortality rates of patients who underwent multivisceral resections were worse than that for patients who did not undergo multivisceral resections.[18] Increased early postoperative mortality rate was the only factor determining the difference between the survival times of these two groups. In addition, the mortality and morbidity rates are higher after emergency surgery than elective surgery.[18]

The invasion of the lymph nodes and the operative technique (en bloc resection, residual tumor, inadvertent perforation of the tumor) are factors that affect survival rates of operated locally advanced colon cancer.

Survival is directly related with the removal of the tumor. In a recent study, the 5-year survival was 42% for patients undergoing multivisceral resections, 51% for patients undergoing curative surgery, and 0% for patients undergoing only palliative surgery.[19] Surgeons should keep this data in mind when deciding whether to remove the tumor or perform a palliative operation. If patients have liver or peritoneal metastasis, they generally do not survive for more than 12 months. Thus, these patients do not benefit from multivisceral resection.[49]

Nodal status is also an important factor that affects 5-year survival. The literature on multivisceral resection shows that the 5-year survival rate is higher for patients without lymph node metastases (average 69%, range 53 to 93%) than for the patients with lymph node metastases (average 22%, range 0 to 45%).[8,10,17,20,22,25,49]

During the multivisceral procedure for locally advanced colon cancer, it is important to achieve a resection with margins that are negative for disease, because incomplete resection is associated with a median survival period of less than 12 months.[14] The literature has shown that extracolonic invasion of colorectal cancer is not a determining factor in prognosis provided that the specimen shows tumor-free resection margins upon histologic examination.[7] If the tumor was transected or if finger dissection was performed, survival significantly decreases. For the node-negative locally advanced cancers, the cure rate is 90% if the margins of the resected specimen are tumor free but is 0% when the cancer is transected.[23,68]

The nature of the adherence to the viscera may be also related to the survival rates. A recent review of the literature revealed that 5-year survival is lower in patients with malignant adhesions than in those with benign adhesions.[17,10,22,49] Another study showed no statistical difference in survival between these two groups.[20] Eisenberg et al. revealed that the difference between the two groups may be related to lymph node status, and when they excluded lymph node positive patients, they found no difference between the malignant and benign adhesions.[25]

The histologic features associated with a good prognosis are generally present in patients without lymph node metastases: well-differentiated neoplasms, large tumor size without skip or discontinuous metastases in the specimen, inflammatory reaction around the tumor, and absence of perineural, lymphatic, or vascular invasion.[9,25]

As a result, if complete en bloc resection is accomplished, overall survival of patients with advanced colon cancer who are treated with multivisceral resection is similar to that of patients who do not require resection of additional organs, and this holds true for every stage and every tumor location.[6,8,17,18,49]

Although en bloc and complete resection techniques affect recurrence rates, many studies have not found any significant difference in recurrence rates of patients treated with multivisceral resections and those who did not require multivisceral resections.[6,18] Hunter et al. noted that local recurrence was significantly more likely in patients after separation of adherent organs (69%) than after en bloc resections (18%). In one series, the evaluation of 58 multiorgan resections showed that the recurrence rate was 100% when the margin was positive. Moreover, recurrence occurred within 8 to 22 weeks in these patients.[68]

Conclusion

Five to 16% of large bowel cancers are adherent to adjacent organs or structures without any evidence of distal metastases. These T4 tumors are called locally advanced cancers, which infrequently present in the right colon and invade the abdominal wall, small bowel, duodenum, liver, pancreas, and urinary and genital organs. Many of these locally advanced lesions, despite attaining large size, are potentially curable by aggressive resection, especially if the regional lymph nodes are free of metastases, as is surprisingly frequent. Many studies have revealed that en bloc resection of such tumors with invaded tissues or organs is associated with a 5-year survival rate of approximately 50%, if the microscopic margins are tumor free. Half of these large tumors are node negative. In that case the 5-year survival rate reaches 80% in some series. These impressive results are achievable when the principles of cancer surgery are implemented. These include meticulous preoperative and intraoperative search for metastases, sharp anatomic dissection, en bloc resection, and minimal manipulation of the tumor. Blunt separation of the structures adherent to the primary tumor should be avoided because adhesions will be malignant in about 50% of cases, and cancer recurrence is almost certain when a tumor is transected. The perioperative morbidity and mortality of multivisceral resection are similar to or slightly more than a regular colectomy. If complete en bloc resection is achieved, the survival of advanced colon cancer patients treated with multivisceral resection is similar to that of patients treated with conventional colectomy. If there is no residual tumor, recurrence rates after multivisceral resection are acceptable.

As a result, extended en bloc resection for localized right colon cancers invading adjacent organs or structures can be undertaken safely and is associated with prolonged survival time and low recurrence rate.

3

References

1. Greenlee RT, Murray T, Bolden S, Wingo PA. Cancer statistics, 2000. *CA Cancer J Clin.* 2000;50:7–33.
2. Posner MC, Steele GD Jr, Mayer RJ. Adenocarcinoma of the colon and rectum. In: Zuidema GD, Yeo CJ, Pemberton JH, eds. *Schackelford's Surgery of the Alimentary Tract.* Vol. 4. 5th ed. Philadelphia: WB Saunders; 2002: 219–236.
3. De Leon ML, Schoetz Jr DJ, Coller JA, Veidenheimer MC. Colorectal cancer: Lahey experience, 1972–1976. An analysis of prognostic indications. *Dis Colon Rectum.* 1987;30: 237–242.
4. Beart RW, Steele GD Jr., Menck HR et al. Management and survival of patients with adenocarcinoma of the colon and rectum: a national survey of the Commission on cancer. *J Am Coll Surg.* 1995;181:225–236.

3

5. Nelson H, Petrelli N, Carlin A et al. Guidelines 2000 for colon and rectal cancer surgery. *J Nat Can Inst.* 2001;93:583–596.
6. Hunter JA, Ryan JA, Art PS. En bloc resection of colon cancer adherent to other organs. *Am J Surg.* 1987;154:67–71.
7. Lopez MJ. Multivisceral resections for colorectal cancer. *J Surg Oncol.* 2001;76:1–5.
8. Curley SA, Evans DB, Ames FC. Resection for cure of carcinoma of the colon directly invading the duodenum or pancreatic head. *J Am Coll Surg.* 1994;179:587–592.
9. Polk HC Jr. Extended resection for selected adenocarcinomas of the large bowel. *Ann Surg.* 1972;175:892–899.
10. Eldar S, Kemeny MM, Terz JJ. Extended resections for carcinoma of the colon and rectum. *Surg Gynecol Obstet.* 1985;161:319–322.
11. Butcher HR Jr, Spjut HJ. An evaluation of pelvic exenteration for advanced carcinoma of the lower colon. *Cancer.* 1959;12:681–687.
12. Spratt JS, Jr. The lognormal frequency distribution and human cancer. *J Surg Res.* 1969;9:151–157.
13. Berrospi F, Celis J, Ruiz E, Payet E. En bloc pancreaticoduodenectomy for right colon cancer invading adjacent organs. *J Surg Oncol.* 2002;79:194–197.
14. Curley SA, Carlson GW, Shumate CR, Wishnow KI, Ames FC. Extended resection for locally advanced colorectal carcinoma. *Am J Surg.* 1992;163:553–559.
15. Bonfanti G, Bozzetti F, Doci R et al. Results of extended surgery for cancer of the rectum and sigmoid. *Br J Surg.* 1982;69:305–307.
16. Devine R, Dozois R. Surgical management of locally advanced adenocarcinoma of the rectum. *World J Surg.* 1992;16:486–489.
17. Gall FP, Tonak J, Altendorf A. Multivisceral resections in colorectal cancer. *Dis Colon Rectum.* 1987;30:337–341.
18. Lehnert T, Methner M, Pollok A, Schaible A, Hinz V, Herfarth C. Multivisceral resection for locally advanced primary colon and rectal cancer, an analysis of prognostic factors in 201 patients. *Ann Surg.* 2002;235:217–225.
19. Gebhardt C, Meyer W, Ruckriegel S, Meier U. Multivisceral resection of advanced colorectal carcinoma. *Langenbecks Arch Surg.* 1999;384:194–199.
20. Heslov SF, Frost DB. Extended resection for primary colorectal cancer involving adjacent organs or structures. *Cancer.* 1988;62:1637–1640.
21. Montesani C, Ribotta G, De Milito R et al. Extended resection in the treatment of colorectal cancer. *Int J Colorectal Dis.* 1991;6:161–164.
22. Hunter JA, Ryan JA, Schultz P. En bloc resection of colon cancer adherent to other organs. *Am J Surg.* 1987;145: 67–71.
23. McGlone TP, Bernie WA, Elliot DW. Survival following extended operations for extracolonic invasion by colon cancer. *Arch Surg.* 1982;117:595–599.
24. Lopez MJ, Monafo WM. Role of extended resection in the initial treatment of locally advanced colorectal carcinoma. *Surgery.* 1993;113:365–372.
25. Eisenberg SB, Kraybill WG, Lopez MJ. Long-term results of surgical resection of locally advanced colorectal carcinoma. *Surgery.* 1990;108:779–786.
26. Yu SK, Cohn I Jr. Tumor implantation on colon mucosa. *Arch Surg.* 1968;96:956–958.
27. Slanetz CA. The effect of inadvertent intraoperative perforation on survival and recurrence in colorectal cancer. *Dis Colon Rectum.* 1984;27:792–797.
28. Fingler SA, Pearl RK. Technical consideration in the surgical treatment of colon and rectal cancer. *Seminars Sug Oncol.* 1994;10:200–207.
29. Grinnell RS. Distal intramucosal spread of carcinoma of the rectum and rectosigmoid. *Surg Gynecol Obstet.* 1954;99: 421–430.
30. Devereux DF, Deckers PJ. Contributions of pathologic margins and Dukes' stage to local recurrence in colorectal carcinoma. *Am J Surg.* 1985;149:323–326.
31. Morikawa E, Yasutomi M, Shindou K et al. Distribution of metastatic lymph nodes in colorectal cancer by the modified clearing method. *Dis Colon Rectum.* 1994;37:219–223.
32. Mallassagne B, Valleur P, Serra J et al. Relationship of apical lymph node involvement to survival in resected colon carcinoma. *Dis Colon Rectum.* 1993;36:645–653.
33. Scott KW, Grace RH. Detection of lymph node metastases in colorectal carcinoma before and after fat clearance. *Br J Surg.* 1989;76:1165–1167.
34. Tagliacozzo S, Tocchi A. Extended mesenteric excision in right hemicolectomy for carcinoma of the colon. *Int J Colorect Dis.* 1997;12:272–275.
35. Toyota S, Ohta H, Anazawa S. Rationale for extent lymph node dissection for right colon cancer. *Dis Colon Rectum.* 1995;38:705–711.
36. Cole WH, Packard D, Southwick HW. Cancer of the colon and special reference to prevention of recurrence. *JAMA.* 1954;155:1549–1553.
37. McGrew EA, Laws JP, Cole HW. Free malignant cells in relation to recurrence of cancer of the colon. *JAMA.* 1954;154:1251–1254.
38. Barnes JP. Physiologic resection of the right colon. *Surg Gynecol Obstet.* 1952;94:722–726.
39. Turnbull RB, Kyle K, Watson FR, Spratt J. Cancer of the colon: the influence of no-touch isolation technic on survival rates. *Ann Surg.* 1967;166:420–427.
40. Wiggers T, Jeekel J, Arends JW et al. No-touch isolation technique in colon cancer: a controlled prospective trial. *Br J Surg.* 1988;75:409–415.
41. Staunas RJ, Schoetz DJ. Extended resection for carcinoma of the colon and rectum. *Surg Clin North Am.* 1993;73: 117–129.
42. Sugarbaker ED. Coincident removal of additional structures in resections for carcinoma of the colon and rectum. *Ann Surg.* 1946;123:1036–1046.
43. Landmann DD, Fazio VW, Lavery IC, Weakley FI, Jagelman DG. En bloc resection for contiguous upper abdominal invasion by adenocarcinoma of the colon. *Dis Colon Rectum.* 1989;32:669–672.
44. Koea JB, Conlon K, Paty PB, Guillem JG, Cohen AM. Pancreatic or duodenal resection or both for advanced carcinoma of the right colon. Is it justified? *Dis Colon Rectum.* 2000;43:460–465.
45. Lopez MJ. Extended resections for colorectal cancer. Multiple organ resections/exenteration. In: Wanebo HJ, ed. *Colorectal Cancer.* Chicago: Mosby-Year Book; 1992.
46. Davies GC, Ellis H. Radical surgery in locally advanced cancer of the large bowel. *Clin Oncol.* 1975;1:21–26.
47. Orkin BA, Dozois RR, Beart RW Jr., Patterson DE, Gunderson LL, Ilstrup DM. Extended resection for locally advanced primary adenocarcinoma of the rectum. *Dis Colon Rectum.* 1989;32:286–292.
48. Newman HK, Stearns MW. Re-exploration for "unresectable" colonic cancer. *Dis Colon Rectum.* 1975;18:576–580.

49. Pittam MR, Thornton H, Ellis H. Survival after extended resection for locally advanced carcinomas of the colon and rectum. *Ann R Coll Surg Engl.* 1984;66:81–84.
50. Izbicki JR, Holsch SB, Knofel WT, Passlick B, Bloechle C, Broelsch CE. Extended resections are beneficial for patients with locally advanced colorectal cancer. *Dis Colon Rectum.* 1995;38:1251–1256.
51. Ledesma EJ, Tseng M, Mittelman A. Surgical treatment of isolated abdominal wall metastasis in colorectal cancer. *Cancer.* 1982;50:1884–1887.
52. Stone HH, Fabian TC, Turkleson ML, Hurkiewicz MJ. Management of acute full-thickness losses of the abdominal wall. *Ann Surg.* 1981;193:612–618.
53. Iwasaki Y, Moriya Y, Miyake H, Akasu T, Fujita S. En bloc surgery for colon cancer: report of a case. *Surg Today.* 2000;30:191–194.
54. Lavery IC. Colon cancer: Surgical technique. In: Mazier WP, Levien DH, Luchtefeld MA, Senagore AJ, eds. *Surgery of the Colon, Rectum and Anus.* Philadelphia: WB Saunders; 1995: 606–616.
55. Karakousis CP, Cheng C, Udobi K, Lascola RJ. Abdomino-inguinal incision in adenocarcinoma of the sigmoid or cecum. Report of two cases. Dis Colon Rectum 1998;41: 1322–1327.
56. Kama NA, Reis E, Doganay M, Gozalan V, Yasti C. Radical surgery of colon cancers directly invading the duodenum, pancreas and liver. *Hepatogastroenterology.* 2001;43: 460–465.
57. Kroneman H, Castelein A, Jeekel J. En bloc resection of colon carcinoma adherent to other organs: an efficacious treatment? *Dis Colon Rectum.* 1991;34:780–783.
58. Ellis H, Morgan N, Wastell C. Curative surgery in carcinoma of the colon involving duodenum. *Br J Surg.* 1972;59: 932–935.
59. Sharma P, Klaasen H. Duodenal seromyectomy in the management of adherent colonic carcinoma in elderly patients. *Can J Surg.* 1997;40:289–293.
60. Harrison LE, Mercant N, Cohen AM, Brennan MF. Pancreaticoduodenectomy for nonperiampullary primary tumors *Am J Surg.* 1997;174:393–395.
61. Yoshimi F, Asato Y, Kuroki Y et al. Pancreaticoduodenectomy for locally advanced or recurrent colon cancer: a report of two cases. *Surg Today.* 1999;29:906–910.
62. Howard TJ, Villanustre N, Moore SA et al. Efficacy of venous reconstruction in patients with adenocarcinoma of the pancreatic head. *J Gastrointest Surg.* 2003;7:1089–1095.
63. Lydigakis NJ, Gurusharan S, Bardoxoglou E et al. Mono-bloc total spleno-pancreatico-duodenectomy for pancreatic head carcinoma with portal-mesenteric venous invasion. A prospective randomized study. *Hepato-Gastroenterology.* 2004;51:427–433.
64. Ye C, Xi PC, Hu XG. Clinical analysis of uncinate process carcinoma of the pancreas. *Hepatobiliary Pancreat Dis Int.* 2003;2:605–608.
65. Susaki M, Kitagawa M, Sakai H, Ikeda G, Machishi H, Umeda K. A case of transverse colon secondarily involving the liver, duodenum, and pancreas. *Surg Today.* 1996;26:42–45.
66. Jensen HE, Balslev I, Nielsen J. extensive surgery in the treatment of carcinoma of the colon. *Acta Chir Scand.* 1970;136:431–434.
67. McSherry CK, Cornell GN, Glenn F. Carcinoma of the colon and rectum. *Ann Surg.* 1969;169:502–509.
68. Gunderson L, Sosin H. Areas of failure found at reoperation following curative surgery for adenocarcinoma of the rectum. *Cancer.* 1971;31:1278–1292.

9 Left Colon

Theodore Saclarides, Heather L. Rossi, and Roderick M. Quiros

Colorectal cancer continues to constitute a major health problem in the United States and other industrialized countries. Approximately 150 000 new cases are diagnosed in the United States each year[1] and roughly 10% of patients who undergo surgery for colorectal cancer have involvement of adjacent organs.[2] Adherence to surrounding viscera may be due to inflammation, fibrosis, or actual malignant invasion, the latter being responsible in 45–75% of such cases.[3,4,5] Dissection between the carcinoma and the adherent structures is not recommended as local recurrence approaches 100% when operative separation occurs.[3] Furthermore, an incomplete positive margin resection is associated with a median survival period of less than 12 months.[3] Although locally advanced carcinomas may metastasize to distant sites, a sub-group of tumors exist that invade adjacent structures and reach large size before metastases occur.[6] Consequently, en bloc radical resection of these lesions may provide long-term survival and even cure in a significant number of these patients. Limited or segmental resection may be considered for palliative care in those patients with metastatic disease.

In 1946, Sugarbaker described a series of 132 patients who underwent curative resections for colorectal cancer. Of these, 32% had en bloc resections of adherent organs with a 45% survival rate at 3 years.[7] Up until this point, direct extension into surrounding organs was generally considered to carry a grave prognosis and constitute surgically incurable disease. However, many authors now support the value of multivisceral resection and favor an aggressive approach when local tumor invasion is suspected.[5,8,9]

☐ Preoperative Preparation

Once a thorough history is obtained, a physical exam is performed. Palpable supraclavicular or inguinal nodes or the presence of hepatomegaly or ascites may preclude further operative intervention. However, tissue confirmation of widely disseminated disease is needed before abandoning potentially curative surgery. Digital rectal exam is performed in all patients. If a tumor is palpated, rigid proctoscopy should be performed to assess degree of circumferential involvement, potential for local (transanal) excision, and likelihood of sphincter preservation. Digital rectal examination may also reveal extraluminal tumor within the cul-de-sac which would also argue against radical curative surgery. Further assessment of the local extent of disease rectal neoplasms can be obtained with rectal ultrasound, whereby the degree of mural penetration and the presence of mesorectal nodal metastases can be determined with confidence. Routine complete blood counts and liver function tests, in addition to carcinoembryonic antigen (CEA), are obtained in all patients. The CEA becomes useful when assessing the patient for tumor recurrence postoperatively. In the absence of obstruction or perforation, the entire lower gastrointestinal tract should be assessed with either a complete colonoscopy or a barium enema to rule out synchronous lesions.

A preoperative abdominal CT and serum transaminases are not always necessary for a patient with normal physical exam (no hepatomegaly). However, systematic CT allows to eventually discover hepatic metastases and suspect adjacent organs invasion. The likelihood of occult liver metastases is low in these patients. However, in the subset of patients where liver metastases are suspected (weight loss, ascites, palpable liver), a physical exam reveals a large fixed abdominal tumor, and/or laboratory values are abnormal, a CT scan can be very useful in preoperative planning to rule out metastatic disease and involvement of adjacent organs.

For elective colon resections, the patient is usually admitted the day of surgery. Preoperatively the patient should be counseled about bowel preparation, which consists of a clear liquid diet the day prior to surgery and a mechanical bowel cleansing (oral cathartics or lavage). The use of oral nonabsorbable antibiotics is associated with significant gastric side effects and many surgeons choose to omit oral antibiotics in favor of intravenous antibiotics given perioperatively. On the morning of surgery, the patient may be given an enema to clear residual stool from the distal colon. The traditional Nichols protocol consists of 1 g of erythromycin base and 1 g of neomycin given at 1300, 1400, and 2300 -hours the day before surgery.[10] If a multiorgan resection is anticipated, the patient is admitted a few days before the operation, depending on his/her general state or specific preoperative examination or preparation.

If a stoma, either temporary or permanent, is being contemplated, it is essential that the site be marked preoperatively, taking into consideration certain important anatomic landmarks. It is advisable to mark both lower quadrants of the abdominal wall in the event that operative circumstances require ileostomy, rather than colostomy, placement. Performing this task before surgery helps the patient prepare emotionally for the possibility of a stoma and certainly is preferable to waking up after anesthesia finding a stoma in place. Frequently, the surgeon must mark the optimum site for a stoma, however, if their services are available, this task is better carried out by a trained enterostomal therapy nurse. The consequences of an improperly placed stoma can be more devastating than the effects of the operation itself, since the patient must live with the limitations imposed upon them which, if they are significant enough, could require further surgery to correct.

In choosing the proper site, one must avoid the groin, the waistline, the costal margins, the umbilicus, skin folds and scars. These all may interfere with appliance adherence and lead to stool leakage and skin breakdown. It is helpful to have the patient lie in the recumbent position and tense the abdominal wall; this helps to highlight the borders of the rectus sheath through which the stoma should be delivered at the time of surgery. The stoma should be placed in the middle of an imaginary triangle whose apices are the umbilicus, anterior superior iliac spine, and the pubis. The patient should then be placed in the upright position to determine whether the proposed site is still visible to them. Obese patients or those with a large pannus may find that the initial site is no longer visible in the upright position, consequently the site should be replaced in a more cephalad direction. It is also helpful to inquire as to the patient's preference for clothing style, since the stoma should ideally be placed below the belt line. Lastly, it is helpful to place the appliance face piece for 24 hours to verify that it adheres to the abdominal wall during routine daily activities and the patient does not manifest signs of an allergic reaction to the appliance or the adhesive.

Since pulmonary embolism (PE) is a leading cause of in-hospital mortality following surgery, proper prophylaxis against deep venous thrombosis (DVT) is essential. A variety of prophylaxis methods are available, the method chosen is determined by patient risk factors. Low risk factors include patient age less than 40 years, minor surgery lasting 30 minutes or less, and no associated conditions such as paralysis, malignancy, obesity, prolonged immobilization, history of varicose veins, or use of estrogens. For these patients, the postoperative incidence of calf DVT is less than 10%, proximal DVT less than 1%, and PE less than 1%. Prophylactic measures for these patients consist simply of early ambulation. Moderate risk factors include patient age greater than 40 years, duration of surgery longer than 30 minutes, and the presence of the associated conditions listed above. For these patients, the incidence of calf DVT is 10–40%, proximal DVT-2–10%, and PE 0.1–0.7%. Prophylaxis may consist of graduated compression stockings, sequential pneumatic compression devices, or low dose heparin (5000 u) administered subcutaneously 2 hours before surgery and every 12 hours thereafter. Rare complications of low-dose heparin include skin necrosis and thrombocytopenia. Patients at highest risk have factors including the moderate factors listed above and those undergoing orthopedic operations, pelvic or abdominal cancer operations, have a prior history of DVT or PE and those with hereditary or acquired coagulopathies such as protein C and S deficiencies, antithrombin III deficiency, or anticardiolipin antibodies. For these patients, the risk of calf DVT is 40–80%, proximal DVT 10–20%, and PE 1–5%. For the patients at highest risk, a combination of graduated compression stockings, sequential pneumatic compression devices, and subcutaneous heparin is recommended. Low molecular weight heparin may be used but this may have a higher incidence of bleeding and is more expensive.[11,12]

Operative Technique

Although regional anesthesia may be used exceptionally for high-risk patients, general endotracheal intubation is the preferred method. After induction, a Foley catheter is placed; postoperatively, it can be removed once the volume status of the patient has stabilized. For operations that involve a pelvic dissection, the Foley catheter should remain in place for up to 5 days. Ureteral catheters are not routinely inserted. They are, however, selectively employed in patients who are undergoing reoperative procedures where scarring and abnormal tissue planes may make identification of the ureters difficult. Ureteral catheters can also be helpful when operating on bulky tumors or tumors that invade the retroperitoneum or kidney. Although ureteral stents aid in identifying the ureters either by palpation or illumination, they should not lull the surgeon into a false sense of security. Furthermore, successful identification of the ureter at one location, e.g., upper abdomen, does not guarantee that the same ureter can be spared from injury at another anatomic location or time during the same operation. It is important to remember that there is no substitute for careful dissection when working around the ureters.

The patient is placed in a supine position and the legs are positioned in stirrups to allow transperineal access to the rectum and pelvis. Pressure points, especially the lateral aspect of the legs, are padded. A midline incision allows easy access to the abdomen and provides excellent exposure with adequate retraction. A midline incision is also ideal if a stoma becomes necessary because it leaves both sides of the abdomen free for placement. Some surgeons prefer a transverse incision. However, this provides somewhat limited access to the abdomen and is less ideal for stoma placement. For better access to the operative site and pelvis, slight Trendelenburg posi-

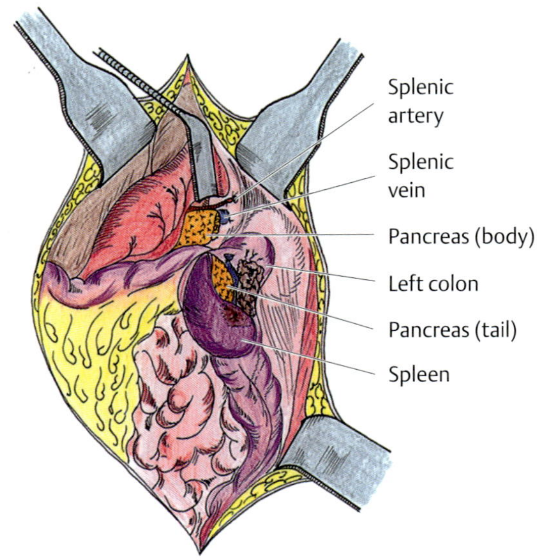

Fig. 9.1 Example of splenic flexure tumor invading the tail of the pancreas. The flexure is mobilized en bloc with the spleen and tail of the pancreas. The body of the pancreas is oversewn or stapled.

3

tioning, rotation of the table, and packing of the upper abdominal viscera with a lap pad will help keep the small bowel out of the operative field.

Once the abdomen is opened, careful and systematic exploration will allow one to determine the extent and involvement by the primary tumor. Adjacent visceral involvement should be assessed to determine if an en bloc resection is possible. The liver and peritoneal surfaces should be assessed for metastatic disease. Small scattered liver metastases should not preclude palliative resection, however, if extensive disease is present, resection may not be advisable.

Multivisceral involvement usually does not come as an unexpected finding. Evidence of this phenomenon may be found preoperatively based either on physical findings of a large mass in the left upper quadrant or midabdomen or on CT scans. If initial operative exploration reveals unexpected fixation to neighboring viscera, the surgeon must be flexible in his/her approach and alter the technique of resection. Certain principles must be followed. First, the surgeon must assume that all points of fixation are due to malignant invasion and not try to create planes of dissection that do not exist. Cutting into tumor dramatically lowers curability. Second, every attempt should be made to resect en bloc all involved structures. The exceptions to this rule are those situations where the risk of radical en bloc surgery outweighs any possible oncologic benefit derived from the procedure. An example is the invasion of the bladder trigone. However, even in this situation, pelvic exenteration can be performed but informed patient consent must be taken into consideration in light of the fact that a urostomy will be needed. Depending on the circumstances, simple fecal diversion can be preferable followed by an attempt at downstaging with radiotherapy and then further surgery after proper patient counseling. Lastly, the extent of colonic resection should be based on our knowledge of the mesenteric blood supply. Anastomotic disruption secondary to ischemia can be avoided if there is proper selection of the distal transverse colon for the proximal margin because of its nearness to a major vascular trunk, namely the middle colic artery. Similarly, for the distal margin of resection, the upper rectum is preferable to the sigmoid colon especially if the inferior mesenteric artery was ligated. The rectum has a dual blood supply, namely the superior rectal artery derived from the inferior mesenteric artery and the middle and inferior rectal arteries derived from the internal iliac arteries.

For large tumors involving the left colon, mobilization of the splenic flexure may be required. Actual splenic involvement by tumor is rare and is seen in less than 1% of cases, therefore a plane of dissection can usually be established. First, division of the splenocolic ligament must be performed to avoid capsular tears from traction during colonic mobilization. If it becomes apparent that there is invasion of the spleen, the splenic artery and vein should be ligated along with the short gastric vessels early during the dissection. Distal pancreatectomy is rarely required (Fig. 9.1). After the splenocolic ligament is taken (in those situations where splenectomy is not required), the gastrocolic omentum is divided beginning at the mid-transverse colon, the lesser sac is entered and dissection proceeds distally to within a short distance of the splenic flexure. One then turns his/her attention to the left colon and the lateral peritoneal reflection is incised. Blunt separation of the left colon and its mesentery on top of Gerota's fascia is performed in a retrograde direction until the plane of dissection enters the lesser sac. The left colon is retracted medially and all loose avascular attachments on top of the kidney are divided (Fig. 9.2). The left ureter is identified along with the gonadal vessels; these are preserved unless directly involved by tumor (Fig. 9.3). If splenic bleeding is encountered, primary suture repair or preferably placement of topical hemostatic agents and packing are performed. If splenic bleeding is refractory to these measures, splenectomy should be carried out and the patient given a polyvalent pneumococcal vaccine postoperatively.

Left hemicolectomy is indicated for lesions of the distal transverse colon, splenic flexure, and descending colon. Mobilization of the splenic flexure should be carried out as outlined above. One should attempt to preserve the right branch of the middle colic artery. The left colic artery should be ligated, if circumstances dictate ligation of the inferior mesenteric artery, the entire distal colon down to the upper rectum should be re-

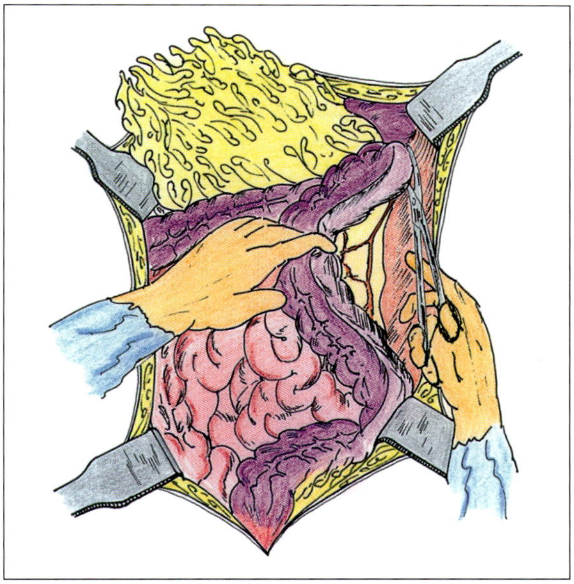

Fig. 9.2 Mobilization of the left colon and splenic flexure. The splenocolic ligament is divided, the lateral peritoneal reflection is incised and the colon is reflected medially.

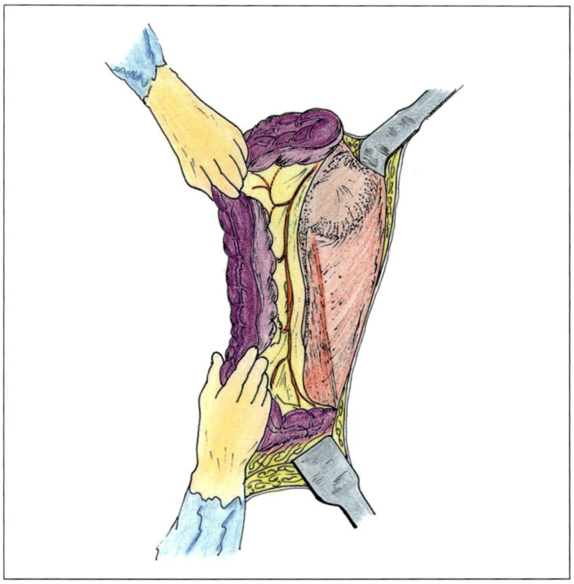

Fig. 9.3 The left colon is bluntly separated from Gerota's fascia exposing the left ureter and the gonadal vessels. Medial retraction of the left colon continues.

sected. If there is any doubt about bowel viability, taking the resection down to the rectum may alleviate these concerns. One should make it a practice of checking capillary refill in the proximal margin, this is accomplished by compressing (not squeezing) the small arterioles with a hemostat as they enter the colonic wall and seeing whether or not they fill with blood. With proper mobilization that may even include the hepatic flexure, there is almost always enough mobility and length to perform a tension-free anastomosis between the mid-transverse colon and the upper rectum. One should avoid closing the mesenteric defect since this may predispose to the creation of a smaller defect that may in fact make it more likely for herniation and obstruction to occur.

Contiguous involvement of abdominal structures proximal to the transverse colon is relatively rare. Landmann et al. reported 17 occurrences over a 20-year period of direct involvement of upper abdominal structures. In order of frequency, the stomach, spleen, and duodenum were most commonly involved followed by the diaphragm, abdominal wall, pancreas, and liver.[13] Because of the magnitude of surgery, major upper abdominal resection is associated with a 12% operative mortality.[14] In a study of 40 patients with locally advanced, adherent colon cancers, Luna-Perez et al. found that neighboring organs were involved in the following order of frequency: small bowel (50%), abdominal wall (43%), ovary (10%), uterus (10%).[4] The following discussion will consider site-specific areas of possible fixation to adjacent organs.

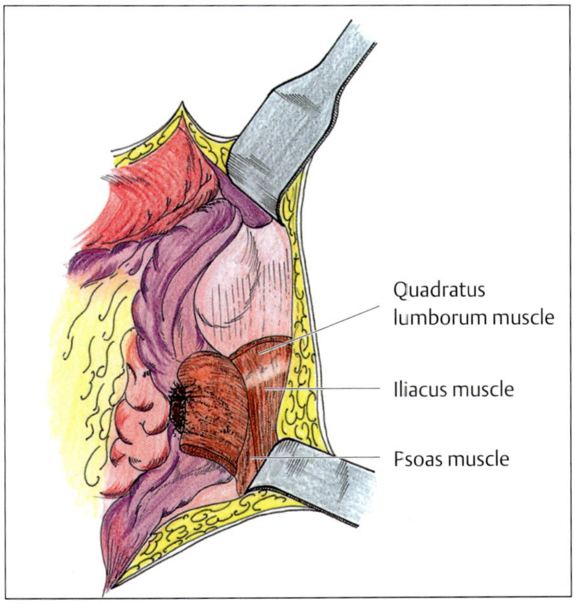

Fig. 9.4 Left colon tumor invading the abdominal wall. The transverse muscle is resected en bloc. The posterior plane with quadratus lumborum, iliacus, and psoas muscles is exposed.

☐ Abdominal Wall

Abdominal wall involvement has a reported incidence of 2.4% and occurs most commonly with tumors arising from the right side of the colon.[15] Left posterior abdominal wall invasion can also occur. En bloc resection involves wide excision of the abdominal wall in continuity with the cancer (Fig. 9.4). The type of recon-

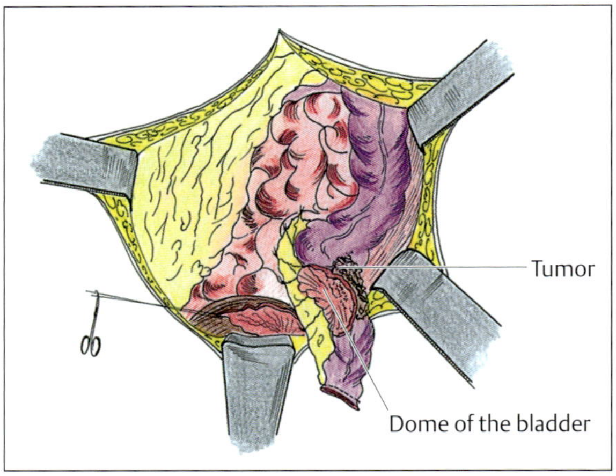

Fig. 9.**5** The dome of the bladder invaded by the tumor is resected with the left colon and sigmoid.

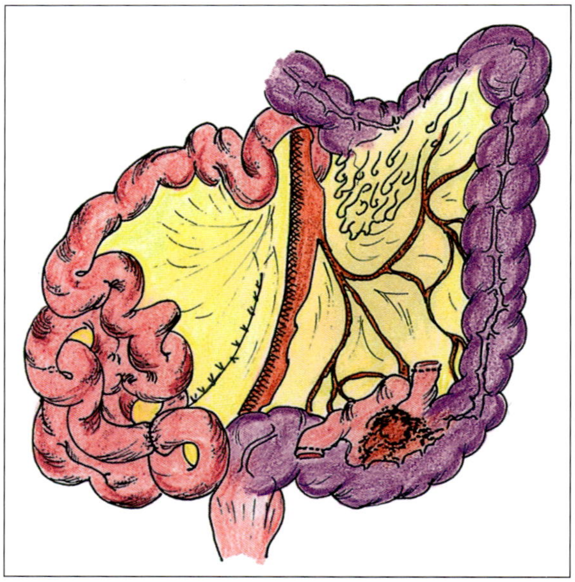

Fig. 9.**6** The small bowel is resected en bloc with the colon. No attempt is made to separate these structures. Small bowel continuity is promptly re-established.

struction depends on the size of the resulting defect. For smaller defects, primary repair without prosthetic material may be possible, otherwise mesh should be inserted, especially for larger defects or if tension is present. Many surgeons would choose to place permanent mesh at a second surgery rather than risk infecting the prosthetic material by inserting it during a bowel operation.

Bladder

Bladder invasion may occur with cancers arising from the sigmoid colon. Men are more frequently affected than women because of the protective effects of the uterus. The portion of the bladder involved will dictate the type of surgical treatment necessary for cure. Partial cystectomy (with primary repair) with en bloc resection of the colon is the preferred treatment for involvement of the dome of the bladder (Fig. 9.**5**). When the cancer invades the trigone, greater consideration should be given to pelvic exenteration. Cure rates are similar between partial cystectomy and the more aggressive approach of anterior exenteration; overall 5-year survival rates of approximately 40% can be expected.[14] Therefore, partial cystectomy with its lower morbidity and mortality is the preferred procedure, however, again the extent of resection is dictated by operative findings.

Small Bowel and Stomach

Involvement or fixation of the small bowel to a colonic tumor is readily apparent. Since small bowel resection can be carried out expeditiously and with minimal morbidity, one should not attempt to separate these structures. Resection of the jejunum and ileum should be carried out early in the course of the dissection so that tearing of the specimen and spillage of tumor cells and fecal matter does not occur when traction is applied to the colon during mobilization. Stapling devices are placed above and below the points of fixation and the small bowel is transected at these areas. A wide mesenteric clearance of the small bowel is not necessary and in fact may render the remaining small intestine ischemic. If there is proximal dilatation of the intestine secondary to obstruction, the staple line can be opened in a small area to permit passage of a sump tube in order to decompress the bowel. Alternatively, intraluminal fluid and air can be advanced in a retrograde direction into the stomach where they can be aspirated with a nasogastric tube. Small bowel diversion is not necessary. Small bowel continuity should be re-established promptly rather than waiting until the end of the tumor resection, this allows time to pass so the anastomotic segment can be inspected once again prior to abdominal closure. The anastomosis can be performed in an end-to-end fashion using a handsewn technique or in a side-to-side fashion with staplers if there is disparity in lumen size (Fig. 9.**6**).

Involvement of the stomach is also readily apparent. If present, a formal resection as for gastric cancer is not required and all that is usually needed is resection of a small portion of the greater curvature. Once the lesser sac is entered proximal and distal to the points of tumor fixation, the necessary extent of gastric resection can be determined. Long surgical stapling devices can be placed across an uninvolved area of the stomach and a portion of the wall amputated (Fig. 9.**7**). The staple line can be reinforced with sutures if there are concerns about hemostasis or security of the staples.

Kidney

Fortunately, direct invasion of the kidney is a rare event. If there is evidence of a renal mass on preoperative CT, it is probably more likely that one is dealing with a second primary tumor. One can almost always establish a plane of dissection on top of Gerota's fascia; this is true for both right and left-sided colonic tumors. If one encounters especially dense adherence of a tumor to Gerota's fascia, he/she should proceed with colon mobilization, although cautiously. These adhesions are likely due to the sometimes dense desmoplastic reaction associated with colon cancer.

Uterus/Adnexa

Direct adnexal involvement should be resected en bloc, this is especially so for women who have completed childbearing. For younger women, the possibility of ovarian fixation to the tumor should always be part of the preoperative discussion especially if CT scanning shows extensive disease within the pelvis. This also holds true if the ovaries appear abnormal even without direct fixation to the tumor. Drop metastases can be a source of future pelvic symptoms secondary to progressive enlargement and compression of adjacent viscera.

Large colonic cancers may adhere to the uterus or fistulize into the vagina, especially if there has been prior hysterectomy. The latter is usually accompanied by symptoms of vaginal pressure and vaginitis from the passage of vaginal gas and stool. Diverticulitis may cause similarly distressing symptoms and every attempt should be made to distinguish this inflammatory condition from cancer since the conduct for surgical treatment will be vastly different. If secondary to diverticulitis, no uterine or vaginal resection is required, all that is needed following colectomy is to separate the organs, curette and close the vaginal opening of the fistula. For cancer, however, surgery involves anterior exenteration for uterine involvement and partial vaginectomy for patients whose cancer has created a fistula.

It is highly advantageous to have knowledge of pelvic organ involvement before embarking on colectomy. Patients can be properly counseled about the loss of their reproductive organs and possible vaginal shortening and the necessary operative allotments can be made with respect to time scheduling and blood product availability. If uterine involvement is found unexpectedly at the time of surgery, pelvic dissection should be kept to a minimum. Perhaps fecal diversion alone followed by radiotherapy and then re-operation may be preferable.

Tumor fixation to the uterus is typically found either at the dome of the fundus or along its posterior wall. En bloc removal of the uterus typically follows colonic

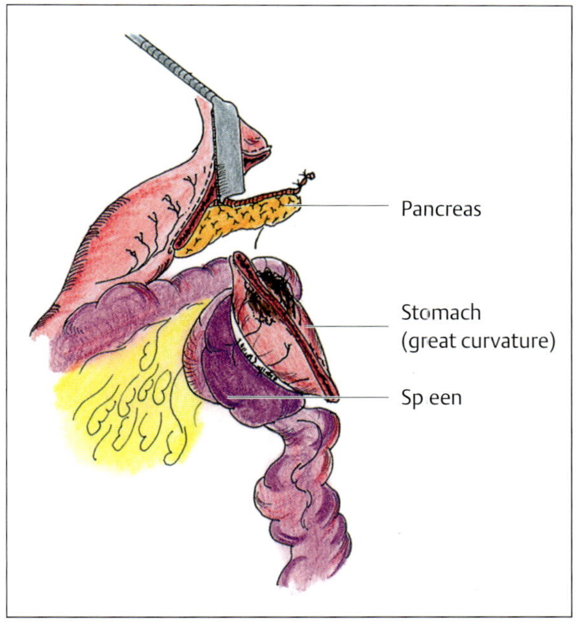

Fig. 9.**7** Tumor of the splenic flexure invading the greater curvature. The flexure is mobilized with the spleen and the greater curvature is stapled.

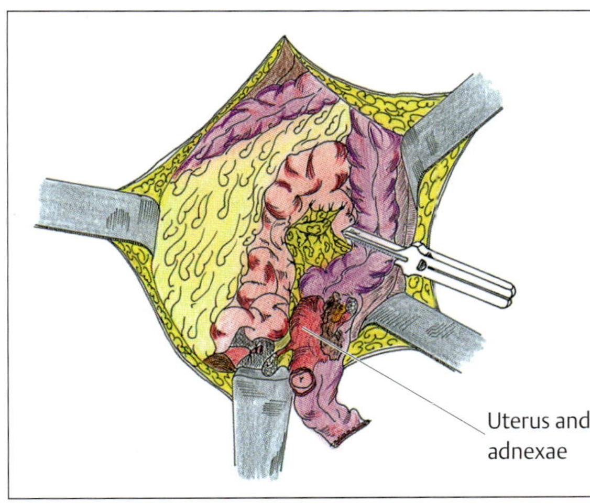

Fig. 9.**8** Sigmoid removed en bloc with the uterus and adnexae. The mesosigmoid is dissected and completely resected.

transection and removal of lymph node bearing tissue in the mesentery (Fig. 9.**8**). It is not necessary to perform all of the components of a radical hysterectomy as one would for gynecologic cancer, i.e., one does not need to take the cardinal ligaments widely as this would predispose to potential urinary bladder dysfunction. Furthermore, one does not need to perform pelvic or paraaortic lymph node dissections. The anterior plane is developed by incising the peritoneum at the cervicovesical fold and the bladder is gently pushed forward. The broad ligaments are penetrated on each side at the level of the cervix and the round ligaments and fallopian tubes are isolated and ligated individually.

The ureters are identified and protected. The infundibulopelvic ligaments on each side are ligated. Upward traction on the uterus is applied and the uterine arteries are sequentially ligated. The specimen is amputated either just below the cervix or at a supracervical location. The cuff is closed; one should attempt to buttress and isolate the closure with omentum especially if a colorectal anastomosis is nearby.

Conclusion

Most colorectal cancers are discovered early enough in their course that fixation to surrounding viscera has not occurred. If tumors have reached a locally advanced stage, signs of fixation may be apparent on physical examination, alternatively multivisceral involvement may be noted on CT scanning. At the time of surgery, separation of neighboring viscera and the colon should not be attempted and an en bloc resection always performed. This reduces local recurrence rates and enhances the likelihood for cure.

References

1. Boring CC, Squires TS, Tong T, Montgomery S. Cancer statistics, 1994. *Cancer J Clin*. 1994;44:7–26.
2. Landercasper J, Stolee RT, Steenlage E, Strutt PJ, Cogbill TH. Treatment and outcome of right colon cancers adherent to adjacent organs or the abdominal wall. *Arch Surg*. 1992; 127:841–846.
3. Curley SA, Evans DB, Ames FC. Resection for cure of carcinoma of the colon directly invading the duodenum or pancreatic head. *J Am Coll Surg*. 1994;179:587–592.
4. Luna-Perez P, Rodriguez-Ramirez SE, Gutierrez De La Barreta M, Zeferino M, Labastida S. Multivisceral resection for colon cancer. *J Surg Oncol*. 2002;80:100–104.
5. Eisenberg SB, Kraybill WG, Lopez MJ. Long-term results of surgical resection of locally advanced colorectal carcinoma. *Surgery*. 1990;108:779–786.
6. Spratt JS, Watson FR, Pratt JL. Characteristics of a variant of colorectal carcinoma that does not metastasize to lymph nodes. *Dis Colon Rectum*. 1970;13:243–246.
7. Sugarbaker ED, Coincident removal of additional structures in resections for carcinoma of the colon and rectum. *Ann Surg*. 1946;123:1036–1046.
8. Gall FP, Tonak J, Altendorf A. Multivisceral resections in colorectal cancer. *Dis Colon Rectum*. 1987;30:337–341.
9. Heslov SF, Frost DB. Extended resection for primary colorectal carcinoma involving adjacent organs or structures. *Cancer*. 1988;62:1637–1640.
10. Nichols RL, Broido P, Condon RE. Effect of preoperative neomycin-erythromycin intestinal preparation on the incidence of infectious complication following colon surgery. *Ann Surg*. 1973;178:453–462.
11. Carter CJ. The natural history and epidemiology of venous thrombosis. *Prog Cardiovasc Dis*. 1994;36:423–438.
12. Hull RD, Raskob GE, Hirsch J. Prophylaxis of venous thromboembolism: an overview. *Chest*. 1986;85(5): 374–383.
13. Landmann DD, Fazio VW, Lavery JC. En bloc resection for contiguous upper abdominal invasion by adenocarcinoma of the colon. *Dis Colon Rectum*. 1989;32:669–672.
14. Staniunas RJ, Schoetz DJ. Extended resection for carcinoma of colon and rectum. *Surg Clin NA*. 1993;73:117–129.
15. Merrill JG, Dockerty MB, Waugh JM. Carcinoma of the colon perforating onto the anterior abdominal wall. *Surgery*. 1950;28:662–671.

Pelvis 4

10 Abdominoinguinal Incision for Pelvic Side Wall Tumors

Constantine P. Karakousis, and Paul H. Sugarbaker

Pelvic tumors with lateral fixation present difficulties in their resection, primarily due to inadequate exposure through conventional abdominal incisions. Inadequate visualization occurs especially with tumors in the lower parts of the pelvis where the anterior abdominal wall converges with the retroperitoneal structures (e.g., along the iliopsoas muscle and iliac vessels). In this area the inferior attachments of the rectus muscle and the inguinal ligament spanning between the anterior superior iliac spine and the pubic tubercle provides the obstacle to adequate exposure. A midline, paramedian, or even an oblique abdominal incision does not provide adequate exposure for these tumors. These conventional incisions render sufficient exposure for the dissection and control of the common iliac vessels proximally, below the bifurcation of the aorta, but do not afford exposure of the terminal portion of the external iliac vessels. Often the tumor interferes with full visibility. In the past these tumors were considered unresectable or were managed with hemipelvectomy.[1]

What is needed for the resection of these tumors is an incision that would simultaneously provide an incontinuity exposure of the abdominal cavity and one or both groins so that both iliac and femoral vessels would be exposed in one field. For this incision, an abdominal component would be needed and an incontinuity inguinal component, i.e., an abdominoinguinal incision. The inguinal ligament would have to be divided to allow uninterrupted exposure and control of the iliofemoral vessels. A lower midline incision provides exposure of the intrapelvic structures. An inguinal incision exposes the external iliac and femoral vessels. A transverse incision connecting the two, by dividing the origin of the rectus abdominis muscle from the pubic crest and the insertion of the inguinal ligament to the pubic tubercle, provides the necessary link that allows a single incontinuity operative field. The abdominoinguinal incision may function much in the same way that the thoracoabdominal incision is used for the upper quadrants of the abdomen.[2,3]

Indications

The indications for the abdominoinguinal incision are: (1) abdominal or pelvic tumors extending over the iliac vessels; (2) tumors in the iliac fossa; (3) primary tumors, possibly involving the iliac vessels or large iliac lymph node metastases; (4) tumors with fixation to the wall of the true pelvis or large obturator nodes; (5) tumors involving the pubic bone with or without extension to the pelvis or adductor group of muscles; and (6) tumors of the groin when they involve the vessels or the lower abdominal wall or extend in the retroperitoneal area.[4,5]

Procedure

Position and Incision (Fig. 10.1)

With the patient in the supine position, a lower midline abdominal incision is outlined from just above the umbilicus to the pubic symphysis. The peritoneal cavity is entered, and exploration is carried out to assess the extent of disease. Preliminary dissection between the tumor mass and visceral pelvic structures may be carried out. Involvement of the latter does not necessarily mean unresectability, of course, since they can often be removed en bloc with the tumor. When there is a question of involvement of the iliac vessels, proximal control is secured; the common iliac vessels are dissected free and vessel loops are passed around them.[6]

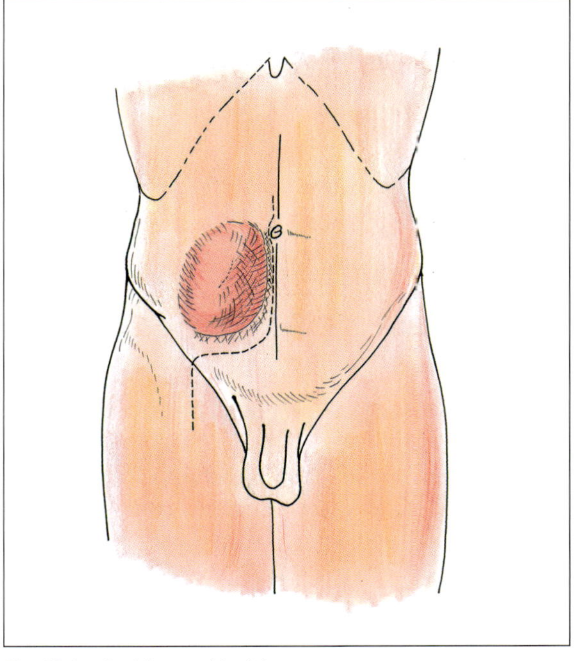

Fig. 10.1 Position and incision.

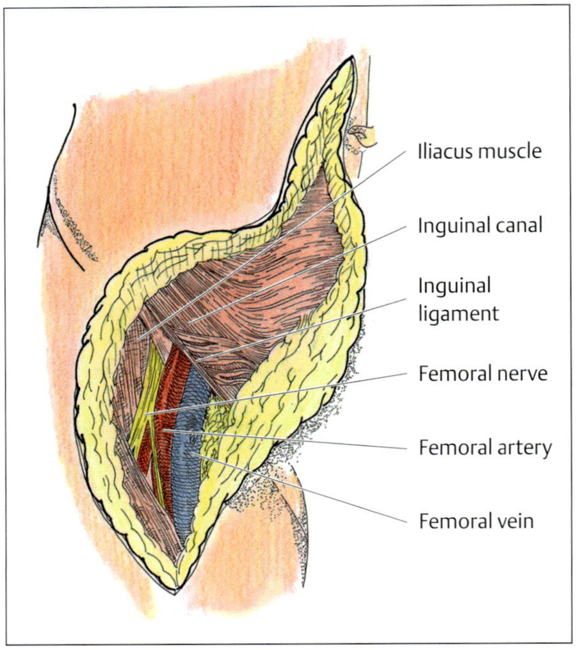

Fig. 10.**2** Incision through inguinal canal.

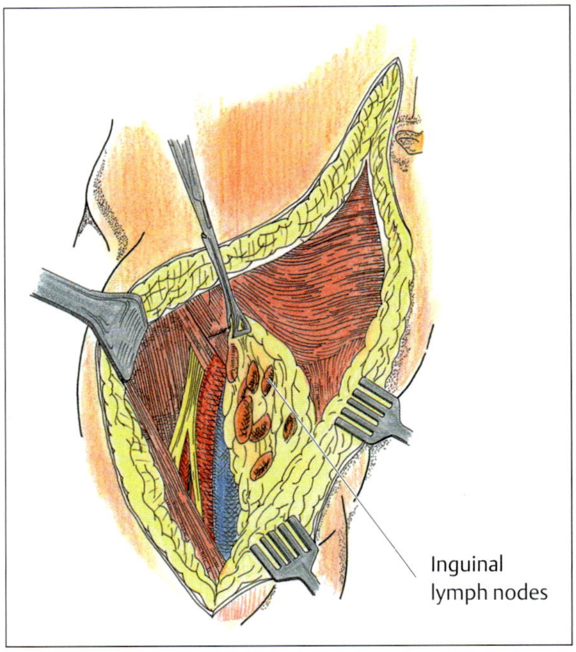

Fig. 10.**3** Dissection of inguinal nodes.

4

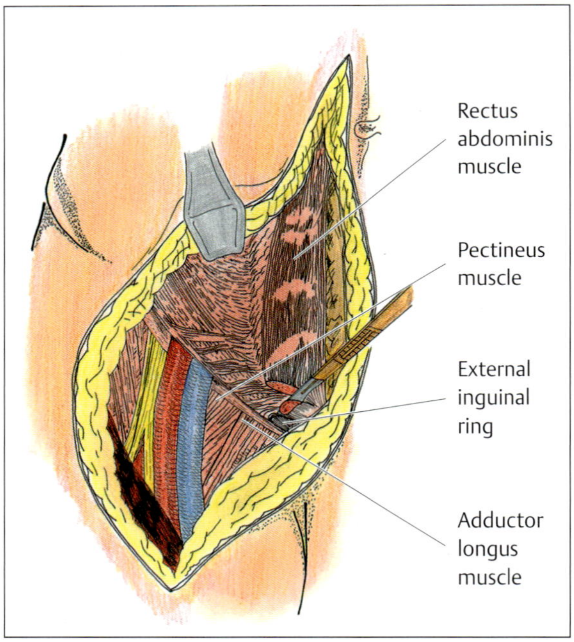

Fig. 10.**4** Division of rectus abdominis muscle.

□ Incision through the Inguinal Canal (Fig. 10.2)

If the decision is made to proceed with the resection, the lower end of the incision is extended transversely to the midinguinal point and then vertically longitudinal to the course of the femoral vessels. The vertical portion of the incision is deepened to expose the common femoral vessels. If necessary distal control with vessel loops is second at this time.

□ Dissection of the Inguinal Nodes (Fig. 10.3)

When the operation is performed for large iliac and/or obturator nodes or if there is clinical or potential microscopic involvement of the inguinal nodes, the vertical portion of the incision is made to extend to the apex of the femoral triangle, flaps are raised as in a groin dissection, and the nodes are mobilized off the femoral vessels, but their proximal continuity with the deep nodes is preserved.[7]

□ Division of the Rectus Abdominis Muscle (Fig. 10.4)

The transverse portion of the incision is deepened to the surface of the anterior rectus sheath which is divided. The rectus abdominis muscle is transected a few millimeters from its origin on the pubic crest. This incision is through its tendinous portion.

□ Opening the Inguinal Canal (Fig. 10.5)

The round ligament in women is divided over the pubic tubercle. In men, if the tumor is not too close to the internal inguinal ring, the spermatic cord can usually be preserved. If the spermatic cord cannot be preserved it is usually necessary to resect the testicle or it will infarct causing postoperative pain. The medial crus of the external inguinal ring is divided close to the pubic

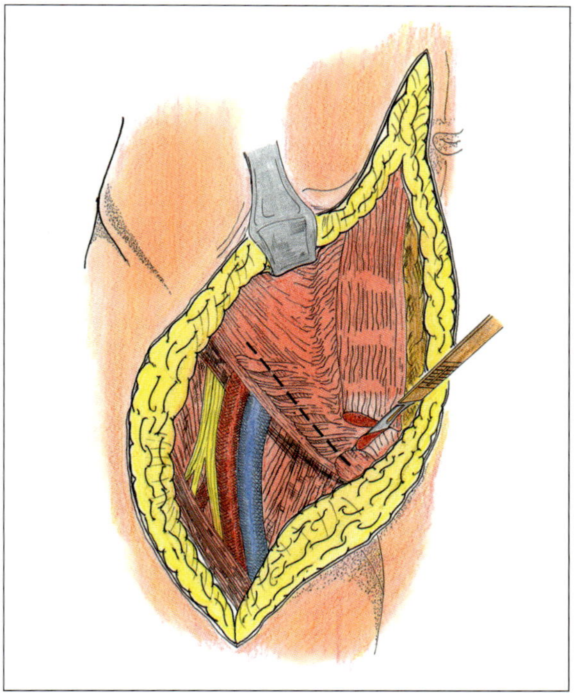

Fig. 10.**5** Opening the inguinal canal.

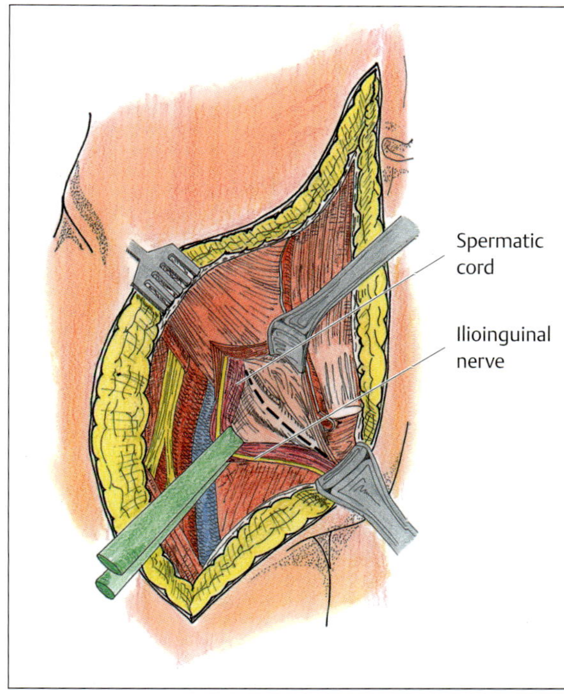

Fig. 10.**6** Incising the floor of the inguinal canal.

tubercle. The external oblique aponeurosis is split from the external inguinal ring lateral as in an inguinal herniorrhaphy.

☐ Incising the Floor of the Inguinal Canal (Fig. 10.6)

The inguinal canal floor is divided in the same direction up to and including the medial border of the internal inguinal ring. In so doing, the spermatic cord is displaced. Alternatively, after division of the medial crus, the inguinal floor may be incised from inside and the cord exposed from within the abdomen. The testicle is extracted from the inguinal canal and scrotum for medial displacement. Deep to the internal inguinal ring the structures of the cord deviate, the vas deferens coursing medially, and the internal spermatic vessels toward a lateral and cephalad direction. Depending on the location of the tumor, the internal spermatic vessels may have to be divided at this level; if the cord structures are divided above the bifurcation of the vas deferens there is a viable ipsilateral testis. Division of the cord at the level of the external inguinal ring does not require ipsilateral orchiectomy but will be accompanied by testicular atrophy.

☐ Exposure of the Pelvic Side Wall (Fig. 10.7)

The inguinal ligament is then divided at the pubic tubercle and dissection carried out on its undersurface

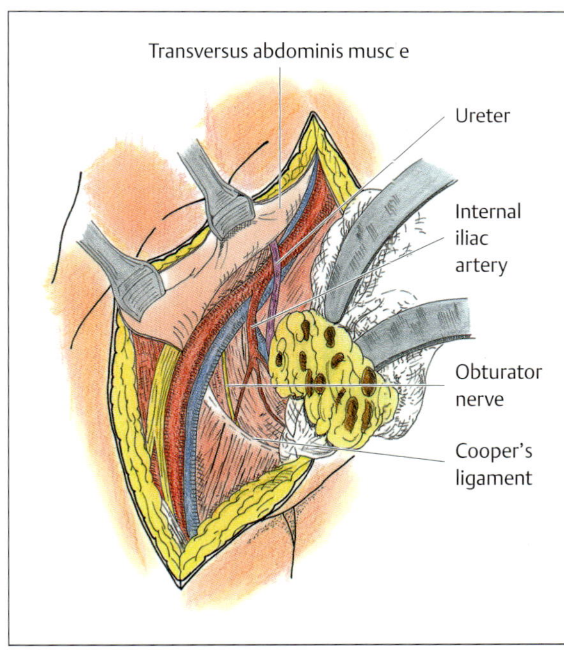

Fig. 10.**7** Exposure of the pelvic side wall.

until the inferior deep epigastric vein and artery are encountered, ligated, and divided. The lateral third of the inguinal ligament is then detached off the iliac fascia. This allows the completion of the abdomino-inguinal incision and provides wide incontinuity exposure of abdomen and pelvis. Further dissection with lymphatic and vascular resection depends on the location of the tumor.

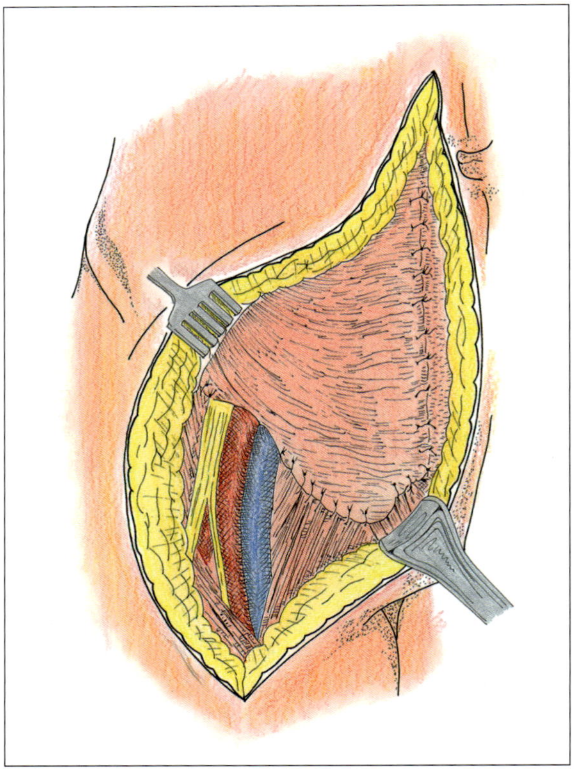

Fig. 10.8 Deep closure.

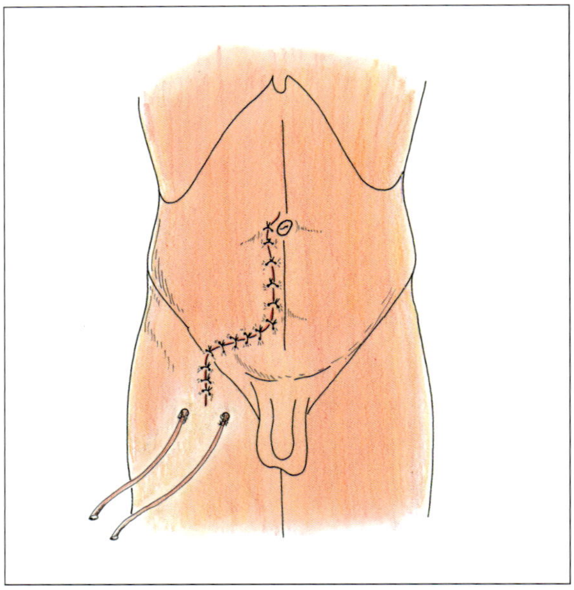

Fig. 10.9 Skin closure.

Deep Closure (Fig. 10.8)

The closure of the abdominoinguinal incision is uncomplicated. Lateral to the vessels the inguinal ligament is approximated to the iliac fascia and medial to the vessels to Cooper's ligament. The rectus sheath and muscle are approximated to their remnants on the pubic crest. A suction drain is placed in the inguinal portion of the incision. A subcutaneous layer of absorbable material may be used. The skin and the midline portion of the incision are closed in a routine fashion (Fig. 10.**9**).

Deep Closure Requiring Mesh (Fig. 10.10)

When a defect in the fascia has been created, it may be covered with a plastic mesh, which also replaces the inguinal ligament. The mesh should not be in direct contact with the vessels. This can usually be done by dividing the sartorius muscle distally at the apex of the femoral triangle and mobilizing the distal end so that the vessels are covered, taking care to avoid devascularization of this muscle.

When the defect in the groin also involves the skin, we have used the contralateral rectus muscle, which is divided proximally and rotated with the posterior sheath attached to it, its blood supply deriving from the inferior epigastric vessels. The muscle is sutured to the defect and skin-grafted immediately.

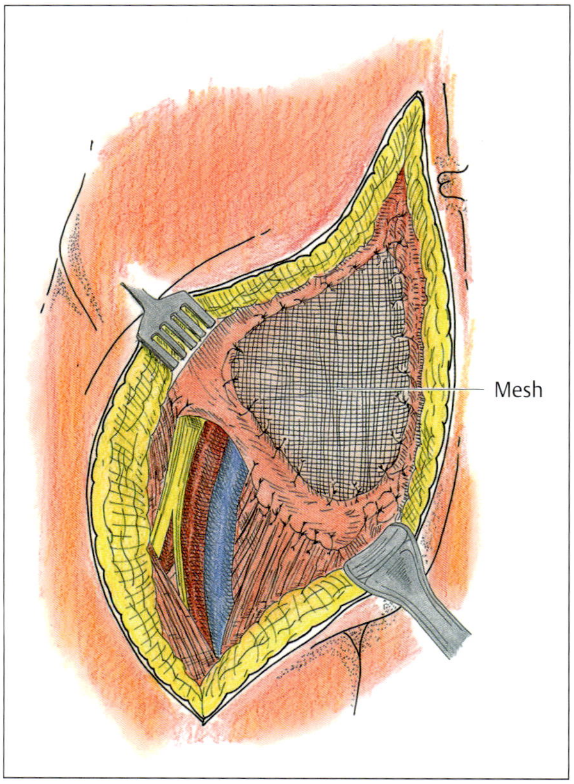

Fig. 10.**10** Deep closure requiring mesh.

Discussion

The authors have extensive experience of the abdominoinguinal incision for a variety of tumors, usually soft tissue sarcomas. The majority of the patients had been operated on once or twice elsewhere, and were found to be unresectable or thought to need a hemipelvectomy. All these tumors, presenting with fixation to the soft tissues of the wall of the pelvis, were resected with the abdominoinguinal incision, with the exception of two patients. They required hemipelvectomy due to extensive nerve involvement. One patient required an abdominoinguinal incision, bilateral extension of the midline abdominal incision to the groin. Tumors involving the innominate bone, with the exception of the medial portion of the pubic bone, are resected with the use of the techniques of internal hemipelvectomy and, if necessary, hemipelvectomy.[8–10]

In the authors' experience, there was one death two weeks postoperatively, which resulted from erosion and hemorrhage of a previously heavily radiated external iliac artery that was in contact with a mesh used to replace a fascial defect. It is important therefore to cover the vessels with the sartorius or rectus femoris muscle when a mesh is placed adjacent to the vessels or when there is concern about flap necrosis (see Chapter 14, Fig. 14.**39**). No instances of postoperative incisional hernia have been noted.

In many situations in which the tumor is not laterally fixed, but when it is large and distal and pressing against the obturator foramen(s) or the obturator areas, one can obtain sufficient exposure with a unilateral or bilateral use of the transverse portion of the full incision. In other words, the lower end of the midline incision is extended transversely from the pubic symphysis to the pubic tubercle, and the ipsilateral rectus sheath and muscle are divided off the pubic crest.

The extent of dissection and resection of lymphatics, arteries, and veins depends on the location of the tumor. If the tumor is simply a pelvic mass extending over and obscuring the iliac vessels, the improved exposure now facilitates the dissection of the mass off the vessels and safe ligation of any tumor-feeding branches. For large nodes the dissection is continued along the surface of the iliac vessels which are skeletonized. For a tumor located in the iliac fossa, the femoral nerve is located lateral to the femoral artery, immediately posterior to the continuation of the iliac fascia. A vessel loop is passed around it. Further cautious dissection along this nerve determines its relation to the tumor and if the nerve can be saved. If the tumor involves the vessels, proximal and distal control are secured and the dissection completed around the tumor mass, with any involved organs removed en bloc. When the specimen is held only by the attachment to the vessels, the patient is heparinized, vascular clamps are placed proximally and distally and the specimen is removed. Vascular reconstruction may be necessary if the common iliac vessels are sacrificed. If either the external iliac vessels alone or the internal iliac vessels alone are sacrificed, vascular reconstruction is rarely necessary.

When the iliofemoral vessels are to be resected, the profunda femoris branches may have to be divided at a distance from the tumor in order to allow the mobilization of the specimen.

For tumors attached to the wall of the lesser pelvis or the obturator fossa, the improved exposure usually allows their resection. For tumors involving the pubic bone, following the completion of the abdominoinguinal incision, the adductor muscles are divided off the pubic bone at an appropriate distance from the tumor, and the anterior and posterior pubic rami are exposed; the former just medial to the acetabulum and the latter medial to the ischial tuberosity. With the help of a right-angle clamp, a Gigli saw is passed around the pubic symphysis, which is divided along with the anterior and posterior pubic rami. The obturator nerve and vessels have to be divided proximally because they course through the obturator foramen. The defect may be replaced with a polypropylene mesh.

For a large tumor located in the groin, covering or involving the entire length of the common femoral vessels and possibly the lower abdominal wall, the abdominoinguinal incision provides incontinuity exposure of the iliofemoral vessels. In making the incision, flaps may have to be raised around the mass. If the lower abdominal wall and inguinal ligament are involved, following transection of the anterior rectus sheath and rectus abdominis muscle off the pubic crest, the incision is continued through the external oblique aponeurosis and internal oblique and transversus abdominis muscles at a sufficient distance from the tumor. The inguinal ligament is divided off the anterior superior iliac spine and the pubic tubercle, and thus the lower abdominal wall muscles and inguinal ligament are removed en bloc with the tumor. The inferior epigastric vessels are divided at the point they proceed behind the rectus muscle. In the illustration, the lateral third of the inguinal ligament was not detached off the iliac fascia, a step providing further exposure.

The abdominoinguinal incision heals well without complications. In the event of a previous transverse incision in the lower quadrant, which may have interrupted the connection to the superior epigastric vessels and the distal portion of intercostal and lumbar branches, a small area of necrosis at the junction of the midline and transverse portions of the incision may occur, since this incision divides the inferior epigastric vessels. In two patients with this condition a small area of ischemic necrosis developed, which, following debridement, healed by secondary intention.

4

The abdominoinguinal incision renders resectable the majority of pelvic tumors with lateral fixation to the soft tissues of the pelvis, and, through improvement in exposure, allows for a safe, deliberate dissection. It is the counterpart of the thoracoabdominal incision for the upper quadrants of the abdomen. The results from the use of this incision obviously depend on the histologic type and stage of the tumor and the expected margin of resection one can thus obtain. It should be used when appropriate consideration is given to the biology of the tumor, the expected margin, and the possible benefits of adjuvant treatments.

Conclusion

The abdominoinguinal incision allows wide exposure and safe resection of tumors in the lower abdomen with fixation to the pelvic side wall. A midline abdominal incision is connected to a longitudinal inguinal incision by separating the inguinal ligament. The pelvic side wall is then directly exposed by ligation of the deep epigastric vessels, detachment of the rectus muscle from its origin on the pubic crest, and division of the inguinal canal along the spermatic cord. This exposure allows safe resections along the iliac vessels without hemorrhage or tumor spillage. The abdominoinguinal incision should be part of the armamentarium of every surgeon willing to accept responsibility for pelvic and pelvic side wall malignancy.

References

1. Karakousis CP. Abdominoinguinal incision and other incisions in the resection of pelvic tumors. *Surg Oncol.* 2000;9:83–90.
2. Karakousis CP. The abdominoinguinal incision in limb salvage and resection of pelvic tumors. *Cancer.* 1984;54: 2543–2548.
3. Karakousis CP. The abdominoinguinal incision: the equivalent of thoraco-abdominal incision for the lower quadrants of the abdomen. *J Surg Oncol.* 1998;69:249–257.
4. Karakousis CP, Cheng C, Udobi K, Lascola RJ. Abdominoinguinal incision in adenocarcinoma of the sigmoid or cecum: report of two cases. *Dis Colon Rectum.* 1998;41: 1322–1327.
5. Karakousis CP. Utility of the abdominoinguinal incision in the resection of lower abdominal tumors. *J Surg Oncol.* 1984;26;176–182.
6. Karakousis CP. Technical aspects of resection of pelvic tumors. *J Surg Oncol.* 1986;31:155–159.
7. Karakousis CP. Ilioinguinal lymph node dissection. *Am J Surg.* 1981;141:299–303.
8. Karakousis CP. Internal hemipelvectomy. *Surg Gynecol Obstet.* 1984;158:279–282.
9. Nambisian RN, Karakousis CP. Bilateral abdominoinguinal incision. *J Surg Oncol.* 1984;25:81–84.
10. Karakousis CP. Abdominoinguinal incision in resection of pelvic tumors with lateral fixation. *Am J Surg.* 1992;164: 366–371.

11 Strategies for Advanced Pelvic Malignancy

Paul H. Sugarbaker

At this point in time, the only curative treatment for solid tumors within the abdomen and pelvis that is associated with long-term survival is complete surgical removal of the cancer with adequate margins.[1–4]The cardinal principle of surgery for resection is en bloc excision of the tumor plus involved adjacent organs and tissues with dissection well clear of the cancerous process. The major factor determining resectability is the extent of invasion to vital structures rather than the size of the tumor. Although preoperative radiologic evaluation is essential, operability can be evaluated definitively only by laparotomy. Even with adherence of tumor to vital structures, with meticulous dissection most of these tumors are resectable. The surgeon must always remember that local recurrence and peritoneal seeding are the major causes of treatment failure and are to be avoided at all cost.[5,6] Tumor debulking may occasionally be beneficial in a palliative way in cases where complete resection is impossible. However, palliative surgery for pelvic cancer carries a high morbidity and limited progression-free survival and should be undertaken with great caution.

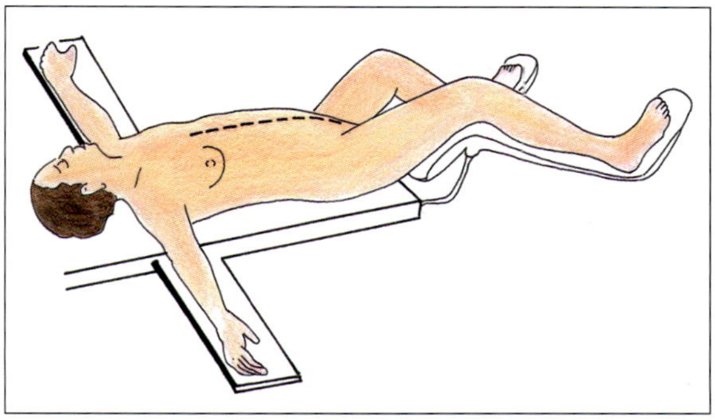

Fig. 11.**1** Patient position for surgical treatment of abdominal and pelvic sarcoma.

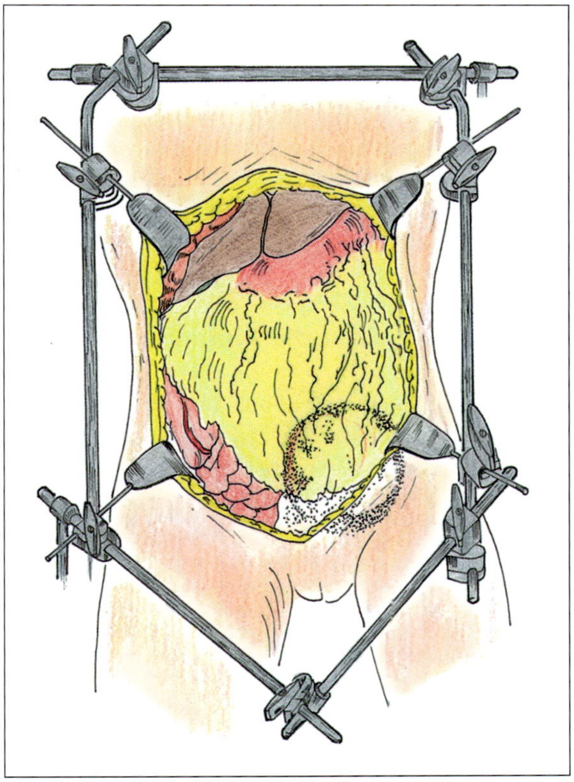

Fig. 11.**2** Exposure for abdominal and pelvic surgery using a self-retaining retractor.

Patient Position and Exposure

One must be prepared for a major surgical event with wide abdominal and pelvic exposure in order to achieve the greatest incidence of success. In most patients extensive abdominal dissections must be performed before the pelvic malignancy can be approached. Positioning of the patients so that surgery through the perineum is possible is often indicated (Fig. 11.**1**). Long abdominal incisions from xiphoid to pubis are usually required and self-retraining retractors that can expose the entire abdomen and pelvis are often indicated (Fig. 11.**2**). Skin is prepared so that a thoracoabdominal or an abdominoinguinal incision can be performed if required.

One must always be cognizant of the surgeon's needs to think three-dimensionally in approaching these deep-seated malignancies. This helps to avoid inadvertent damage to vital structures. In order to build within the surgeon's mind a three-dimensional appreciation of the vital structures in the abdomen, one should always strive to open the abdomen and set up the self-retaining retractor system in the same way. This means that the iliac arteries and veins, the ureters, etc., have a particular spatial orientation within the surgeon's mind. A standard exposure of the abdominal cavity through a midline incision with uniform placement of the self-retaining retractor can assist the surgeon in his goal of avoiding hemorrhage and inadvertent damage to vital structures.

Reoperative Surgery

Frequently in a tertiary referral center, one sees patients with pelvic malignancy after one or more prior attempts at the surgical removal of the cancer.[7] In these patients, removal of the recurrent cancer may be delayed many hours because exposure of the tumor mass may be difficult and time consuming. Cancer within the old abdominal incision, extensive abdominal adhesions, tumor that has regrown within scar tissue, fibrosis that accompanies the local recurrence of cancer, and alterations of normal anatomy by prior reconstructions may require patience and advanced technical skills to bring about the complete exposure of the malignant process.[8,9]

Always Open Old Incisions

Even though opening an old incision is difficult and may result in small or large bowel damage, rarely should a new incision be made into the abdomen in performing reoperative surgery. New incisions will cause additional adhesions and may severely jeopardize primary wound healing of the abdominal wall. It is usually necessary to excise old incisions because they can contain malignant foci embedded within the scar tissue. The surgeon routinely plans to completely excise the old scar tissue in the skin, subcutaneous tissue, and fascia as the abdomen is opened.

4

Safe Entry into the Abdominal Cavity

Opening the abdomen without damage to the small bowel in a patient who has had several prior surgical procedures in order to remove a pelvic malignancy may be difficult and time consuming. One should realize that entering an abdomen with multiple adhesions requires a strong upward traction of the abdominal wall in order to avoid inadvertent small bowel or large bowel enterotomy. Adair clamps should be used to pull up on the skin or abdominal fascia as the abdomen is entered (Fig. 11.**3**). Pushing down in order to spread the scar that makes up the old abdominal incision is to be avoided.

Surgical Approach to Intraabdominal Adhesions

Small bowel adhesions present a special problem in management. Small bowel enterotomy resulting in fistula formation after reoperative procedures is a major problem that will be encountered. The experienced surgeon will adhere to several principles in lysing small bowel adhesions:

- Tactile sense should be added to visual perceptions in the dissection of the adhesions (Fig. 11.**4**). This requires the use of ball-tipped electrosurgery. Fibrous adhesions and fat are morseled between the thumb and index finger of the nondominant hand. Important pressure may need to be applied. Ball-tip electrosurgery electroevaporates (carbonizes) residual tissue on the small bowel surface as this tissue is splayed out on the middle finger.
- Absolute hemostasis must be maintained at all times in dissecting small bowel adhesions. One must realize that bleeding that occurs while dissecting small bowel adhesions indicates that the surgeon is in an improper plane. Fat with blood vessels contained within should only be divided in the abdomen and pelvis when the surgeon is transecting omentum, retroperitoneal structures, or perirectal fat. Bleeding that is encountered while taking down intestinal adhesions indicates that the surgeon is entering

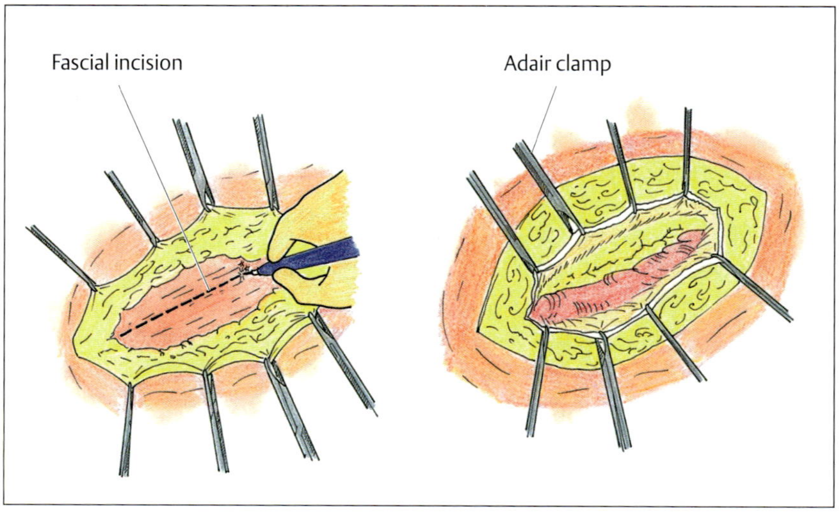

Fig. 11.**3** Opening the old abdominal incision by pulling upward on skin (*left*) or fascial edges (*right*) using Adair clamps.

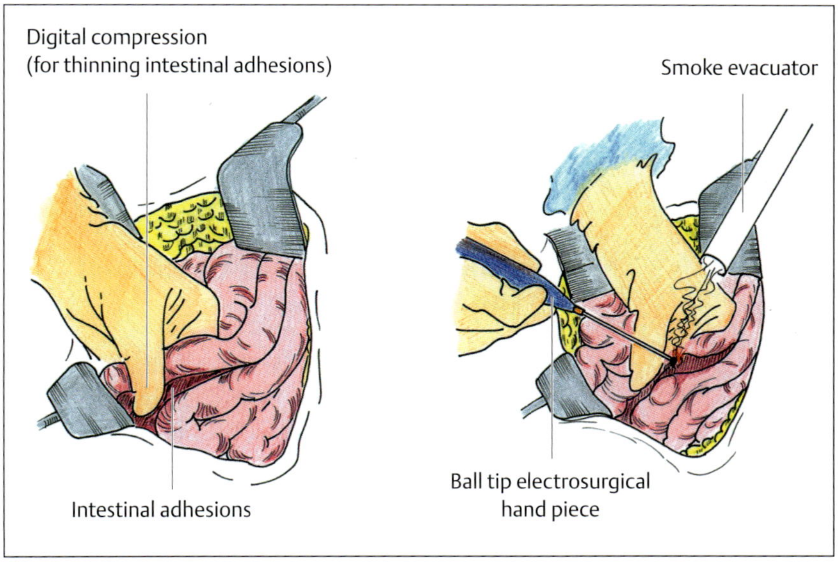

Fig. 11.**4** Dividing abdominal adhesions. Pressure between thumb and index finger is used to thin out the adhesion between two loops of smal bowel. Ball-tip electrosurgery is used to divide and evaporate the adhesion (*right*). Division of adherent tissue on small bowel surfaces on the middle finger of the nondominant hand adds tactile to visual perceptions (*left*).

into the small or large bowel mesentery and this should be avoided.

- Large volume saline irrigation should be used frequently. Even small amounts of blood can interfere with adequate visualization of delicate tissue planes for further dissection. If absolute hemostasis is combined with frequent irrigation the translucent nature of the tissues will be preserved throughout the dissection and inadvertent damage to vital structures or to blood vessels should not occur.
- Fat or scar tissue should never be left behind on small bowel surfaces. This scar tissue may frequently contain entrapped tumor cells. If miscellaneous tissues remain on bowel surfaces, confusion may arise in subsequent dissection. There is only one small bowel surface that contains fat on its antimesenteric border, and this is at the terminal ileum.
- Broad traction (as compared to point traction) should be maintained. The small bowel should be splayed out so that the plane of dissection for the ball-tipped electrosurgical handpiece is clearly visualized.
- Complete removal is the rule when dealing with intraabdominal adhesions. Generally, all adhesions must be lysed and then resected. The complete anatomy of the large and small bowel is visualized prior to beginning the definitive resection.

In the reoperative setting opening old abdominal incisions and the dissection of abdominal adhesions without damage to the bowel must be mastered by the cancer surgeon. Use of electrosurgery with the ball-tip is indicated because it allows tactile sensations to be added to visual perceptions in the dissection. This makes the process safer and certainly expedites the opening of the abdomen, lysis of intraabdominal adhesions, and clarification of the dissection required for radical excision of the recurrent malignancy.

□ Abdominal and Pelvic Exploration

In performing surgery on patients with advanced pelvic malignancy, the complete (both visceral and parietal) abdominal and pelvic surfaces must be visually inspected to look for tumor deposits.[10] This means that all abdominal adhesions must be lysed as part of the complete exploration. The omentum, likewise, must be dissected free and inspected to determine whether it contains sarcoma nodules. The presence of carcinomatosis or sarcomatosis is of great importance in the decision-making process in patients undergoing reoperative surgery. If there was tumor spillage at the time of earlier surgery, then implants are expected to be revealed with the abdominal exploration.

If the patient can be made disease-free in the presence of peritoneal surface spread, then the benefits of intraperitoneal chemotherapy should be considered. The adhesions are completely dissected as part of the oncologic procedure to allow uniform distribution of chemotherapy. From a purely technical point of view, complete lysis and resection of all abdominal adhesions is not an absolutely necessary step in complete resection of abdominal and pelvic sarcoma. However, from an oncologic perspective, complete lysis and resection of all adhesions followed by early postoperative intraperitoneal chemotherapy is an absolute requirement for the prevention of subsequent carcinomatosis or sarcomatosis.

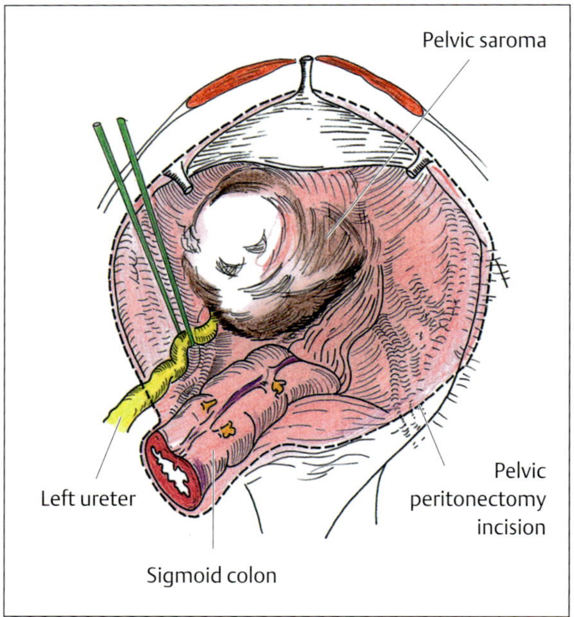

Fig. 11.5 Pelvic peritonectomy is useful to completely excise a pelvic sarcoma, especially if there is sarcomatosis or recurrent tumor at the resection site.

Centripetal Dissection

"Centripetal dissection" requires repeated dissection in a circular manner around the principal tumor mass. Dissection continues at a particular site only if there is clear visualization of the operative field. The surgeon should repeatedly circle the tumor mass completing the superficial dissections before the more difficult deep ones are attempted ("Do what is easy first."). He moves around and around the cancer, only working where he has good exposure, where he is loosing no blood, where he is unlikely to damage vital structures, and where the dissection is proceeding with a clear margin. If any of these criteria for safe progress are not met, the surgeon should move his dissection to a different area. The tumor mass is generally circled many times prior to delivering the intact specimen. In summary, centripetal dissection avoids at all times major hemorrhage or damage to vital structures by limiting dissection to areas that allow clear visualization of the operative field. A circular pattern of progressively deeper dissection results from this approach.

Avoid Trauma to the Tumor Surface Especially with Sarcoma

In the removal of pelvic sarcomas, one must always be aware of possible major hemorrhage from surface vasculature. Blood vessels in the sarcoma pseudocapsule are large, thin-walled, easily traumatized, and difficult to control once bleeding has occurred. Once one disrupts the tumor vasculature, bleeding is likely to be brisk. One should dissect away from the tumor in normal tissues as much as possible. If strong traction on the sarcoma mass is required, this should be allowed only after all other dissection is completed.

Maintain Hemostasis throughout the Procedure

One must always pay continuous attention to hemostasis, because inadequate hemostasis interferes with subsequent exposure. Blood in the operative field obscures the identification of additional bleeding points. Hemostasis must be achieved with electrocoagulation, ligatures, or clips as the dissection proceeds. The translucent nature of the tissues within the surgical field can be maintained by meticulous hemostasis and frequent irrigation.

Use of Peritonectomy Procedures

Very often in the reoperative setting the surgeon must be willing to dissect in a preperitoneal or retroperitoneal plane rather than moving through the peritoneal cavity itself. Peritonectomy procedures go beneath scar tissue to achieve a negative margin of resection.[11–15] Tumor at a resection site will almost always be beneath the peritoneal surface. An effective way to safely approach these recurrent tumor masses is by going beneath the peritoneal layer into a deeper plane away from the tumor mass (Fig. 11.**5**). Pelvic peritonectomy should be pursued in the reoperative setting with recurrence at the resection site and for invasive tumors being resected for the first time.

Utilize "Piecemeal" Excision

Often freeing up of a pelvic tumor mass will progressively obscure the plane of dissection. This will compromise the safety of subsequent dissection because of inadequate visualization, inadequate hemostasis, or an unnecessarily narrow margin of excision. Large tumor masses will become more and more difficult to extirpate as the dissection proceeds. As the anatomic site for further dissection is more deeply obscured by a large mass of tumor, the surgeon may be tempted to resort to dangerous blunt pelvic dissection to continue resection.

In this situation, piecemeal excision of the sarcoma is an important part of the operative procedure. Superficial components of the tumor may be removed prior to continuing the dissection of a deeper aspect of the tumor. Piecemeal excision using an electrosurgical loop

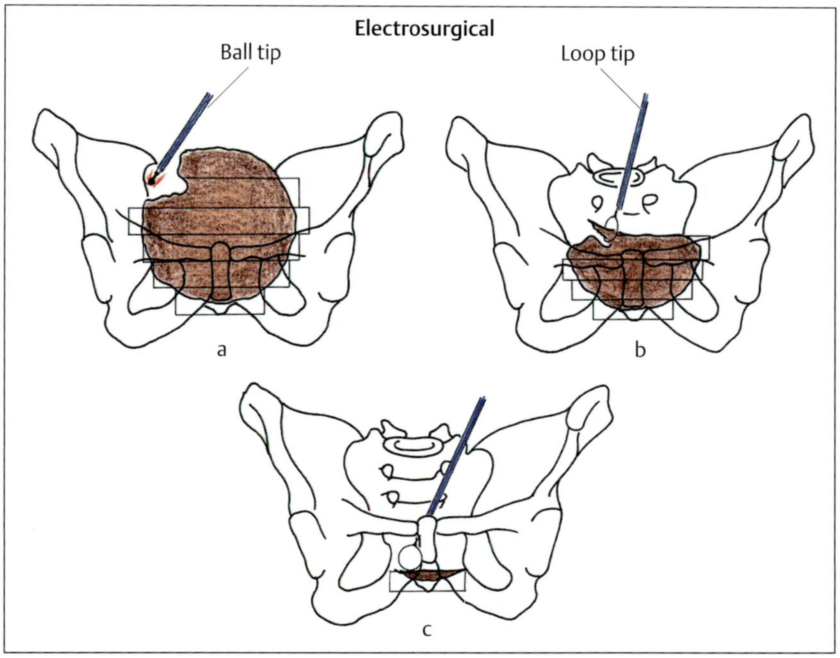

Fig. 11.6 Piecemeal excision of abdominal or pelvic sarcoma.

on pure cut is usually the best way to remove portions of the tumor prior to its complete resection (Fig. 11.**6**).

Piecemeal excision of a large tumor mass is much safer for the patient than is dissection with inadequate visualization. However, one must do everything possible to guard against the intraabdominal dissemination of cancer cells. The surrounding structures must be protected with laparotomy pads and towels. The electrosurgical loop at high voltage on pure cut removes fillets of tumor with minimal spillage of viable malignant cells. After each level of tumor is resected, thorough irrigation of the operative field is required.

☐ Guard Against Frustration toward the End of a Difficult Resection

The surgeon should realize that the greatest number of surgical misadventures occur just a few minutes prior to final removal of the tumor mass. Additional patience must be demonstrated just prior to complete removal. The final dissection is often performed over the tumor mass with reduced visualization. One must avoid the division of a vital structure such as a ureter or damage to a major blood vessel such as the left common iliac vein which results in profuse hemorrhage. Many serious intraoperative errors in cancer resection occur just prior to the removal of a large specimen.

Table 11.**1** Rationale for pelvic tissue transplants

1. Fill pelvic space
2. Provide vascularity to ischemic, irradiated tissues
3. Encircle and thereby protect anastomoses within the pelvis
4. Provide vascularity to minimize infectious complications
5. Provide a new abdominopelvic partition to prevent small bowel loops from becoming entrapped within the pelvis
6. Exclude bowel from the perineal incision so that intestinal function is maintained despite infection and/or breakdown of this incision

☐ Transplants of Primary Vascularized Tissue

After the removal of a pelvic malignancy and the organs involved by this tumor, a large space may be left behind. This is especially true in the pelvic exenteration procedure. Poor wound healing must always be expected in patients who have had radiation therapy. Pelvic tissue transplants have both immediate and long-term beneficial effects (Table 11.**1**). Tissue transplants bring much needed vascularity into the ischemic, irradiated tissues within the pelvis. Nonirradiated, well-vascularized tissue will greatly promote wound healing. Anastomoses can be protected from localized sepsis in the postoperative period. By displacement of blood and fluid infection will be minimized by the vascularized tissue occupying space within the pelvis.

Long-term benefits are realized since the pelvic tissue transplant will create a new abdominopelvic partition. This partition will not allow small bowel to be-

Table 11.**2** Techniques used for pelvic reconstruction

Pelvic tissue transplantation	Abdominopelvic partitions
Omentum	Omentum pedicle
Rectus abdominis muscle flap (unilateral or bilateral)	Uterus
Posterior gluteal flap	Bladder
Lateral thigh flap	Uterus
Gracilis muscle flap	"Leaf" of sigmoid colon or small bowel mesentery
Free flaps	Prosthetic mesh
Prosthetic material	

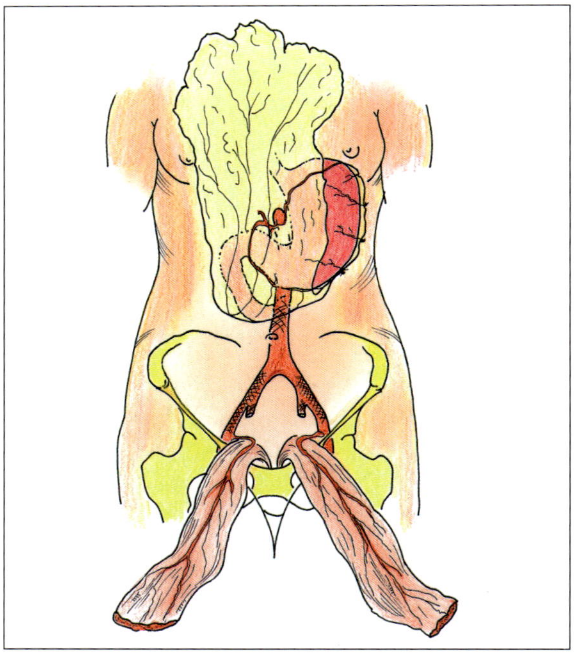

Fig. 11.**7** Primarily vascularized tissue tranplants may be harvested from three sources for abdominal and pelvic surgery. They are the greater omentum, right rectus muscle and left rectus muscle. One or all three sources may be appropriate.

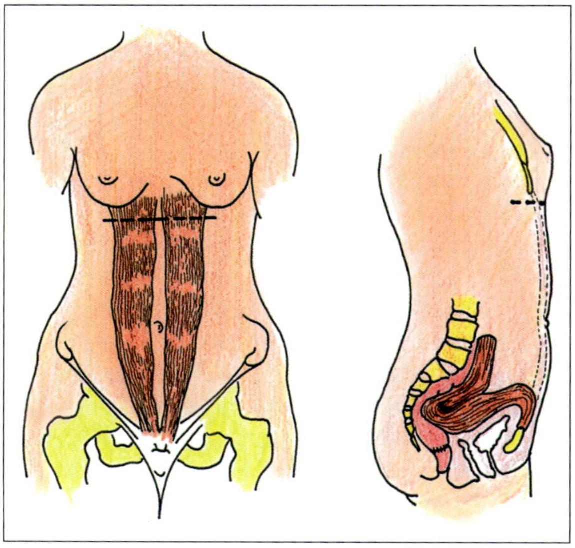

Fig. 11.**8** Primarily vascularized tissue transplant of rectus abdominis muscles. These are especially needed if the patient had prior radiation therapy to the pelvis.

come entrapped within the pelvis. Also, should infection or breakdown of the perineal incision occur, small bowel will be excluded from this infection focus. Even though the perineal incision is open and requires intensive wound care, nutrition via the enteral route can proceed because of the new abdominopelvic partition (Table 11.**2**).

Within the abdomen there are two prominent sources of primarily vascularized tissue. These are the omentum and the rectus abdominus muscles. The rectus abdominus muscles based on the deep inferior epigastric vessels can be harvested either bilaterally or unilaterally (Fig. 11. **7**). The omentum can be harvested so that its gastroepiploic pedicle is based on the left gastroepiploic vessels and the short gastric vessels on the left side of the stomach. More frequently the omental pedicle is based on the right side from the right gastroepiploic vessels. In both instances the numerous branches of the gastroepiploic vessels to the greater curvature are ligated and the gastroepiploic arcade is preserved. These large masses of freshly vascularized tissue are indicated in four clinical situations:

The primarily vascularized tissue is frequently used to fill empty space in the abdomen or pelvis (Fig. 11.**8**). This tissue is often placed into an irradiated abdominal gutter or into the irradiated pelvis. This greatly facilitates healing and serves to displace fluid accumulation and reduce the likelihood of pelvic sepsis.

A second use of pedicle flaps is to create a new abdominopelvic partition. This tissue barrier does not allow small bowel to become entrapped in the pelvis, resulting in subsequent intestinal obstruction or fistulization. Other sources of tissue can also be used in construction of an abdominopelvic partition. Bladder, uterus, leaf of sigmoid mesentery, and prosthetic materials have been used successfully (Fig. 11.**9**).

A third common indication for a primarily vascularized tissue transplant is coverage of cancerous tissues that have been incompletely excised. Residual disease is walled off from the remainder of the abdominal or pelvic cavity by the primarily vascularized tissue transplant. This will greatly improve long-term function by preventing cancerous invasion of the small bowel and the resultant intestinal obstruction.

A fourth indication for these primarily vascularized tissue transplants is to cover vascular grafts, reconstructed vessels, or urinary tract reconstruction. Omentum or muscle draped over a suture line will protect against false aneurysm, graft infection, and late blow out (Fig. 11.**10**).

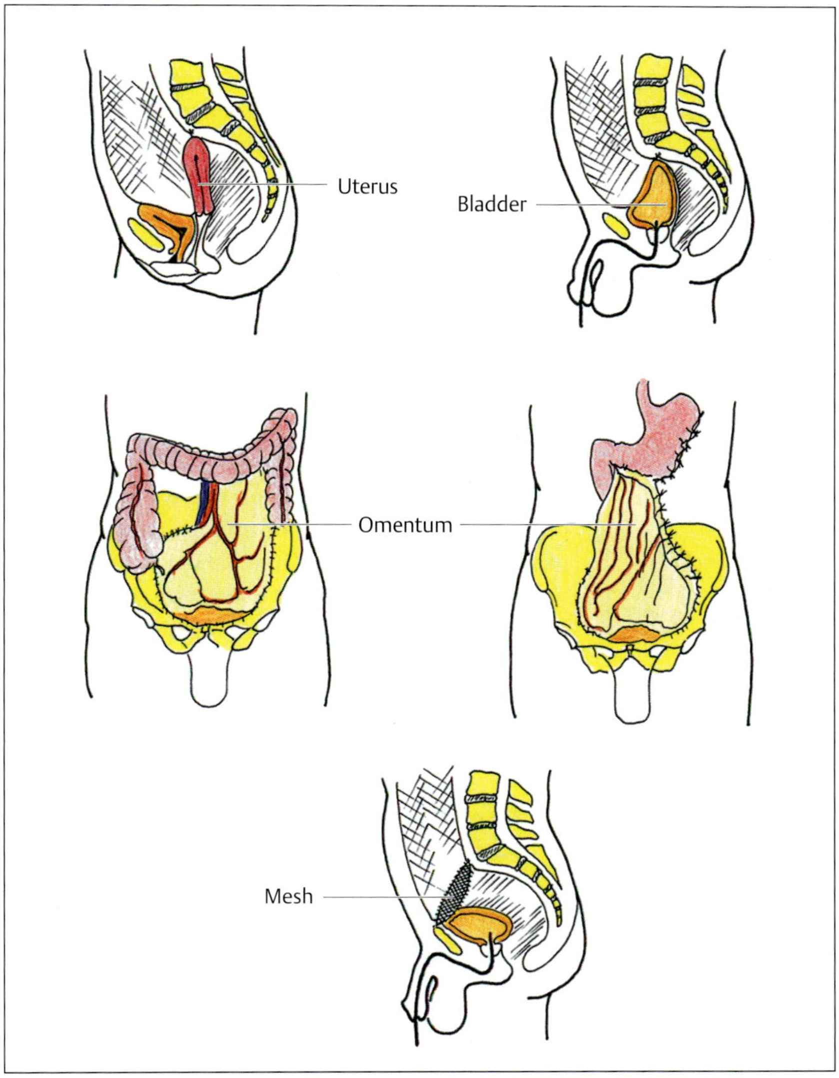

Fig. 11.**9** Methods to construct abdominopelvic partitions.

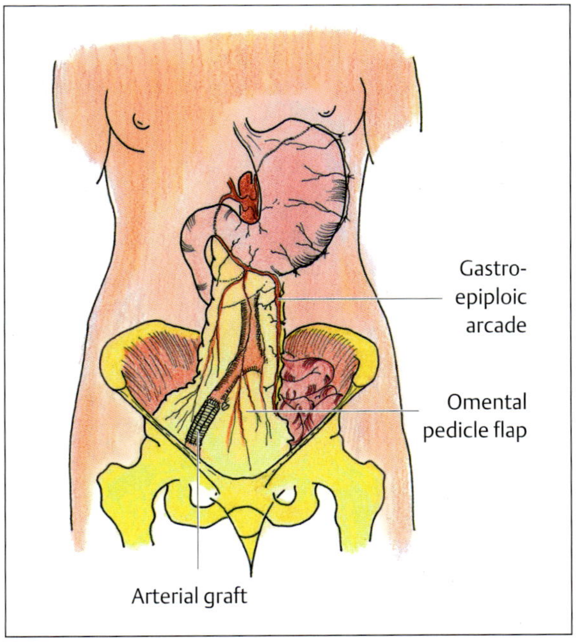

Fig. 11.**10** Omental pedicle flap used to cover arterial or urinary tract reconstruction. This technique is especially valuable for covering irradiated structures.

Peritonectomy and Intraperitoneal Chemotherapy

Another strategy of great value in selected patients concerns the treatment and prevention of resection site recurrence and peritoneal surface implantation.[16,17] Heated intraperitoneal chemotherapy employed intraoperatively is effective in reducing the high incidence of resection site recurrence and peritoneal surface dissemination that so frequently occurs after cancer resection.[18–21] Elimination of cancer seeding by peritonectomy and the resulting improvement in local-regional control has an effect on the survival of patients with sarcomatosis or with local recurrence. Standardized orders for heated intraoperative intraperitoneal chemotherapy are shown in Table 11.**3**. Figure 11.**11** shows the tubes and drains required to deliver early postoperative intraperitoneal chemotherapy. Figure 11.**12** shows the methodology for safe intraoperative delivery of heated cisplatin and doxorubicin via the intraperitoneal route.

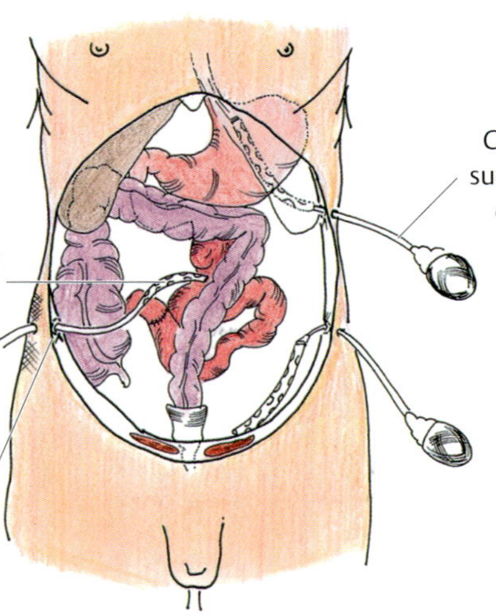

Fig. 11.**11** Tubes and drains used for early postoperative intraperitoneal chemotherapy.

After intraabdominal heated chemotherapy is complete, the abdomen is suctioned dry of fluid. The abdominal wall is then reopened and the retractors repositioned prior to performing anastomosis. It should be reemphasized that no suture lines are constructed until after the chemotherapy perfusion is complete.

The indications for intraperitoneal chemotherapy are shown in Table 11.**4**. Tumor spillage should in all instances be accompanied by intraoperative intraperitoneal chemotherapy.[22] Prevention of peritoneal carcinomatosis or sarcomatosis is a surgeon's responsibility. This cannot be relegated to later systemic chemotherapy treatment by the medical oncologist. Once cancer cells are imbedded in scar tissue they are not treatable by any technique.

Immediate Postoperative Abdominal Lavage

In patients with peritoneal carcinomatosis from large bowel cancer, early postoperative intraperitoneal 5-fluorouracil is always recommended.[23] The catheters that were positioned for intraperitoneal chemotherapy for drug instillation and abdominal drainage must be kept clear of blood clots and tissue debris. To accom-

Table 11.**3** Mitomycin C orders for adenocarcinoma and cisplatin plus doxorubicin orders for heated intraoperative intraperitoneal chemotherapy

Mitomycin orders	1. For pseudomyxoma peritonei and adenocarcinoma from appendiceal, colonic, and rectal cancer; add mitomycin C ______ mg to 2 L of 1.5% dextrose peritoneal dialysis solution. Dose of mitomycin C for males 12.5 mg/m^2; dose of mitomycin C for females 10 mg/m^2.
	2. Use 33% dose reduction for heavy prior chemotherapy, marginal renal function, age greater than 60, extensive intraoperative trauma to small bowel surfaces, or prior radiotherapy.
	3. Send 1 L of 1.5% dextrose peritoneal dialysis solution to test the perfusion circuit.
	4. Send 1 L of 1.5% dextrose peritoneal dialysis solution for immediate postoperative lavage.
	5. Send the above to operating room ______ at ______ o' clock.
Cisplatin and Doxorubicin orders	1. For gastric and ovarian cancer, mesothelioma and sarcoma; add cisplatin ______ mg to 2 L of 1.5% dextrose peritoneal dialysis solution. Dose of cisplatin 50 mg/m^2.
	2. Add doxorubicin ______ mg to same 2 L of 1.5% dextrose peritoneal dialysis solution. Dose of doxorubicin 15 mg/m^2
	3. Use 33% dose reduction for heavy prior chemotherapy, marginal renal function, age greater than 60, extensive intraoperative trauma to small bowel surfaces, or prior radiotherapy.
	4. Send 1 L of 1.5% dextrose peritoneal dialysis solution to test the perfusion circuit.
	5. Send the above to operating room ______ at ______ o' clock.

From: Sugarbaker PH. Intraperitoneal chemotherapy and cytoreductive surgery. Manual for Physicians and Nurses. 3rd ed. Grand Rapids: Ludann Company; 1998.[22]

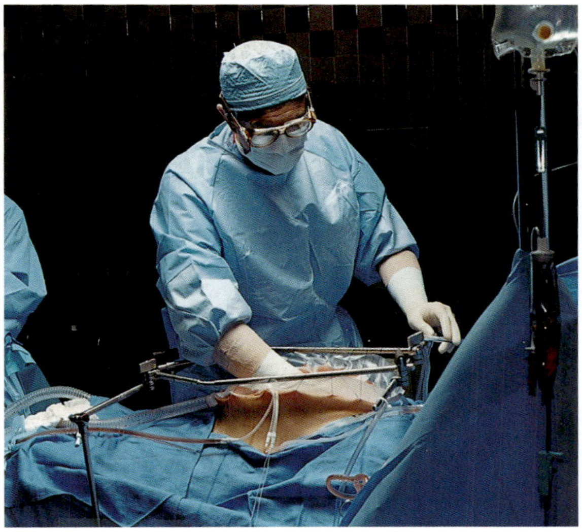

Fig. 11.**12** Coliseum technique: heated intraoperative intraperitoneal chemotherapy using a self-retractor. After placement of tubes, drains, and temperature probes, the skin edges are elevated onto the frame of a self-retaining retractor with the use of a running suture. A plastic sheet incorporated into the sutures covers the abdomen and prevents splashing or loss of chemotherapy aerosols into the environment. A smoke evacuator pulls air from beneath the plastic sheet through a charcoal filter. A slit in the plastic sheet allows the surgeon's hand access to the abdomen and pelvis. Continuous manipulation of all viscera guarantees that all surfaces will have uniform exposure to heat and chemotherapy.

plish this, an abdominal lavage is started in the operating room. This lavage utilizes the same tubes and drains that were positioned for heated intraoperative intraperitoneal chemotherapy. Large volumes of fluid are rapidly infused and then drained from the abdomen after a short dwell time. The standardized orders for immediate postoperative abdominal lavage are given in Table 11.**5**. All intraabdominal catheters are withdrawn before the patient is discharged from the hospital.

Early Postoperative Intraperitoneal 5-Fluorouracil

The standardized orders for early postoperative intraperitoneal 5-fluorouracil are presented in Table 11.**6**. After the patient stabilizes postoperatively and after the drainage from the immediate postoperative abdominal lavage is no longer bloodstained, the 5-fluorouracil instillation begins. In some patients who have extensive small bowel trauma from lysis of adhesions, the early postoperative 5-fluorouracil is withheld for fear of fistula formation. During the first 6 hours of intraperitoneal 5-fluorouracil administration, the patient turns every 30 minutes from the right to left side to maximize drug distribution through gravitational effects.

Table 11.**4** Indications for heated intraoperative intraperitoneal chemotherapy (HIIC)

Rupture or perforated cancer
Tumor spillage
Small volume peritoneal carcinomatosis or sarcomatosis after resection of primary sarcoma and peritonectomy of implants
Small volume local residual disease
After complete cytoreduction of carcinoma or sarcoma recurrence
Positive cytology
Lymph nodes positive at the margin of excision

Table 11.**5** Immediate postoperative abdominal lavage

Day of Operation
1. Run in 1000 mL 1.5% dextrose peritoneal dialysis solution as rapidly as possible. Warm to body temperature prior to instillation; clamp all abdominal drains during infusion.
2. No dwell time.
3. Drain as rapidly as possible through the Tenckhoff catheter and abdominal drains.
4. Repeat irrigations every 1 h for 4 h, then every 4 h until returns are clear; then every 8 h until chemotherapy begins.
5. Change dressing covering Tenckhoff catheter and abdominal drain sites using sterile technique once daily and as necessary.
6. Standardized precautions must be used for all body fluids from this patient.

Table 11.**6** Early postoperative intraperitoneal chemotherapy with 5-fluorouracil

Postoperative days 1–5
1. Add to _____ mL 1.5% dextrose peritoneal dialysis solution:
2. _____ mg 5-fluorouracil (650 mg/m^2, maximal dose 1300 mg)
3. 50 mEq sodium bicarbonate.
4. Intraperitoneal fluid volume: 1 L for patients 2.0 m^2, 1.5 L for >2.0 m^2.
5. Drain all fluid from the abdominal cavity prior to instillation, then clamp abdominal drains.
6. Run the chemotherapy solution into the abdominal cavity through the Tenckhoff catheter as rapidly as possible; dwell for 23 h and drain for 1 h prior to next instillation.
7. Use gravity to maximize intraperitoneal distribution of the 5-fluorouracil; instill the chemotherapy with the patient in a full right lateral position; after ½ h, direct the patient to turn to the full left lateral position; change position right to left every ½ h; if tolerated, use 10° of Trendelenburg position; continue turning for the first 6 h after instillation of chemotherapy solution.
8. Continue to drain abdominal cavity after final dwell until Tenckhoff catheter is removed.
9. Use 33% dose reduction for heavy prior chemotherapy, age >60, or prior to radiotherapy.

Second-Look Surgery

Patients are maintained on systemic chemotherapy after discharge from the hospital. After approximately 6 months of systemic treatment, the patient is recommended for a second-look procedure.[24] At the time of second-look surgery, the abdomen is widely opened and all the peritoneal surfaces are visualized with a complete takedown of all adhesions. Additional cytoreduction is performed and additional visceral peritonectomies may be required.[25] If a complete cytoreduction can be achieved, the heated intraoperative intraperitoneal chemotherapy is used again. With carcinoma early postoperative intraperitoneal 5-fluorouracil is also recommended after the reoperation. In some patients, the disease may suggest a "chemotherapy failure." In this situation, a change in the drugs used for intraperitoneal chemotherapy is recommended. Usually a regimen of intraperitoneal cisplatin and doxorubicin is utilized.

References

1. Sugarbaker PH. Managing the peritoneal surface component of gastrointestinal cancer. Part 1. Patterns of dissemination and treatment options. *Oncology.* 2004;18:51–59.
2. Sugarbaker PH, Yu W, Yonemura Y. Gastrectomy, peritonectomy and perioperative intraperitoneal chemotherapy: the evolution of treatment strategies for advanced gastric cancer. *Semin Surg Oncol.* 2003;21:233–248.
3. Sugarbaker PH. Review of a personal experience in the management of carcinomatosis and sarcomatosis. *Jpn J Clin Oncol.* 2001;31:573–583.
4. Piso P, Bektas H, Werner V et al. Improved prognosis following peritonectomy procedures and hyperthermic intraperitoneal chemotherapy for peritoneal carcinomatosis from appendiceal carcinoma. *Eur J Surg Oncol.* 2001;27: 286–290.
5. Yonemura Y, Fujimura T, Fushida S et al. A new surgical approach (peritonectomy) for the treatment of peritoneal dissemination. *Hepatogastroenterology.* 1999;46:601–609.
6. Elias D, Liberale G, Manganas D, Lasser P, Pocard M. Surgical treatment of peritoneal carcinomatosis. *Ann Chir.* 2004;129:439–443.
7. Sugarbaker PH. Management of peritoneal-surface malignancy: the surgeon's role. *Langenbecks Arch Surg.* 1999; 384:576–587.
8. Sugarbaker PH. Successful management of microscopic residual disease in large bowel cancer. *Cancer Chemother Pharmacol.* 1999;43:15–25.
9. Yonemura Y, Bandou E, Kinoshita K et al. Effective therapy for peritoneal dissemination in gastric cancer. *Surg Oncol N Am.* 2003;12;635–648.
10. Sugarbaker PH. New responsibilities in the management of colorectal cancer with peritoneal seeding. *Cancer Invest.* 2002;20:1118–1120.
11. Sugarbaker PH. Peritonectomy procedures. *Ann Surg.* 1995;221:29–42.
12. Glehen O, Mithieux F, Osinsky D et al. Surgery combined with peritonectomy procedures and intraperitoneal chemohyperthermia in abdominal cancers with peritoneal carcinomatosis: a phase II study. *J Clin Oncol.* 2003;21: 799–806.
13. Fujimura T, Yonemura Y, Nakagawara H et al. Subtotal peritonectomy with chemohyperthermic peritoneal perfusion for peritonitis carcinomatosa in gastrointestinal cancer. *Oncol Rep.* 2000;7:809–814.
14. Cavaliere F, Di Filippo F, Botti C et al. Peritonectomy and hyperthermic antiblastic perfusion in the treatment of peritoneal carcinomatosis. *Eur Surg Oncol.* 2000;26: 486–491.
15. Sarnaik AA, Sussman JJ, Ahmad SA, Lowy AM. Technology of intraperitoneal chemotherapy administration: a survey of techniques with a review of morbidity and mortality. *Surg Clin N Am.* 2003 12:849–863.
16. Glehen O, Cotte E, Schreiber V, Sayag-Beaujard AC, Vignal J, Gilly FN. Intraperitoneal chemohyperthermia and attempted cytoreductive surgery in patients with peritoneal carcinomatosis of colorectal origin. *Br J Surg.* 2004;91: 747–754.
17. Sugarbaker PH. Cytoreduction including total gastrectomy for pseudomyxoma peritonei. *Br J Surg.* 2002;89:208–212.
18. Guner Z, Schmidt U, Dahlke MH, Schlitt HJ, Klempnauer J, Piso P. Cytoreductive surgery and intraperitoneal chemotherapy for pseudomyxoma peritonei. *Int J Colorectal Dis.* 2005;20:155–160.
19. Cavaliere F, Di Filippo F, Cosimelli M et al. The integrated treatment of peritoneal carcinomatosis. A preliminary experience. *J Exp Clin Cancer Res.* 1999;18:151–158.
20. Begossi G, Gonzalez-Moreno S, Ortega-Perez G, Fon LJ, Sugarbaker PH. Cytoreduction and intraperitoneal chemotherapy for the management of peritoneal carcinomatosis, sarcomatosis and mesothelioma. *Eur J Surg Oncol.* 2002;28: 80–87.
21. Sugarbaker PH, Chang D. Results of treatment of 385 patients with peritoneal surface spread of appendiceal malignancy. *Ann Surg Oncol.* 1999;6:727–731.
22. Sugarbaker PH. *Management of Peritoneal Surface Malignancy using Intraperitoneal Chemotherapy and Cytoreductive Surgery. A Manual for Physicians and Nurses.* 3rd ed. Grand Rapids, Michigan: The Ludann Company; 1998.
23. Glehen O, Osinsky D, Cotte E et al. Intraperitoneal chemohyperthermia using a closed abdominal procedure and cytoreductive surgery for the treatment of peritoneal carcinomatosis: morbidity and mortality analysis of 216 consecutive procedures. *Ann Surg Oncol.* 2003;10:863–869.
24. Esquivel J, Sugarbaker PH. Second-look surgery in patients with peritoneal dissemination from appendiceal malignancy: analysis of prognostic factors in 98 patients. *Ann Surg.* 2001;234:198–205.
25. Sugarbaker PH. Peritonectomy procedures. *Surg Oncol N Am.* 2003;12:703–727.

12 Pelvic Surgery

Harold J. Wanebo and Ihor N. Ponomarenko

Resection of locally advanced or recurrent pelvic tumors is particularly challenging because of technical difficulties posed by the bony confines of the pelvis, complex physiologic considerations, and considerable risk of major complications. This is frequently compounded in the setting of prior surgery, chemotherapy, and radiotherapy. Oncologic control requires a multimodality approach including microscopically clear resection margins and, if warranted, radiation or chemotherapy. Other important considerations are the potential for preservation of function and the patient's ability to tolerate the procedure and undergo rehabilitation.[1–5]

Options for resection are determined largely by the nature and location of the tumor. The management of a primary pelvic tumor, whether of epithelial or mesenchymal origin, is governed by the extent of involvement of adjacent structures. For example, a limb-sparing internal hemipelvectomy can be used for primary tumors localized to the lateral pelvis.[1–3,5] On the other hand, a full hemipelvectomy is usually required for secondary (recurrent) tumors of this area due to frequent invasion of the surrounding soft tissues.[1,6–8] Primary tumors of the posterior pelvis can usually be managed by sacral resection with preservation of the rectum.[9–13] Secondary tumors are generally more extensive, thus requiring composite resection of viscera, soft tissue, and bone.[10,13–17] This type of resection has also been referred to as an extended pelvic exenteration or an abdominosacral resection (ASR).[18]

In the case of rectal cancer, 40 to 55% of patients are at risk of recurrence.[19] Advances in primary control such as preoperative chemoradiation and total mesorectal excision (TME) have been shown to decrease local recurrence from approximately 40% to as low as 5%.[20]

Primary surgical treatment is not yet standardized however, and recurrence remains a significant problem. Interestingly, in half of the patients with local recurrence, disease is isolated to the pelvis; there is no evidence of distant spread.[21] This group is thus potentially curable by reoperation and en bloc resection. In rare situations where extremely aggressive resections and amputations may be necessary,[14] adequate neuromuscular function can be preserved in most patients. However, with resulting significant fixed impairments such as anorectal and urogenital dysfunction and lower extremity weakness, aggressive rehabilitation will be required.

Radical pelvic surgery is performed primarily with curative intent in patients without evidence of extrapelvic or distant spread. In patients with hepatic metastases, involvement of the extrapelvic lymphatics, or gross invasion of the sacral promontory, the risks of the procedure may outweigh its potential benefit. In our experience, the patients undergoing radical pelvic resection for palliation of symptoms all died within a year. Such patients may be candidates for other modes of palliation, including brachytherapy and isolated chemotherapy perfusion.

Preoperative Evaluation and Preparation

Pain is a common presentation in patients presenting with isolated pelvic disease, who may be relatively young and otherwise healthy. With respect to the risks of radical surgery though, this patient may have already undergone several rounds of surgery, radiation, and chemotherapy. The main objectives of the preoperative evaluation are to determine resectability, exclude metastasis, and assess the patient's general medical status. Radical pelvic surgery imposes a heavy burden on the reserves of various organ systems. Hence, a thorough assessment of the severity of comorbidities including diabetes, cardiovascular disease, pulmonary, hepatic, and renal insufficiencies is of vital importance. Given the potential postoperative sequelae requiring significant rehabilitation, evaluation of psychologic status, psychosocial support system, and preoperative teaching are also critical. These factors in patient selection have been addressed in detail elsewhere.[6–8,15,17,22–26] A complete clinical examination should include documentation of baseline neuromuscular function of the lower extremities, paying particular attention to any deficits caused by the tumor. Rectal and vaginal examinations if possible are helpful in assessing the extent of the tumor, its fixation to the lateral wall, and possible involvement of anterior pelvic viscera.

Essential imaging studies include a computed tomography (CT) scan of the abdomen and pelvis, plain X-rays of the chest and lumbosacral spine, a bone scan, and magnetic resonance imaging (MRI). A plain chest radiograph is usually sufficient to rule out lung metastasis, although a chest CT scan may be required in the presence of suspicious but equivocal findings.The CT scan demonstrates the local extent of the tumor and may also reveal enlarged periaortic nodes and liver metastases. A bone scan and possibly a positive-radionuclear scan (PET scan) are important to exclude marrow involvement. In the presence of a positive PET scan, an MRI may help define whether there is anatomic marrow invasion. MRI T2-weighted sagittal views are helpful in planning operative strategy by delineating the relationship of the tumor to the sacrum and especially in demonstrating the upper limits of the tumor. If suspicious areas are seen on imaging, CT-guided needle biopsy can provide tissue diagnosis. In some cases of primary sacral cancer, an open biopsy may be necessary. Laparoscopy provides direct evaluation of peritoneal metastases. Arteriography is selectively performed only with extensive tumors. In patients with rectal carcinoma, evaluation of the colon with colonoscopy (via rectum or colostomy) or contrast enema is important for detection of synchronous lesions which would alter the extent of the resection. Cystoscopy is useful in evaluating the extent of urinary bladder involvement and the finding of limited dome involvement may allow for a partial cystectomy with preservation of function, whereas invasion of the trigone will undoubtedly require total cystectomy with urinary diversion.

Regarding nonsurgical treatment, patients with large primary sarcomas are candidates for preoperative radiation or chemotherapy, whereas those with chordomas usually receive postoperative radiation. For sarcomas, we use 3000 to 3500 cGy of radiation, given in 10 to 15 fractions and doxorubicin, 30 mg/day for 3 days, given by continuous infusion, as a radiation sensitizer. Patients with locally advanced or recurrent rectal adenocarcinomas or epidermoid anorectal carcinomas also receive preoperative chemoradiation, unless they have previously undergone radiation therapy. For rectal adenocarcinomas, 45 to 50 Gy of radiation is administered in 20–25 fractions along with sensitizing 5-fluorouracil, 750 $mg/m^2/day$ for 5 days or 250 mg/ M^2/d by continuous infusion during the period of radiation. Patients with advanced epidermoid carcinoma receive preoperatively up to 50 Gy of radiation in 15 fractions plus 5-fluorouracil, 750 $mg/m^2/day$ for 5 days and mitomycin, 15 $mg/m^2/day$ for 1 day.

Patients who still have the rectum in continuity with the gastrointestinal tract are instructed to change their diet to clear liquids 48 hours before the operation. The day before surgery, standard mechanical bowel preparation begins with the drinking of a standard solution until the rectal effluent becomes clear. Two doses of antibiotics, neomycin and metronidazole, are also given orally. One must guard against fluid and electrolyte losses during bowel preparation by ensuring adequate oral intake or with supplementary intravenous fluid. A broad spectrum antibiotic with activity against gram-negative and anaerobic bacteria is given parenterally just prior to incision.

□ Operative Technique

Chapter 11 describes the surgical strategies for primary or recurrent pelvic malignancy. Chapter 10 considers the abdominoinguinal approach for pelvic sidewall tumors. They complement the following description.

□ Tumors Primarily Involving Posterior Pelvis or Pelvic Sidewalls

For the purpose of this discussion, the technique of an ASR is presented here because it encompasses most of the problems encountered in managing pelvic cancer. Inclusion of the sacrum can be considered to be the posterior margin of an extended pelvic exenteration. We perform a two-stage procedure including a 24 to 36 hour intermission in the intensive care unit (ICU). Others have described it as a single stage procedure, entirely in the lithotomy position.[27] The abdominal stage basically entails determination of resectability, lymph node dissection, urinary and fecal diversion as indicated, and vascular isolation of the tumor. The actual resection is reserved for the sacral stage. The procedure is well detailed in Joel Bauer's *Colorectal Surgery Illustrated.*[28]

For the abdominal stage, the patient is positioned in lithotomy and ureteral stents are placed. Careful positioning is important because of the rare but serious leg complications that can occur especially with procedures of this length.[29] The procedure starts with entry into the abdomen through a generous lower midline incision extending from the pubic symphysis to approximately 10 cm above the umbilicus. A meticulous exploration is done to rule out extrapelvic disease which precludes curative resection and is therefore a contraindication. This includes peritoneal seeding, unresectable metastases to the liver, extra-pelvic lymphadenopathy (i. e., paraaortic or external iliac), or involvement of the sacral promontory.

If no extrapelvic disease is found, exposure of the pelvis is obtained by packing the small bowel up into the middle and upper abdomen with use of a self-retaining retractor. If the rectum is still intact and must be resected, the site of transection in the sigmoid colon is selected by taking into consideration the adequacy of the length and blood supply of the remaining left colon for forming a permanent colostomy without tension or ischemia. The mesocolon is serially clamped, divided, and ligated from the selected transection site to the level of the sacral promontory and the sigmoid is transected with a linear gastrointestinal stapler. The upper rectum is mobilized with sharp dissection. Dense adhesions between the tumor and bowel or bladder should be considered cancerous and necessitate removal of the tumor-attached organ or at least the site of attachment. To avoid jeopardizing a curative resection, dissection must be avoided in the area where the tumor appears to invade the sacrum.

Aortoiliac node dissection is started at the level of the aortic and caval bifurcations and continues along the common and external iliac arteries; it includes the internal iliac, the obturator, and the hypogastric nodes (Fig. 12.**1**). These lymph nodes are submitted for histopathologic study separately from the main specimen. Extensive nodal involvement in the lower pelvis generally precludes continuing the resection, but the presence of enlarged but easily resectable obturator nodes does not. If the ureters are free of tumor, they are dissected and fixed anteriorly to the lateral pelvic wall just below the external iliac artery and vein to prevent injury during the posterior dissection. If the bladder and distal ureters are involved but considered resectable, the ureters are divided, the bladder is dissected free from the lateral side walls but left attached to the posterior tumor. An ileal conduit is constructed in a standard fashion (Fig. 12.**2**). An involved uterus or ovaries are treated similarly.

If the tumor extends into the internal iliac artery or vein, these are bisected from the parent vessel (common iliac artery or vein) and attached to the tumor and posterior pelvis (to be resected from above; Fig. 12.**3**). In general, tumor involvement of the common iliac artery or vein is considered nonresectable for primary or recurrent rectal, anorectal, or gynecologic cancer. For primary sarcoma of the pelvis, however, localized sarcoma demonstrating vascular invasion may be resected by composite resection with reconstruction as dictated by specific circumstances.

Pelvic devascularization is optimized during the abdominal stage because of easier exposure and it facilitates hemostasis during the sacral stage. This is accomplished by transecting and ligating with sutures the internal iliac arteries and veins (Fig. 12.**3**). An effort should be made to ligate the internal iliac artery beyond the first branch to preserve vascularization of the skin and muscle flaps to be used for closure of the posterior wound. The middle sacral artery and vein and individual branches to the tumor mass are divided if found in the plane of dissection. If the bladder is to be preserved it is important to maintain at least one cystic artery. There is also important vascular inflow from retropubic vessels and these attachments should not be disturbed.

The peritoneal floor is restored with Vicryl mesh, preferably with an interposed omental pedicle or local peritoneal flap to protect the bowel from fistula formation (Fig. 12.**4**).[30] A transpelvic rectus abdominis mus-

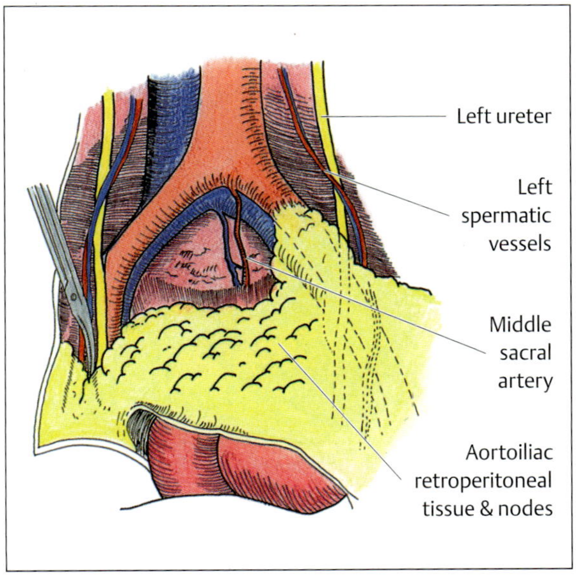

Fig. 12.**1** Aortoiliac and obturator node dissection.

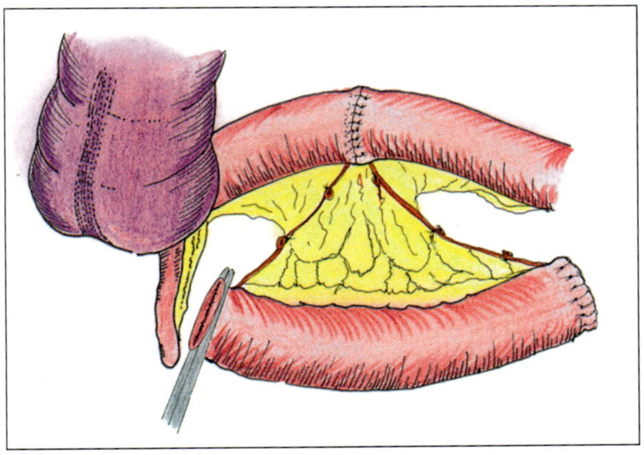

Fig. 12.**2** Ileal conduit and ureteral anastomosis.

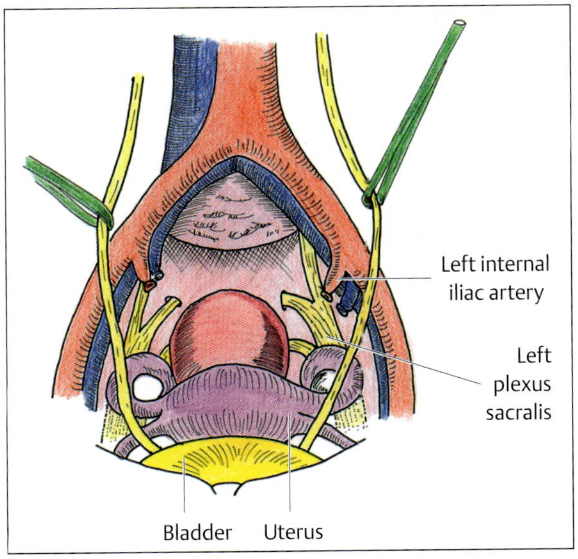

Fig. 12.**3** Pelvic devascularization.

4

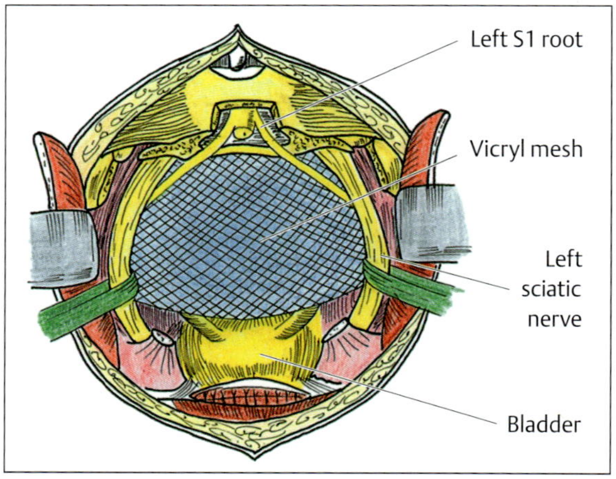

Fig. 12.**4** Vicryl mesh, peritoneal, or omental sling is developed to prevent posterior herniation of bowel.

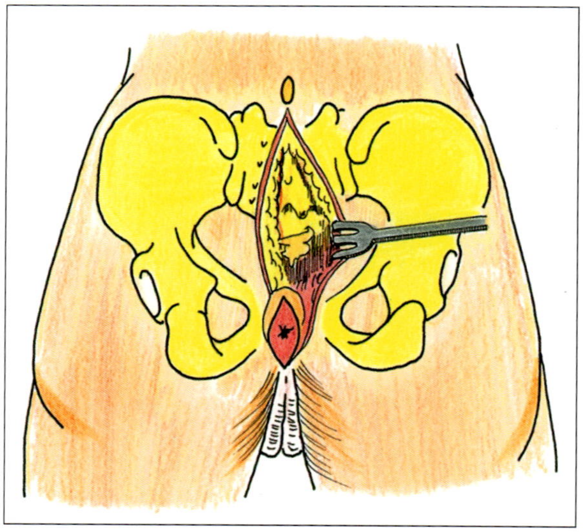

Fig. 12.**5** Posterior skin incision.

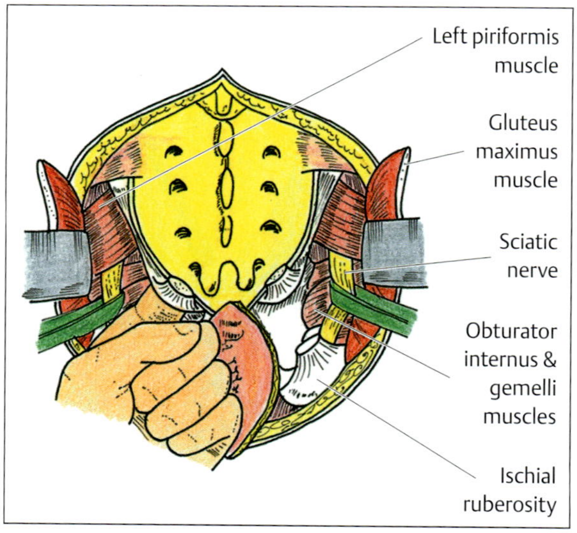

Fig. 12.**6** Identification of sciatic nerves. Sacrotuberous and sacrospinous ligaments are incised. Surgeon's finger "breaks through" endopelvic fascia to assess proper site for sacral osteotomy.

4

culocutaneous rotation flap can be used to fill the resulting pelvic dead space and close the perineal wound. This can help minimize healing complications, especially if the area had previously undergone radiotherapy.[31] The closed end of the ileal loop is sutured to paravertebral tissues proximal to the periosteum of the sacral promontory to prevent twisting of the mesentery. Before closure of the abdominal incision, the distal end of the ileal loop and the divided end of the sigmoid colon are exteriorized through openings at the predesignated areas of the abdominal wall. The distal ends of the ureteral stents are also brought out through the ileostomy.

After satisfactory hemostasis has been achieved, the abdominal incision is closed. If oozing persists despite meticulous hemostasis, the pelvis is packed with laparotomy sponges, which are removed during the sacral part of the procedure. After closure of the abdominal incision, the stomas are matured with interrupted 4–0 Vicryl sutures. The ureteral stents are transfixed to the skin surrounding the stoma of the ileal loop and left in place for 5 to 7 days; they are removed only after anastomotic integrity has been documented by means of a retrograde contrast study.

Upon completion of the abdominal stage, the patient is allowed to equilibrate and is to become optimized in the ICU for approximately 24 hours. The sacral stage of the procedure begins with the patient being placed in the prone position. A posterior sacral incision is made from the spinous process of L5 to the perineum. The lower part of the incision has an elliptical course so it can include the anus and urethra, depending on which pelvic organs are to be removed. Full-thickness flaps are raised at the level of the sacral periosteum to the lateral extent of the sacrum (Fig. 12.**5**). The gluteus maximus and medius muscles are dissected from their sacral origins with maintenance of a fascial cuff on the muscles for the subsequent midline wound closure.

The sciatic nerve is located by retracting the gluteus maximus and underlying piriformis muscles superiorly at the lateral aspect of the middle portion of the sacrum. The nerve lies superficial to the obturator internus and gemelli muscles as it courses inferolaterally midway between the ischial tuberosity and the greater trochanter. During the dissection, it is encircled with a vessel loop for ease of identification (Fig. 12.**6**). To access the pelvis, the sacrotuberous and sacrospinous ligaments are incised at the level of their attachments to the ischial tuberosity and ischial spine. A finger is then inserted medially to the sciatic nerve and advanced deeply beneath the piriformis muscles and through the underlying endopelvic fascia. With this maneuver, the surgeon "breaks through" the endopelvic fascia to reach the anterior surface of the sacrum in the area of the pelvic dissection performed during the abdominal procedure. This approach directs the subsequent sacral osteotomy and ensures an adequate margin proximal to the tumor. Further dissection is carried out around the sacrum by incising the piriformis muscles and the soft tissues surrounding the sciatic nerve.

A laminectomy is performed at the planned level of sacral transection, usually between L5 and S1, to help dissect the nerve roots and ligate the terminal end of the dural sac. The proximal sacral roots are identified and an effort is made to preserve them by dissecting them free from the portion of the sacrum to be resected. After the resection line on both sides of the sacrum is determined, an osteotome or oscillating saw is used to transect the bone while the surgeon's finger is positioned anteriorly to protect the intraabdominal contents (Fig. 12.**7**). For resections above the level of S3, greater effort is required as the line of resection is continued laterally through the sacroiliac joints. Care is taken not to injure the lumbar component of the sciatic nerve. The sacral components of the nerve are dissected if necessary. The sacrum, pelvic sidewall, and tumor-bearing structures are removed en bloc (Fig. 12.**8**). Hemostasis is obtained after initial packing of the wound to gain temporary control of bleeding. The region is examined carefully and any residual tumor or devitalized tissue is removed. If the presence of residual tumor is suspected, the margins are examined histologically by frozen section. Additional margins are serially obtained until there is frozen section confirmation that margins are free of tumor. When possible, a 2-cm margin is desirable. It is important to examine the specimen carefully with the pathologist. It is also helpful to perform biopsies at the periphery of the resection sites that correspond to high risk areas observed after examination of the specimen.

Closed-suction drains are placed bilaterally and the sacral wound is closed. If the fascial origin of the gluteus maximus has been preserved, the muscles are approximated in the midline with heavy nonabsorbable monofilament suture, thereby forming a new pelvic floor. A relaxing incision at the level of the lateral insertion of the gluteus maximus on the greater trochanter may be necessary to allow additional medial advancement of the muscle (Fig. 12.**9**). The subcutaneous tissue is approximated with interrupted absorbable sutures and the skin with staples. Depending on the extent of the resection and the status of the patient, reconstruction with musculocutaneous flaps may be performed at the time of resection or delayed for a few days.

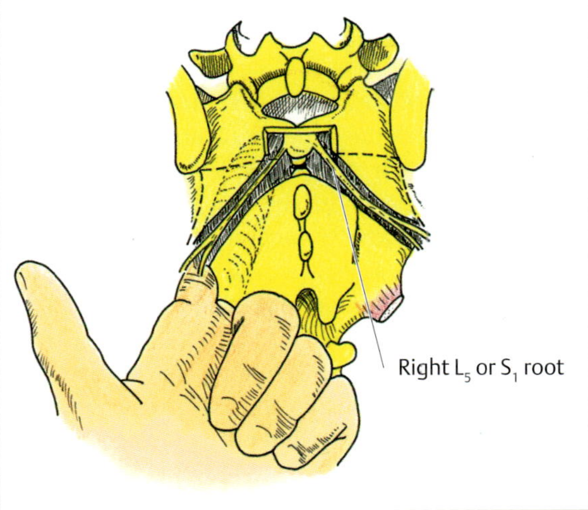

Fig. 12.**7** Laminectomy (L5–S1) with dissection and preservation of selected sacral root (usually S1 or more distal if possible).

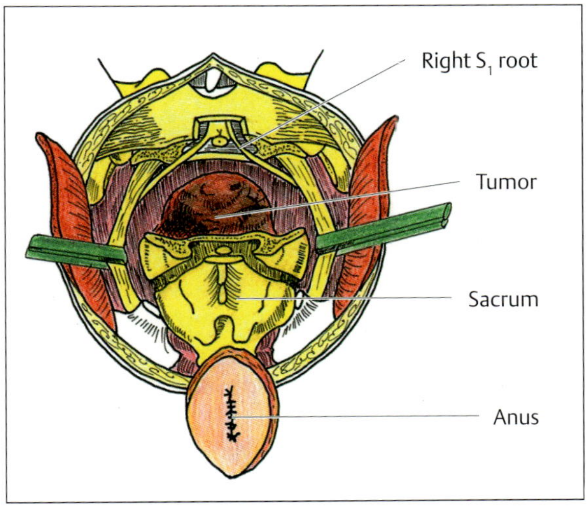

Fig. 12.**8** The sacrum, pelvic sidewalls, and tumor are removed en bloc along with the attached structures (bladder, retained rectum) as indicated.

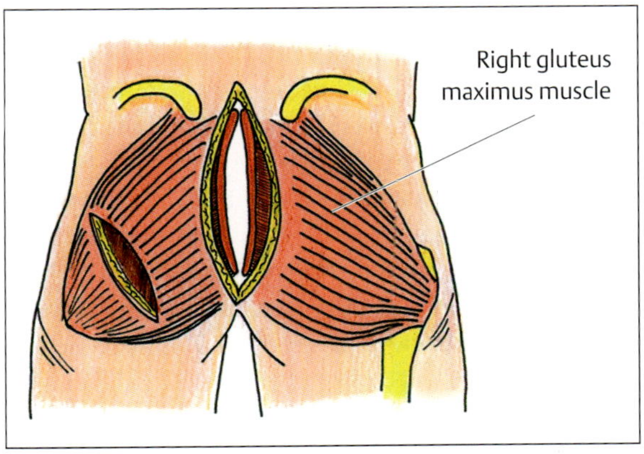

Fig. 12.**9** The gluteus maximus muscles are approximated to midline forming a new pelvic floor. To allow greater medial advancement of the muscle, it may be necessary to incise the lateral insertions of the gluteus maximus on the greater trochanter.

4

Complications, Mortality and Morbidity

The potential complications of extended radical pelvic operations include the same spectrum of problems occurring after major abdominal surgery. In addition, complications related to the urinary diversion, the stomas, and the sacral resection can arise. However, these patients are at greater risk because they have a healing disadvantage from prior surgery and radiation therapy.

The long anesthesia and operative time coupled with the vast extent of dissection and exposure results in an extensive intravascular volume deficit. Bleeding, third space and insensible fluid losses requiring massive replacement represents a difficult, sometimes overwhelming challenge. It is this stress that matters most in patient selection. Close intraoperative and postoperative hemodynamic monitoring is essential. We usually use autotransfusion intraoperatively. Fatal postoperative hemorrhage has been reported after radical pelvic surgery.[22,25,32] Death from uncontrolled bleeding, however, should be preventable with proper handling of the pelvic vasculature and establishment of good hemostasis during the procedure. When satisfactory hemostasis cannot be accomplished, packing of the pelvis, followed by a return to the operating room 2 or 3 days later to remove the pack, is safe and effective. Another potential problem in this setting is the development of abdominal compartment syndrome resulting in respiratory compromise, renal dysfunction, and hemodynamic instability. Emergent decompressive laparotomy is required.

Patients undergoing radical pelvic surgery are also prone to cardiopulmonary complications caused by massive fluid shifts, rapid administration of large volumes of fluid, and substantial continuing postoperative fluid loss.[22,23,25,32,33] Close monitoring, with appropriate fluid replacement and correction of electrolyte imbalances plays a critical part in preventing cardiac problems. A sufficient urine output indicates not only the adequacy of hydration and renal function but also the patency and integrity of the ureteral anastomosis.

Wound infections have been an important cause of morbidity, particularly in earlier series.[6,22,23,25,33] Infections and flap separation after ASR occur markedly more often in patients undergoing the procedure for recurrent disease and in those who had received high doses of radiation preoperatively. Large open granulating wounds contribute to sepsis and volume deficit. Pelvic abscesses and collections such as lymphoceles and urinomas should be initially managed nonoperatively with percutaneous drainage.

Intestinal obstruction is a common early postoperative complication that may cause considerable morbidity if it is not diagnosed quickly and treated properly.[6,22,23,25,33] The principal predisposing factors are the empty, deperitonealized pelvis and the presence and position of the urinary-diversion conduit.[22,24,26,34] The empty pelvis is also the source of enteroperineal fistulas.[24,25–37] Delay in the surgical management of early postoperative intestinal obstruction runs the risk of entering the pelvis after the formation of adhesions which increases surgical mortality and morbidity.[38] In such situations, sound surgical judgment dictates that if the bowel cannot be dissected free of the pelvis safely, the obstruction should be relieved by an intestinal bypass procedure.[22,36,37,39] Preoperative radiotherapy facilitates local control at the expense of morbidity associated with operating on irradiated tissue. Because the incidence of intestinal obstruction is significantly higher in patients given preoperative irradiation, particularly in those without pelvic reconstruction, it is advisable to perform pelvic reconstruction with use of omental or myocutaneous flaps or colonic advancement in these patients.[24,26] Immediate or delayed reconstruction by mucocutaneous flaps is associated with fewer healing complications than primary closure in this subset of patients that have undergone radical pelvic surgery or received preoperative radiation.[40] Similarly, obliteration of the pelvic defect should be done in patients likely to undergo postoperative radiation to prevent descent of the small bowel into the pelvis where it will be exposed to the radiation.[41] Gracilis, rectus abdominis, tensor fascia lata, and inferior gluteal flaps have all been used successfully to fill pelvic defects.[42–44] The potential for reducing pelvic adhesions by barrier agents such as Interceed/GoreTex is an additional consideration that merits exploration.

The lower urinary tract is vulnerable during pelvic surgery depending on the extent and proximity of dissection, preoperative radiotherapy, and extent of disease. Ureteral stents do not prevent these injuries, but do aid in early recognition and thus prompt correction. Dehiscence of intestinal and ureteral anastomoses has been reported[22,23,33] and appears to be more frequent after preoperative radiation. It can be minimized by using nonirradiated ileum or colon for formation of the ileal conduit.[22]

Other early complications that have been reported include fecal and urinary fistulas, urinary tract infections, hydronephrosis, retraction or separation of the stomas, thrombophlebitis, pulmonary embolism, evisceration, psychosis, cerebrovascular accident, prolonged ileus, atelectasis, and pneumonia.[16,22,23,25,28,33] Lower extremity complications such as deep venous thrombosis, perineal neuropathy, and compartment syndrome are rare but serious complications of prolonged pelvic surgery in the lithotomy position.[28]

Late complications occur quite often, making evident the importance of continued surgical follow-up. Late intestinal obstruction and enteroperineal fistula formation have been reported and surgical management of these problems entails a considerable risk.[22] The surgical therapy used is the same as that for early similar complications. Again, if the risk associated with dissection of the small intestines from the pelvis is high, an intestinal bypass procedure should be done. Although it is unlikely that an enteroperineal fistula will close after a bypass procedure, leaving a draining fistula in the perineum may be the proper choice if the risk involved in dissecting the small intestine from the pelvis is prohibitive.[22] Extensive resections of the small bowel should be avoided because they may lead to short bowel syndrome.

Pyelonephritis occurs as a late complication and is usually easily controlled with the proper antibiotics if there is no mechanical obstruction at the ureteral anastomosis that is causing stasis. If obstruction is present, it should be corrected surgically. Extensive dissection of the ureter in patients who have undergone radiation therapy incurs the risk of ischemic damage to the ureter and possible resultant ureteral fibrosis or fistulas. Acute episodes of ureteral obstruction in such patients may initially be managed by percutaneous nephrostomy to permit controlled urinary decompression; this allows time to assess the problem and plan elective reconstruction.

Other late complications include perineal, paracolostomy and incisional hernias.[22,25] They are usually amenable to surgical repair with use of conventional techniques, synthetic mesh or myocutaneous flaps.[22,43,45,46]

Follow-Up

The degree of surveillance required to detect early recurrence in an asymptomatic patient and whether it makes a difference in subsequent cure potential is controversial.[47] We believe that intense postoperative follow-up must be maintained in these patients. Careful history-taking with focus on recurrence of pain and other symptoms, serial physical exams, serum chemistries including carcinoembryonic antigen (CEA), and selected imaging studies must be monitored on a 3-month interval for the first 3 years. A postoperative pelvic CT should be obtained to serve as a baseline. Follow-up CT examination may indicate the need to obtain CT-directed biopsy to confirm recurrence or metastasis.

Results

In a review of the 53 patients who had resection for recurrent rectal cancer with curative intent, overall survival was 30% with a median of 32 months (Fig. 12.**10**, Table 12.**1**).[49] Preoperative CEA of less than 5 ng/ml was statistically significant in overall survival. The type of surgery for the primary tumor was significant. Patients who had an original abdominoperineal resection (APR) had worse disease-free survival vs. anterior resection (AR). Also there was no predictive value for primary tumor stage or free interval. Another group of eight patients underwent ASR resection for palliation of symptoms including: painful ulcerated, draining tumors. Four patients had sacral marrow involvement and three had distant metastases. Median survival was less than 12 months. Considering these results, patients at our institution are only resected with curative intent.

The extent of resection with respect to the level of the sacrum and the involved adjacent organs is shown in Table 12.**2**. Six patients had disease low enough (S4–5) that only an anterior approach was necessary.

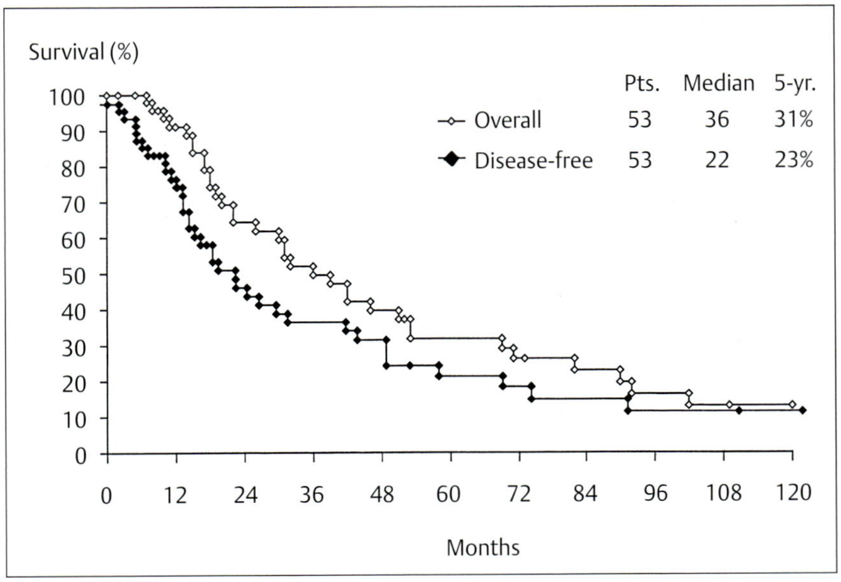

Fig. 12.**10** Overall and disease-free survival compared in 53 patients treated for recurrence by abdominosacral resection. Pts: number of patients; median: median survival time; 5-yr: five-year survival.

Table 12.**1** Prognostic factors related to survival after abdominosacral resection of pelvic recurrent rectal cancer

		Overall Survival			Disease-Free Survival		
	No Pts	**Median (months)**	**Five-year (%)**	**P-value**	**Median (months)**	**Five-year (%)**	**P-value**
Type of primary surgery*							
APR	30	22	18	0.01	14	13	>0.01
AR	19	53	41		43	28	
Preoperative CEA*							
>10 ng/ml	31	53	42	0.15	48	34	0.05
10 ng/ml	21	31	29.7	0.9	18	0	
Dukes stage of primary cancer							
Dukes B	23	42	37	0.9	29	20	0.9
Dukes C	23	31	29.7		18	0	
Free interval							
12 months	18	46	36	0.81	26	31	0.65
>12 months	35	36	30		22	21	

Median = median survival time; Five-year = five-year survival rate; APR = abdominoperineal resection; AR = anterior resection; CEA = carcinoembryonic antigen. *Significance according to disease-free survival: APR vs. AR, P 0.001; CEA 10 ng/ml, P 0.05

Table 12.**2** Level of resection and other organs resected

Surgery	**No. of patients (total = 53)**
Level of sacral resection	
L5–S1	1
High S1 or S1–2	32
Mid S2 or S3	14
Low S4–5*	6
Added resection	
Pelvic vessels-side wall	2
Pelvic lymph node dissection	53
Other organs resected	
Rectum	21
Bladder**	27
Partial bladder resection	6
Prostate/seminal vesicles	19
Vagina	9
Total abdominal hysterectomy	10
Segmental bowel resection	11

* Four patients resected via anterior approach. **All required ileal conduit

Table 12.**3** Pathologic extent of disease in pelvic resection group

Extent of tumor invasion	**No of patients (total = 53)**
Organ invasion	
Sacrum	
– Periosteum/cortex/ligament	30
– Marrow	7
– Plus side wall	8
Bladder/ureters	27
– With prostate/seminal vesicles	9
– With uterus/vagina	6
Pelvic lymph nodes (53 dissections; aortoiliac, -internal iliac and obturator nodes)	
– Lymph nodes negative	51
– Obturator nodes positive	1
– Para-aorta nodes positive	1
Surgical margins (histologic)	
– Clear	39
– Close (2 mm)	6
– Margin involved/marrow invasion	8

All patients in this curative group underwent pelvic node resection. Only seven patients had a partial bladder resection. In one case, a segmental resection of the common iliac artery and vein was performed. Table 12.**3** shows the pathology reviews of the specimens including extent of invasion and margin status.

Cumulative recurrence rate at 1, 3, and 5 years was 32, 66, and 80% respectively. Forty-four patients (76%) had recurrence after a mean of 22 months (median 14 months). Recurrence was local in 27%, distant in 52%, and local and distant in 20%. Re-resection or other therapies were done in 10 patients. Local-regional therapies included re-resection with or without pelvic perfusion, cryoablation, or radiofrequency ablation. Actual cure is suggested in eight patients who survived more than 90 months without evidence of disease.[49]

Our results are similar to those of others. Takagi et al.[50] reported on ASR in seven patients with localized recurrence of rectal cancer. Three of the patients died of recurrent disease, two were alive with recurrent disease in the lungs and pelvic wall, and two were alive without evidence of recurrence. Temple and Ketcham[27] performed single-stage ASR in 12 patients (nine of whom had rectal cancer) and reported a median disease-free survival time of 24 months and a 5-year disease-free survival rate of 18%. Because of the extent and complexity of this type of surgery, the term perioperative mortality should include 60 days, not the traditional 30. In our current series, two patients died of septic complications after 60 days and one patient died 5 months later of relapsing pneumonia. In the series by Mannaerts, two patients died of chronic infection and necrosis of the perineal wound at 3 and 4 months, respectively.

Survival varied according to the origin and histologic characteristics of the tumor. Of the 18 patients with primary cancers of the posterior pelvis, 16 were high grade sarcomas and two were chordomas. Nine were alive without evidence of disease 14 to 136 months after surgery. The estimated 5-year survival rate was 52%.

ASR is associated with considerable morbidity (Table 12.**1**).[48] In a series reported by Wanebo et al.,[6] the mean operative time was 18.5 hours and the mean blood loss was 10 000 mL. The overall long-term hospital mortality rate was 7.8% (6 of 76 patients). Two patients died within 48 hours of surgery. One patient died of platelet-induced coagulopathy and myocardial infarction 24 hours after resection for pelvic recurrence of rectal cancer. Another patient died of a myocardial infarction 48 hours after sacrectomy for a chordoma. Delayed deaths occurred at 35, 40, 52, and 90 days. Three of the patients died after resection for recurrent rectal cancer—one from a cerebrovascular accident and two from sepsis and multisystem failure. The fourth patient died with multiple small bowel fistulas, wound breakdown and sepsis 90 days after resection of a recurrent bladder cancer involving the symphysis pubis.[48] In an updated review of our ASR experience, including 53 patients with recurrent rectal cancer, 92% of the recurrences were isolated to the pelvis and 94% had prior radiation therapy. Interestingly, only one patient had prior liver resection for metastasis. Every patient had a complication: cardiovascular 35%, pulmonary 27%, gastrointestinal 27%, urologic 79%, musculoskeletal and neurologic 14%, sepsis 50%, and wound infection or dehiscence 70%.[49]

Major morbidity occurred more often in patients undergoing resections for advanced or recurrent rectal or epidermoid cancer than in those having resections for primary pelvic tumors. This was probably because the operation for primary cancer was shorter and most of the patients had not previously undergone radiation therapy. Of the 18 patients with primary tumors, only two had wound-related complications whereas among those with advanced or recurrent disease, six with epidermoid carcinoma and 22 with rectal adenocarcinoma had wound problems. Other complications in patients with primary tumors were intraoperative coagulopathy, postoperative hemorrhage, intestinal fistulas, urinary fistulas, urinary retention, urinary incontinence, renal failure, myonecrosis, and deep vein thrombosis (Table 12.**1**). There were no infectious complications.

Of the 58 patients having ASR for epidermoid or rectal cancer, 10 had cardiopulmonary insufficiency requiring prolonged intubation, six had postoperative hemorrhage necessitating another operative procedure, and five had renal failure. Wound infections occurred in 12 patients and flap separation in 16. Other complications in this group included myocardial ischemia, pneumonia, intestinal fistulas, urinary tract fistulas, small bowel obstruction, hydronephrosis, perineal nerve palsy, and deep vein thrombosis (see Table 12.**1**). Although six patients had documented deep vein thrombosis, no recognized episodes of pulmonary embolism occurred.

Less favorable results have been obtained with ASR for advanced epidermoid carcinoma of the anorectum. Although early epidermoid carcinomas are generally highly responsive to radiation and chemotherapy, advanced, bulky tumors are less responsive and require extensive resections to obtain local control.[51] In the series by Wanebo et al.,[51] of eight patients who had resection for epidermoid cancer with curative intent, six died of disease between 7 and 28 months after surgery and only one was alive without evidence of disease at 153 months. Because patients with recurrent epidermoid cancers of the cervix rarely present with isolated pelvic bone invasion, they are seldom candidates for major resections with curative intent.

In a recent series by Weber et al.,[52] 23 patients with locally advanced anal or recurrent rectal cancer were treated with preoperative radiotherapy, resection, and intraoperative electron radiation. At 19 to 54 months of follow-up, nine patients were alive, four with disease. Mean survival was 32.9 months. Kaplan–Meier survival for all patients was 82% at 1 year and 73% at 2 years. Fifty seven percent (13/23) of patients had another local recurrence develop at a mean of 17.2 months. Thirty five percent (8/23) developed metastases at a mean of 16.3 months.

An important objective of resection of advanced and recurrent pelvic tumors is relief from the unrelenting symptoms caused by such lesions. The results achieved with respect to this goal have been satisfactory. In a series described by Wanebo et al.,[39] 97% of the patients with long-term follow-up (>6 months) experienced relief of the initial symptoms of pelvic, perineal, or lower back pain. Takagi et al.[50] reported pain relief in all seven patients they treated with ASR for localized recurrence of rectal cancer. Appreciable pain relief was observed in 7 of 12 patients given sacropelvic resection by Pearlman et al.[15] Touran et al. reported good palliation in all 12 patients who had abdominosacral resection. Temple and Ketcham[27] also observed excellent palliation of pelvic pain in all nine of their patients who underwent curative resection for local recurrence.

Isolated pelvic perfusion has been used either to palliate unresectable tumors or as an attempt to enable resectability. In a series of 25 patients, Wanebo et al.[38,53,54] describe a closed balloon-occlusion technique for aortic and caval control. The amount of leakage to the systemic circulation was 28–38%. Ten of 15 patients treated for palliation had symptomatic pain relief. Of the 10 preoperative patients, one of five rectal cancer patients had a complete response and four out of five of patients with other types of malignancies had partial responses.

Patients' functional capacity after resection depends on the extent and level of the sacral resection. We found that those who had sacral resections at or distal to the level of S3 retained normal bladder and anorectal function. Bilateral resections above the S3 level compromised both anorectal and urogenital function. Unilateral resection of S1–S3 nerve roots will result in mild urinary dysfunction. In general, for anatomic reasons, female patients were less likely to have urinary retention. Patients with resections at the S1/S2 level could manage urologic function by practicing the Crede method at defined times. Male patients with high sacral resections (through the S1 level) also required periodic catheterization. In some patients, treatment with ephedrine lessened incontinence. Placement of a periurethral device for control of persistent incontinence was necessary in one patient after resection of a sacral chondrosarcoma. Impairment of anorectal function can be managed by rectal irrigation every other day. Kegel exercises may aid rectal tone. A penile implant can be placed in men with impotence.

Twelve of 34 patients (35%) had persistent postoperative pain, typically new phantom pain or causalgia and local symptoms related to delayed wound healing. In 7 of the 12 patients, the symptoms improved during ensuing months, often with administration of amitriptyline or carbamazepine. Although long-term neurologic sequelae were unusual, many patients did have short-term lower extremity symptoms, including unsteadiness, diminished lower leg strength, and sensory deficits in the foot. Serious locomotive dysfunction was evident only in those who had resections involving the S1 and S2 roots bilaterally. Bilateral S1 nerve root resection results in complete bladder denervation and loss of plantar flexion but does not compromise walking. Although resection of S1 could affect pelvic ring stability and therefore walking potential, this has not been a problem in any patients having resections through S1. The preservation of the L5–S1 joint appears to ensure adequate stability. Functional outcomes are shown in Table 12.**3**. Overall, 66% of the patients returned to their previous lifestyle and 43% returned to work. In general, function was impaired for only about 3 months. All patients were referred for rehabilitation and usually required aggressive outpatient therapy.

Our results show that radical surgery for locally advanced yet isolated pelvic tumor is the only chance for cure and improvement of quality of life in these patients. Curative resection may result in 5-year survival rates of 20 to 50%.[55–59] En bloc resection of the involved sacrum along with the exenteration of pelvic viscera is a modification that has evolved in an effort to avoid dissection through "cancerous adhesions."[60–62] Although it may be tempting to dissect the tumor off of the bone in the plane of the presacral fascia, our series showed that the sacrum was pathologically involved in 52%. The literature shows colorectal tumor invasion of adhesions in 24 to 100%. Numerous studies have shown that the 5-year survival decreases from 45–60% to 17–23% if the tumor is torn or adhesions are dissected.[61–63]

□ Conclusion

Technical advancements have been made in imaging, staging, patient selection, perioperative critical care, free flaps, brachytherapy, and even more experimental techniques such as perfusion. Thus, in these times of minimally invasive surgery, ASR is a radical but still realistic option in certain patients. Pelvic recurrence of rectal cancer can be resected safely with the expectation of long-term survival. Careful patient selection based on known risk factors can identify those most likely to benefit from resection versus those best served by nonresectional palliation.

The importance of careful follow-up of patients who have undergone extended radical pelvic surgery cannot be overestimated. In many of them, recurrence or metastases, late postoperative complications, psychologic or marital problems develop. The surgeon should play a major role in coordinating the follow-up and managing the problems that arise. Despite the profound anatomic and functional changes associated with extended radical pelvic surgery, patients with proper support and rehabilitation can adjust and live meaningful, productive lives.

□ References

1. Ariel IM, Shah JP. The conservative hemipelvectomy. *Surg Gynecol Obstet*. 1977;144:406–413.
2. Eilber FR, Grant TT, Saka D, Morton DL. Internal hemipelvectomy. Excision of the hemipelvis with limb preservation. An alternative to hemipelvectomy. *Cancer*. 1979;43: 806–809.
3. Enneking WE. Pelvis. In: Enneking WE, ed. *Musculoskeletal Tumor Surgery*. Vol 1. New York: Churchill Livingstone; 1983: 483.
4. Karakousis CP. The abdominoinguinal incision in limb salvage and resection of pelvic tumors. *Cancer*. 1984;54: 2543–2548.

5. Karakousis CP, Vezeridis MP. Variants of hemipelvectomy and their complications. *Am J Surg.* 1983;145:273–277.
6. Wanebo HJ, Koness RJ, Turk PS, Cohen SI. Composite resection of posterior pelvic malignancy. *Ann Surg.* 1992;215:685–693.
7. Wanebo HJ, Temple WJ, Popp MB, Dowil CE, Yablonski M. Combination regional therapy for extremity sarcoma: A tricenter study. *Arch Surg.* 1990;125:355–359.
8. Wanebo HJ, Turk PS. Abdominal sacral resection for recurrent cancer of the rectum. In: Bauer JJ, ed. *Colorectal Surgery Illustrated.* Chicago: Mosby-Year Book; 1993: 241.
9. Gunterberg B, Kewenter J, Petersen I et al: Anorectal function after major resections of the sacrum with bilateral or unilateral sacrifice of sacral nerves. *Br J Surg.* 1976;63: 546–554.
10. Karakousis CP. Sacral resection with preservation of continence. *Surg Gynecol Obstet.* 1986;163:270–273.
11. MacCarty CS, Waugh JM, Coventry MB, O'Sullivan. Sacrococygeal chordomas. *Surg Gynecol Obstet.* 1961;113 :551–554.
12. MacCarty CS, Waugh JM, Mayo CW, Coventry MB. The surgical treatment of presacral tumors: A combined problem. *Proc Mayo Clin.* 1952;27:73–84.
13. Sundadresan N, Huvos AG, Krol G, Lane JM, Brennan M. Surgical treatment of spinal chordomas. *Arch Surg.* 1987; 122:1479–1482.
14. Miller TR, MacKenzie AR, Randall HT et al. Hemicorporectomy. *Surgery.* 1966;59:998–993.
15. Pearlman NW, Donohue RE, Stiegmann GV, Ahnen DJ, Sedlacek SM, Braun TJ. Pelvic and sacropelvic exenteration for locally advanced or recurrent anorectal cancer. *Arch Surg.* 1987;122:537–541.
16. Wanebo HJ, Marcove RC. Abdominal sacral resection of locally recurrent rectal cancer. *Ann Surg.* 1981;194: 458–471.
17. Wanebo HJ, Gaker DL, Whitehill R, Morgan RF, Constable WC. Pelvic recurrence of rectal cancer: Options for curative resection. *Ann Surg.* 1987;205:482–495.
18. DeSaia PJ, Creasman WT. *Clinical Gynecology Oncology.* 5th ed. St Louis: Mosby; 1997.
19. Pilipshen SJ, Heilweil M, Quan SH Stemberg SS, Enker WE. Patterns of pelvic recurrence following definitive resections of rectal cancer. *Cancer.* 1984;53:1354–1362.
20. MacFarlane JK, Ryall RDH, Heald RJ. Mesorectal excision for rectal cancer. *Lancet.* 1993;341:457–460.
21. Rao AR, Kagan AR, Chan PM, Gilbert HA, Nussbaum H, Hitz BL. Patterns of recurrence following curative resection alone for adenocarcinoma of the rectum and sigmoid colon. *Cancer.* 1981;48:1492–1495.
22. Bricker EM, Kraybill WG, Lopez MJ, Hohnston WD. The current role of ultraradical surgery in the treatment of pelvic cancer. *Curr Probl Surg.* 1986;23:869–953.
23. Eisenberg SB, Kraybill WG, Lopez MJ. Long-term results of surgical resection of locally advanced colorectal carcinoma. *Surgery.* 1990;108:779–786.
24. Jakowatz JG, Porudominsky D, Riihimaki DU et al. Complications of pelvic exenteration. *Arch Surg.* 1985;120: 1261–1265.
25. Kraybill WG, Lopez MJ, Bricker EM. Total pelvic exenteration as a therapeutic option in advanced malignant disease of the pelvis. *Surg Gynecol Obstet.* 1988;166:259–263.
26. Lopez MJ, Kraybill WG, Downey RS, Johnston WD, Bricker EM. Exenterative surgery for locally advanced rectosigmoid cancers. Is it worthwhile? *Surgery.* 1987;102 644–651.
27. Temple WJ, Ketcham AS. The closure of large pelvic defects by extended compound tensor fascia lata and inferior gluteal myocutaneous flaps. *Am J Clin Oncol.* 1982;5:573–577.
28. Baur JJ, ed. *Colorectal Surgery Illustrated: a Focused Approach.* St Louis: Mosby; 1993: 395.
29. Peters P, Baker SR, Leopold PW, Taub NA, Burnand KG. Compartment syndrome following prolonged pelvic surgery. *Brit J Surg.* 1994;81:1128–1131.
30. Martin FE, Boyd SD. Artificial urinary sphincter in patients following major pelvic surgery and/or radiotherapy: are they less favorable candidates? *J Urol.* 1995;153: 1188–1193.
31. De Hass WG, Miller MJ, Temple WJ et al. Perineal wound closure with the rectus abdominus musculocutaneous flap after tumor ablation. *Ann Surg Oncol.* 1995;2:400–406.
32. Boey J, Wong J, Ong GB. Pelvic exenteration for locally advanced colorectal carcinoma. *Ann Surg.* 1982;195: 513–518.
33. Eldar S, Kemeny MM, Terz JJ. Extended resections for carcinoma of the colon and rectum. *Surg Gynecol Obstet.* 1985; 161:219.
34. Jaffe BM, Bricker EM, Butcher HR Jr. Surgical complications of ileal segment urinary diversion. *Ann Surg.* 1968;167: 367–376.
35. Devereau DF, Sears HF, Ketchem AS. Intestinal fistula following pelvic exenteration surgery: Predisposing causes and treatment. *J Surg Oncol.* 1980;14:227–234.
36. Lifshitz S, Johnson R, Roberts JA, Buchsbaum HJ. Intestinal fistula and obstruction following pelvic exenteration. *Surg Gynecol Obstet.* 1981;152:630–632.
37. Polk HC, Butcher HR Jr, Bricker EM. Perineal fecal fistula following pelvic exenteration. *Surg Gynecol Obstet.* 1966; 123:308–312.
38. Kiselow M, Butcher HR Jr, Bricker EM. Results of the radical surgical treatment of advanced pelvic cancer: A fifteen-year study. *Ann Surg.* 1967;166:428–436.
39. Khoo AK, Skibber JM, Nabawi AS et al. Indications for immediate tissue transfer for soft tissue reconstruction in visceral pelvic surgery. *Surgery.* 2001;130:463–469.
40. Wheeless CR Jr. Small bowel bypass for complications related to pelvic malignancy. *Obstet Gynecol.* 1973;42: 661–666.
41. Devine RM, Dozois RR. Surgical management of locally advanced adenocarcinoma of the rectum. *World J Surg.* 1992;16:486–489.
42. Miller LB, Steele G, Cady B, Wolfort FG, Bothe A Jr. Resection of tumors in irradiated fields with subsequent immediate reconstruction. *Arch Surg.* 1987;122:461–466.
43. Palmer JA, Vernon CP, Cummings BJ, Moffat FL. Gracilis myocutaneous flap for reconstructing perineal defects resulting from radiation and radical surgery. *Can J Surg.* 1983;26:510–512.
44. Ledesma EJ, Bruno S, Mittelman A. Total pelvic exenteration in colorectal disease: A 20-year experience. *Ann Surg.* 1981;194:701–703.
45. Leuchter RS, Lagasse LD, Hacker NF, Berek JS. Management of postexenteration perineal hernias by myocutaneous axial flaps. *Gynecol Oncol.* 1982;14:15–22.
46. Porell WJ, Parsons L. Perineal hernia repair with nylon mesh. *Surgery.* 1958;43:447–451.
47. Enker WE, Kramer RG. The follow-up of patients after definitive resections for large bowel cancer. *World J Surg.* 1982;6:578–584.
48. Vezeridis MP, Wanebo HJ. Sacral resection of posterior pelvic malignancy. *Cancer Invest.* 1995;13:375–380.

49. Wanebo HJ, Belliveau J, Begossi G, Levy A. Isolated chemotherapeutic perfusion of the pelvis for advanced rectal cancer. *Colorectal Dis.* 2003;5:508–514.
50. Takagi H, Morimoto T, Hara S, Suguki R, Horio S. Seven cases of pelvic exenteration combined with sacral resection for locally recurrent rectal cancer. *J Surg Oncol.* 1986;32:184–188.
51. Wanebo HJ, Furgell W, Constable W. Multimodality approach to surgical management of locally advanced epidermoid carcinoma of the anorectum. *Cancer.* 1981;47: 2817–2826.
52. Weber KL, Nelson H, Gunderson LL, Sim FH. Sacropelvic resection for recurrent anorectal cancer. A multidisciplinary approach. *Clin Orthop.* 2000;372:231–240.
53. Turk PS, Belliveau JF, Darnowski JW, Weinberg MC, Leenen L, Wanebo HJ. Isolated pelvic perfusion for unresectable cancer using a balloon occlusion technique. *Arch Surg.* 1993;128:538–539.
54. Wanebo HJ, Chung MA, Levy AI, Turk PS, Vezeridis MP, Belliveau JF. Preoperative therapy for advanced pelvic malignancy by isolated pelvic perfusion with the balloon-occlusion technique. *Ann Surg Oncol.* 1996;3:295–303.
55. Turk PS, Wanebo HJ. Results of surgical treatment of nonhepatic recurrence of colorectal carcinoma. *Cancer.* 1993; 71:4267–4277.
56. Yeung RS, Moffat FL, Falk RE. Pelvic exenteration for recurrent colorectal carcinoma: a review. *Cancer Investigation.* 1994;12:176–188.
57. Ogunbiyi OA, McKenna K, Birnbaum EH, Fleshman JW, Kodner IJ. Aggressive surgical management of recurrent rectal cancer-is it worthwhile? *Dis Colon Rectum.* 1997; 40:150–155.
58. Meterissian SH, Skibber JM, Giacco GG, El-Naggar AK, Hess KR, Rich TA. Pelvic exenteration for locally advanced rectal carcinoma: factors predicting improved survival. *Surgery.* 1997;121:479–487.
59. Law WL, Chu KW, Choi HK. Total pelvic exenteration for locally advanced rectal cancer. *J Am Coll Surg.* 2000;190: 78–83.
60. Lehnert T, Methner M, Pollok A, Schaible A, Hinz V, Herfarth C. Multivisceral resection for locally advanced primary colon and rectal cancer. An analysis of prognostic factors in 201 patients. *Ann Surg.* 2002;235:217–225.
61. Sugarbaker PH, Corlew S. Influence of surgical techniques on survival in patients with colorectal cancer. *Dis Colon Rectum.* 1982;25:545–557.
62. Gall FP, Tonak J, Altendorf A. Multivisceral resections in colorectal cancer. *Dis Colon Rectum.* 1987;30:337–341.

Peritoneum 5

13 Peritonectomy for Carcinomatosis, Sarcomatosis, and Mesothelioma

Paul H. Sugarbaker

Peritoneal seeding is a frequent cause of surgical treatment failure and subsequent death of patients with abdominopelvic malignancies. The clinical presentation of peritoneal carcinomatosis, sarcomatosis, or mesothelioma may occur concomitant with the primary tumor or as recurrence in a patient with a prior resection of cancer. In the former, dissemination of cancer cells is spontaneous and dependent upon the anatomic site, histology, size, and depth of invasion of the primary malignancy. In the latter instance cancer spread is usually caused by a lack of containment during surgery.[1] Tumor emboli released from severed lymphatic channels, traumatized narrow margins of resection, and retained venous blood, implant on peritoneal surfaces and within the resection site. Progression of implants is promoted by the wound healing process. In a large proportion of patients this surface dissemination occurs in the absence of lymphatic and hematogenous metastasis so that its eradication can result in long-term survival. New knowledge regarding the pathobiology of the peritoneal surface dissemination of abdominopelvic malignancy has permitted the development of treatment strategies to attack a clinical situation previously managed only by palliative care.[2] The utilization of peritonectomy procedures combined with perioperative intraperitoneal chemotherapy offers a new paradigm to prevent and to treat cancer on peritoneal surfaces. As a result of these new modalities peritoneal carcinomatosis, sarcomatosis, and mesothelioma can be treated with curative intent.

With prevention and curative treatment of peritoneal surface malignancy as an accepted goal, a modification of the surgical approach to the patient with abdominal and pelvic cancer develops. A surgical approach directed at the complete eradication of the disease requires new technical skills that allow safe and effective peritonectomy procedures that fulfill the intent of the treatment. Our purpose is to describe this current strategy for prevention and treatment of peritoneal surface malignancy with an emphasis on the technical details utilized in the performance of peritonectomy procedures.

□ Patient Position and Incision

For patient safety throughout a prolonged surgical procedure, careful positioning is required. We advocate the lithotomy position with open legs, thighs flexed at 15° on the abdomen and legs flexed 30° on the thighs (see Fig. 11.**1**, chapter 11). The legs are supported with St. Mark leg holders (AMSCO, Erie, PA) surrounded by alternating pressure devices (SCB Compression Boots, Kendall, Boston, MA), and protected from decubitus lesions by egg crate foam padding. The weight of the lower extremity is on the heel and not on the calf or popliteal crease.

The incision must be from the xiphoid to symphysis pubis; the xiphoid is excised. When combined with a self-retaining retractor (Thompson Surgical Instruments, Traverse City, MI), such an incision allows access and free continuous visualization of the abdominal and pelvic cavity (see Fig. 11.**2**, chapter 11). This exposure of the operative field facilitates complete lysis of adhesions and thorough peritoneal cavity exploration. In reoperative surgery the xiphoid to pubic incision includes a wide excision of the prior surgical scar from the skin to the peritoneum, including the umbilicus. Unless there is a wide resection of prior incisions many recurrences take place in the prior incision.[3] For this reason old incisions, as opposed to new incisions, are preferred.

□ Lysis of Adhesions, Exploration, and Retraction

Currently, a major proportion of treatment for peritoneal surface malignancy is directed at recurrent disease. This timing should change as therapeutic strategies to prevent carcinomatosis and sarcomatosis become accepted and surgeons definitively interrupt further progression of primary disease presenting with seeding. In the patients operated in a recurrent disease setting, adhesions are a common problem during reoperative intervention. Adhesions alter the normal anatomy and prevent adequate exploration required to assess the extent of disease. Therefore, complete lysis of adhesions is the necessary initial dissection of the abdomen and pelvis. When entering the abdominal cavity, elevation of the abdominal wall using strong traction from skin hooks will minimize the possibility

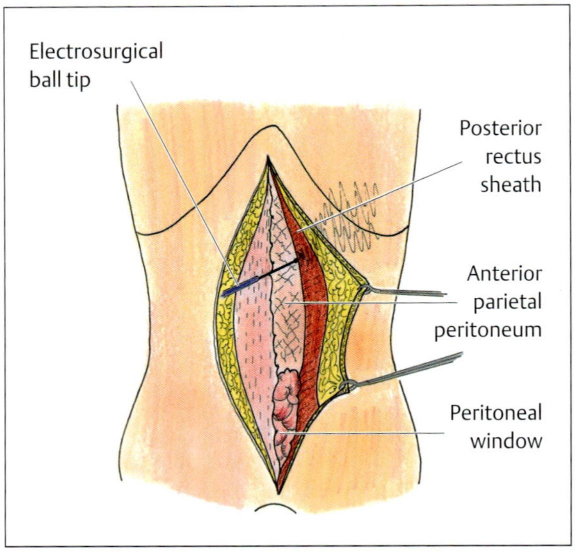

Fig. 13.**1** Abdominal wall under tension to allow lysis of adhesions between the abdominal wall and the underlying bowel and preservation of the rectus abdominis muscle.

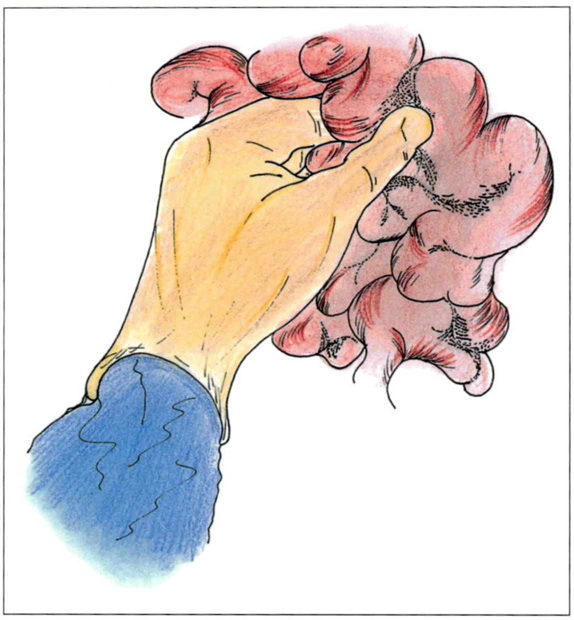

Fig. 13.**2** The lysis and resection of intestinal adhesions requires finger and ball-tip electrosurgical dissection, irrigation, and smoke evacuation.

of damage to small bowel loops adherent to the abdominal incision (Fig. 13.**1**). Care must be taken to preserve the rectus abdominis muscles. These muscles will be needed postoperatively for patient mobilization and respiratory function. However, sacrifice of the posterior rectus sheath may facilitate a more rapid entrance beyond the scar associated with the prior incision. The abdominal wall must be cleared of viscera for a distance of 7–10 cm from the edges of the abdominal incision; following this the self-retaining retractor is inserted and will facilitate enterolysis. Compression of tissues between thumb and index finger will thin out abdominal adhesions between bowel and abdominal wall or between bowel loops. This compression is a form of blunt dissection that can avoid damage to intestinal structures by adding tactile sensation to visualization in order to separate loops of intestine (Fig. 13.**2**).

As a requirement of complete exploration, resection of the gastrohepatic and gastrocolic ligaments must be performed. Exploration of the omental bursa is not possible unless it is widely opened.

Seromuscular tears are frequent during dissection in patients with many adhesions. These tears are marked with a single stitch and repaired definitely after intraoperative chemotherapy has been completed. Since adhesions in progressive abdominal-pelvic cancer are likely to contain tumor foci, the fibrous tissue is not merely divided but is resected and then collected for histopathologic examination. This complete clearance of adhesions is essential not only for a proper decision regarding the surgical procedure but also for the uniform distribution of intraperitoneal chemotherapy.

There are great advantages for mechanical retraction in performing peritonectomy procedures. The Thompson self-retaining retractor is the most useful and versatile instrument (see Fig. 11.**2**, Chapter 11). It allows multiple angles of retraction to be applied at variable strengths on the abdominal wall. Also, a second tier of retraction to remove viscera from an operative site can greatly facilitate dissection or suturing. The major function of the self-retaining retractor is a sustained complete visualization of the entire operative field that allows for centripetal dissection.

Electrosurgical Dissection

After division of the skin with a scalpel, all subsequent dissection is performed with electroevaporative surgery.[4] This methodology requires a ball-tipped electrosurgical handpiece. The preferred tip diameter is 0.3 cm and the tip is extended 10 cm beyond the hand control device (Fig. 13.**3**). The ball-tip is powered by a high-voltage electrosurgical generator. For dissection one commonly uses maximal pure cut. The pure-cut mode electroevaporizes the tissues that are in contact; this eliminates the accumulation of tissue debris as occurs with coagulation current. The buildup of coagulated tissue and distortion of normal anatomy obscures visualization of the dissection site. Because of the high voltage, the electroevaporation of tissue produces a copious amount of smoke that interferes with visualization of the operative field. The smoke is an important health hazard that needs to be eliminated from the operating room environment. To evacuate the smoke, a laser-smoke evacuator is necessary for electroevaporative surgery.

In addition to excess smoke production requiring a smoke vacuum, to prevent heat damage, frequent intermittent saline irrigation at the site of tissue dissection is necessary. Heat necrosis is of great value at the margin of dissection to minimize disease progression. Heat necrosis of a tubular structure can cause fistula formation that results in excessive morbidity and mortality. Frequent saline cooling is essential.

A major advantage of ball-tip electrosurgical dissection is the creation of a lens-shaped (lenticular) defect as a result of the electroevaporation of the tissue (Fig. 13.**4**). If strong traction is maintained at the plane of dissection, visualization of vital structures occurs before injury occurs. In contrast, the defect created by a blade-tip is linear so that a visual monitor of the structures at the deepest extent of the dissection is not possible. Consequently the risk of damage to vital structures is much greater with blade dissection than with ball-tip dissection.

Long-term local control of peritoneal implants as a result of ball-tip electrosurgical dissection is related to the growth pattern of the tumor. Adenocarcinoma is an infiltrative process and electrosurgery may only remove the superficial portion of the tumor mass. Although small implants are minimally invasive, deeper resection of large adenocarcinoma implants can provoke severe damage to the underlying structures. In contrast cystadenocarcinoma (adenomucinosis) or low-grade sarcomas may have an expansive growth with minimal invasion of the underlying tissues. The ball-tip dissection can resect the tumor mass leaving behind little or no residual tumor. The long-term success of intraperitoneal chemotherapy in maintaining control of peritoneal surface malignancy may depend on the mass of residual malignancy that remains following cytoreduction. Microscopic residual disease is reliably controlled by intraperitoneal chemotherapy; control of macroscopic or gross residual disease is not usually maintained (Fig. 13.**5**).

During dissection pure-cut electroevaporative surgery provides absolute hemostasis of small vessels up to 1.0 mm in diameter. Coagulation current can control vessels from 1.0 to 3.0 mm in diameter. Electrosurgery is most effective in providing hemostasis if the vessel is compressed by upward traction by the index finger of the nondominant hand. The vessel walls are reliably sealed together if the blood has been eliminated from within the lumen. Larger vessels are first visualized by electrosurgical dissection, and then clearly defined from surrounding fat by "thumb and index finger compression." Once clearly visualized the larger vessels are ligated in continuity and divided. The same technique is also applied to large lymphatic vessels. Absolute hemostasis and lymphostasis combined with frequent large

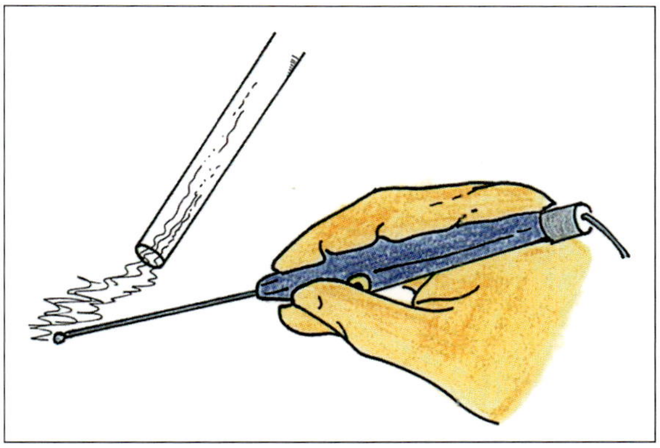

Fig. 13.**3** Ball-tip electrosurgical device.

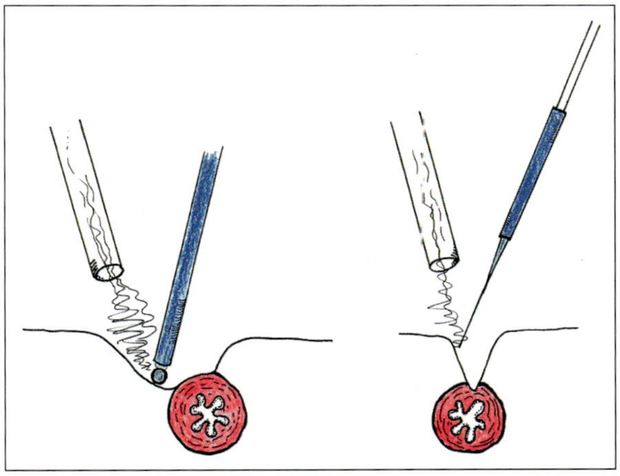

Fig. 13.**4** Comparison of the operative defect created by ball-tip and blade-tip electrosurgery.

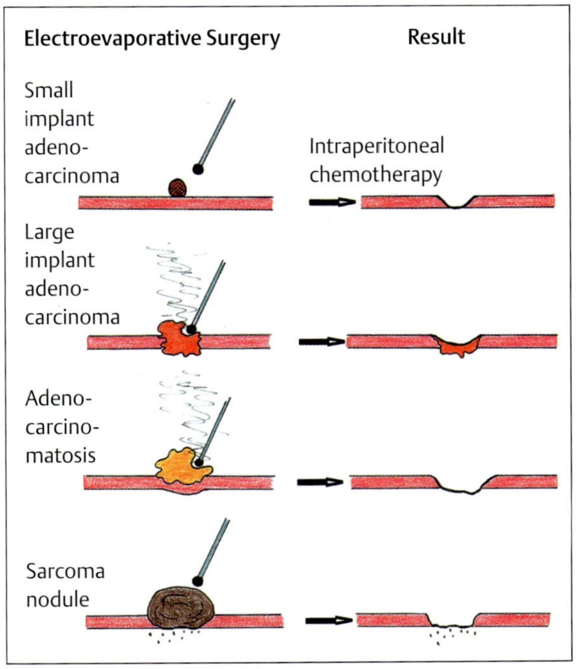

Fig. 13.**5** Long-term local control expected after ball-tip electrosurgical dissection and perioperative intraperitoneal chemotherapy with different peritoneal surface tumors.

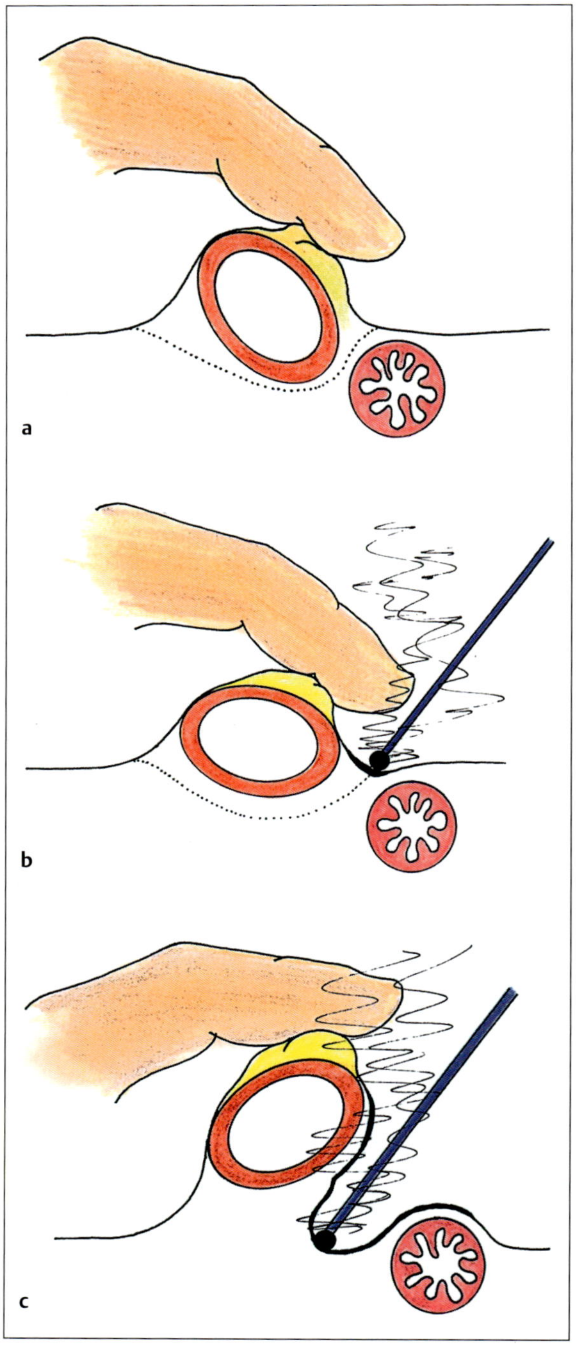

Fig. 13.**6** A narrow margin of dissection may be a cancer-free margin if a thin layer of heat necrosis occurs from the electro-evaporative surgery.

volume irrigation and suction are responsible for a clean operative field and clear visualization of all vital structures. The translucent nature of the tissues should be maintained by eliminating blood from the operative field. The result should be minimal blood loss and no disruption of cancerous masses as the centripetal dissection proceeds.

In some instances a generous free margin of dissection is not possible in performing peritonectomy. Ball-tip electrosurgical dissection destroys tumor foci encountered at the interface of cancerous peritoneum and normal tissue during peritonectomy by causing a heat necrosis layer up to 1.0 mm in thickness from the dissection margins. This margin of heat necrosis provides a small but usually adequate tumor free margin that often results in curative peritonectomy (Fig. 13.**6a–c**). If narrow margins of dissection are attempted using scissor or knife dissection the margins of the peritonectomy are extensively tumor contaminated so that perioperative intraperitoneal chemotherapy is less likely to eradicate residual cancer cells. Peritonectomy can only be maximally effective using electroevaporative surgery.

Irrigation and Suction

Irrigation and suction should be repeated continuously during electrosurgical dissection. Although heat necrosis may provide an essential cancer-free margin of dissection, electrosurgical dissection may provoke heat damage to vital structures, especially tubular structures. Repeated saline irrigation cools dissected tissues and clears tissue debris and blood from the operative field. If blood is repeatedly cleared from within the operative field the translucent nature of the tissues is preserved. This results in minimal inadvertent damage to vital structures. Strong and complete suction is essential to evacuate blood, fibrin, and saline that continuously accumulate within the operative field.

At the end of surgery, copious irrigation of the abdominal cavity with a solution of 1% hydrogen peroxide may help in reducing the number of cancer cells trapped within blood clots. Also, residual blood within the abdomen and pelvis will cause postoperative adhesions. Free cancer cells and tumor emboli that are retained within the operative site may progress rapidly stimulated by growth factors modulating the wound healing process.

The electroevaporation caused by electrosurgery results in copious smoke production. The release of these carbonized tissues into the air creates a health hazard within the operating room environment. Also, smoke obscures clear visualization of the operative field. Especially in deep dissections as in the chest, under the diaphragm, or in the pelvis, smoke will obscure the operative field and makes surgery unsafe. A smoke evacuator is an essential tool necessary for electroevaporative surgery.

Peritonectomy Procedures

The most fundamental technique of cytoreductive surgery is the peritoneal stripping procedure. With this methodology all of the parietal peritoneum of the abdo-

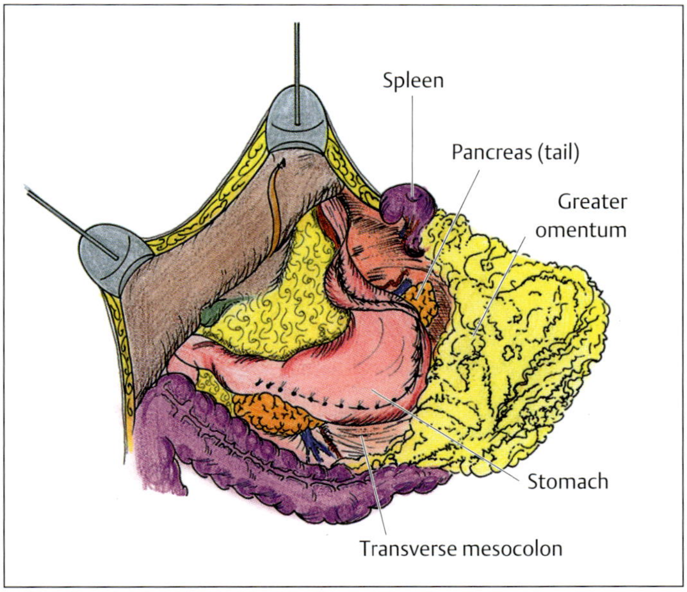

Fig. 13.7 Dissection of the greater omentum.

men and pelvis involved by tumor is stripped away. The implants on visceral peritoneum are individually electroevaporized if they are small and diffuse. If large tumor nodules are present on small bowel surfaces this portion of the intestine must be resected. The surgeon's goal must be to remove all visible evidence of cancer implants in order to maximize the benefits of perioperative intraperitoneal chemotherapy. The long-term results of local-regional chemotherapy are optimized if the volume of residual cancer is minimal. The following paragraphs describe the surgical technique of peritonectomy.

☐ Techniques

Greater Omentectomy and Splenectomy

The greater omentum is resected in order to free the midabdomen of large volume disease and to improve visualization of the residual abdominal cavity. The greater omentum is elevated and separated from the transverse colon using electroevaporative surgery (Fig. 13.**7**). The dissection continues beneath the peritoneum that covers the anterior aspect of the transverse mesocolon in order to expose the anterior peritoneal surface of the pancreas. All branches of the gastroepiploic vessels on the greater curvature of the stomach and the short gastric vessels are transected. The last step of this procedure is the resection of the spleen. This allows exposure and complete dissection of tumor implants on the anterior fascia of the pancreas.

Left Upper Quadrant Peritonectomy

In order to strip peritoneum and tumor from the undersurface of the left hemidiaphragm, the dissection of the peritoneum is begun from the posterior sheath of the rectus muscle. The dissected peritoneum is secured and traction maintained with the help of clamps at 10-cm intervals (Fig. 13.**8**). In performing the left upper quadrant peritonectomy, the following structures are exposed: the undersurface of the left hemidiaphragm muscle, left adrenal gland, distal portion of the pancreas, and cephalad one half of the perirenal fat. The completed left upper quadrant peritonectomy is shown in Figure 13.**9**.

Right Upper Quadrant Peritonectomy

As in the left upper quadrant peritonectomy, the right upper quadrant peritonectomy begins by stripping peritoneum from the posterior rectus sheath beginning at the edge of the abdominal incision. Dissection is favored by strong traction with clamps and performed with electrosurgery to prevent blood loss (Fig. 13.**10**). The dissection is continued up to the bare area of the liver. At this point, the eradication of the tumor on the anterior surface of the liver may occur in two different ways. If there are isolated patches of tumor, it is possible to electroevaporize them with the distal 2 cm of the ball-tip bent and freed from insulation (hockey stick configuration). If the tumor involves a major portion of the Glisson's capsule, the best approach involves a dissection beneath tumor through the capsule itself. If possible, the specimen should be maintained intact. Dissection continues laterally on the right stripping

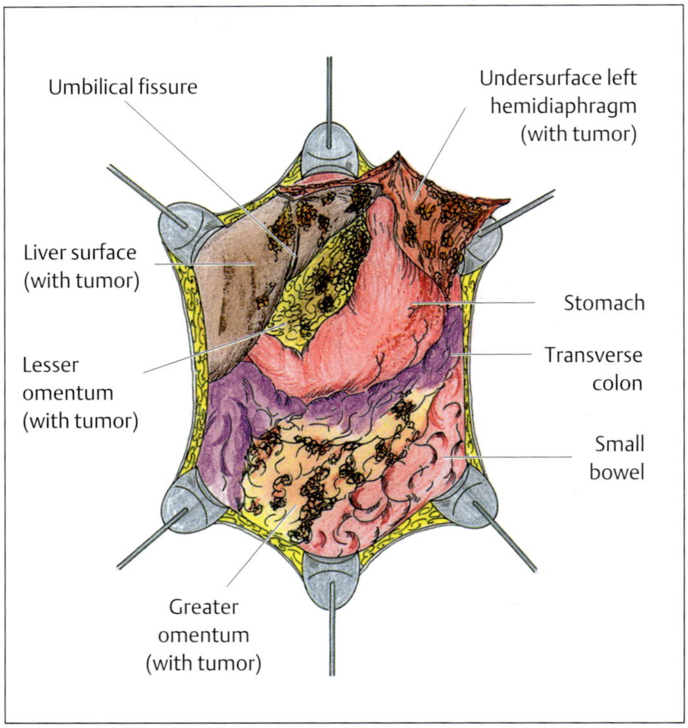

Fig. 13.**8** Abdominal cavity after greater omentectomy and splenectomy.

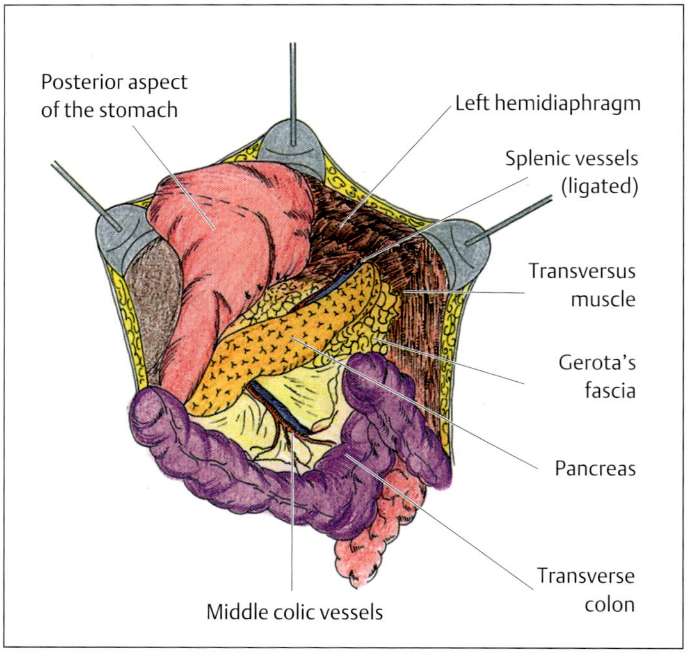

Fig. 13.**9** Stripping of the left upper quadrant peritoneum completed.

the peritoneum away from the right perirenal fat and thereby freeing the right subhepatic space (Morrison's pouch) of tumor (Fig. 13.**11**). In this area the surgeon must be careful not to damage the inferior vena cava and the caudate lobe veins that pass between the vena cava and segment I of the liver. At the end of the procedure, it is possible to see the right upper quadrant freed from peritoneum and tumor between the right costal margin and the liver displaced medially. As shown in Figure 13.**12**, the following structures are visualized at the completion of the right upper quadrant peritonectomy: the undersurface of the right hemidiaphragm with anterior branch of the phrenic artery and vein, right hepatic vein, inferior vena cava, right adrenal gland, and the cephalad one half of the perirenal fat surrounding the right kidney.

Sometimes during performance of left and/or right upper quadrant peritonectomy, tumor may be invasive into the central tendon of the diaphragm. In this situation it is necessary to resect the peritoneum together

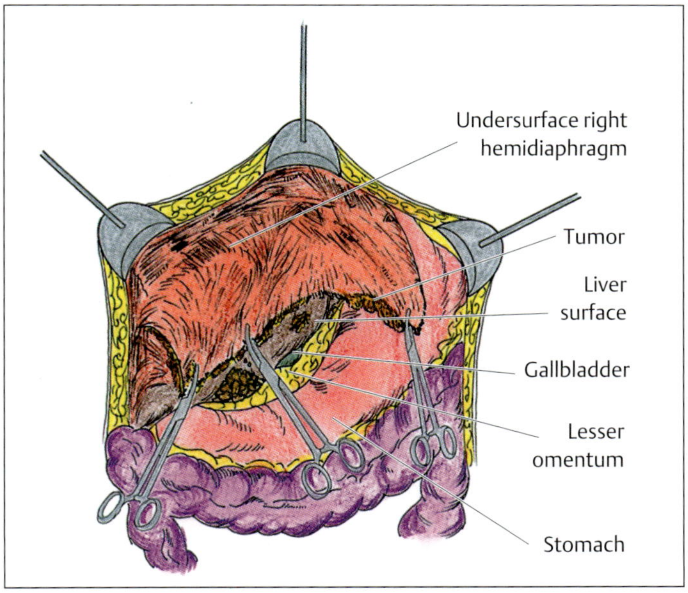

Fig. 13.**10** Stripping of the right upper quadrant peritoneum.

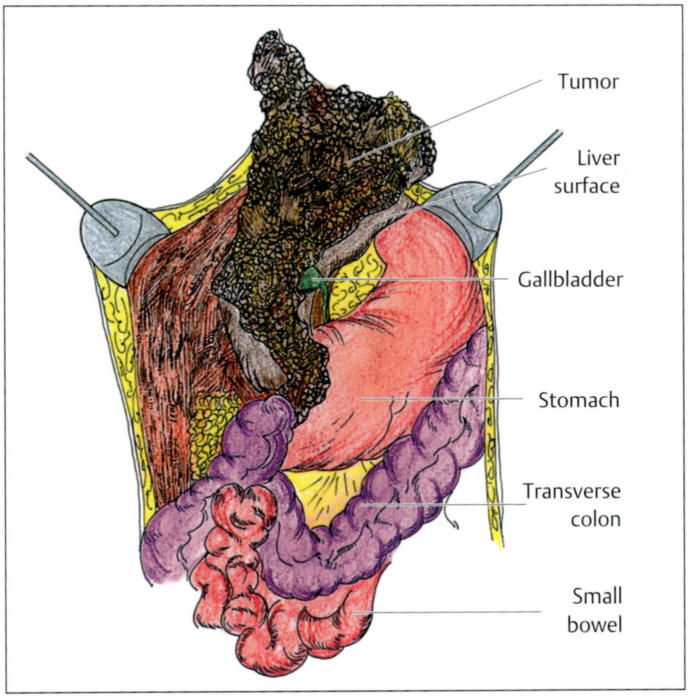

Fig. 13.**11** Resection of the Glisson's capsule involved by the tumor in the right upper quadrant.

with a generous portion of the central tendon involved by the tumor. Reconstruction is carried out after intraoperative chemotherapy of the peritoneum and pleural space in order to avoid implantation of tumor cells within the pleural space.

Pelvic Peritonectomy with Resection of the Rectosigmoid Colon, Uterus, Fallopian tubes, and Ovaries

Even though all anatomic structures within the pelvis are fused together by malignancy, a complete extirpation of the disease is possible in most patients (Fig. 13.**13**). The pelvic peritonectomy begins with the centripetal dissection of peritoneum from the posterior aspect of the lower abdominal incision. The dissection proceeds towards the bladder avoiding the muscular layer of this structure (Fig. 13.**14**). The urachus is divided at the superior aspect of the bladder and used for traction. Traction is important in this phase of dissection because of the high risk of bladder injury; strong traction on the bladder helps to define the proper plane of dissection. In the female with uterus in place, the round ligaments are electrosurgically transected at the level of the internal inguinal ring. Peritoneal stripping is continued within the false and true pelvis taking care to

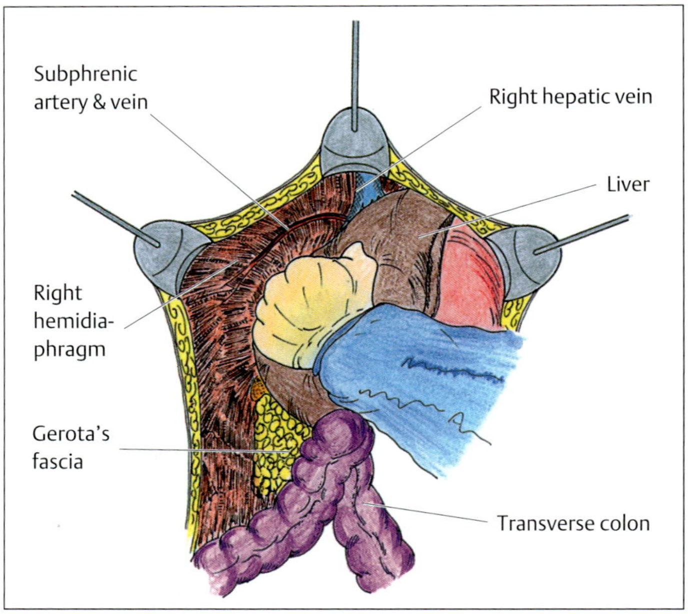

Fig. 13.**12** Stripping of the right upper quadrant peritoneum completed.

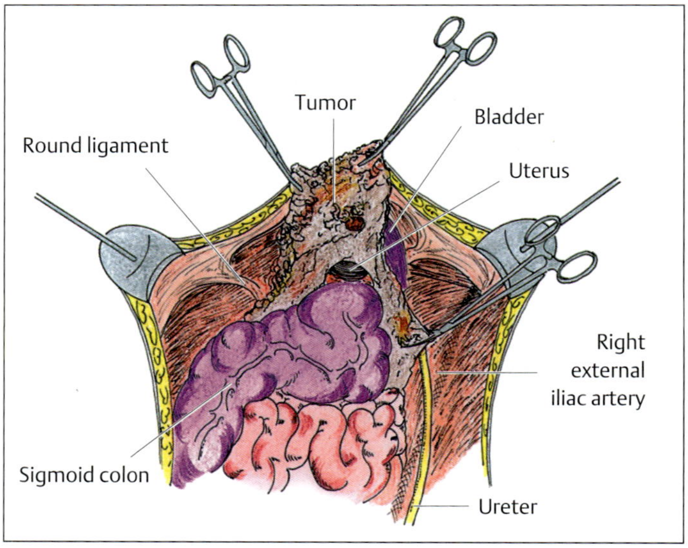

Fig. 13.**13** Female pelvis with anatomic structures fused together by mucinous tumor.

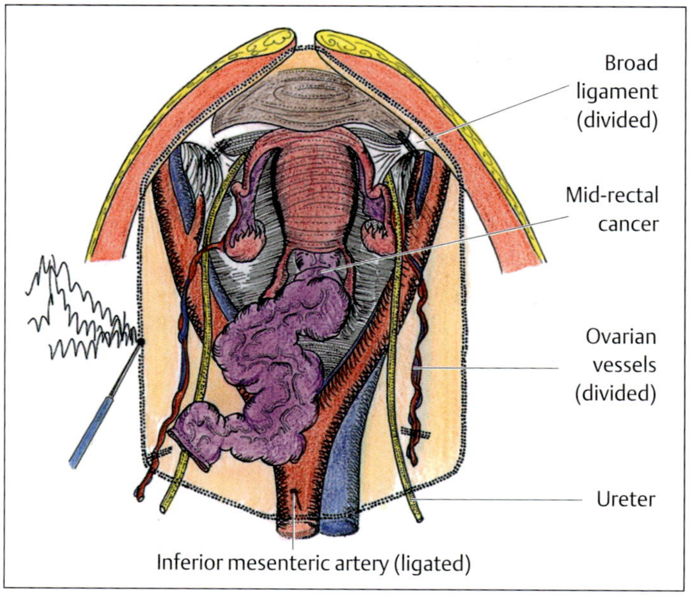

Fig. 13.**14** Pelvic peritonectomy. Centripetal division of peritoneum at the limits of a complete pelvic peritonectomy.

isolate the ovarian vessels and spare the ureters. The ovarian vessels are followed up to the lower pole of the kidney where they are ligated and transected. In order to secure the uterine arteries and veins traction is placed on the uterus to separate these vessels from the ureter. Digitoclasis of tissues lateral to the uterus and along the course of the ureter may help separate the uterus from the surrounding tissues. Transection of the obliterated umbilical artery at the level of the ureter will help separate these tissues. Suture ligatures are placed around the uterine artery directly above the ureter and then more centrally near the uterus. These ligatures are tied prior to the division of the uterine arteries with the uterus in full view. Again with traction on the uterus the end of the cervix is palpated through the intact vagina before the anterior aspect of this structure is divided using electroevaporative surgery. Bleeding points anteriorly can be electrocoagulated; laterally the vaginal branches of the uterine artery are secured using long Allis clamps to elevate the corners of the vagina. The posterior aspect of the vagina is transected beneath the cul-de-sac of Douglas.

The rectosigmoid dissection begins by releasing the root of the small bowel mesentery from the retroperitoneum. The peritoneum that constitutes the ligament of Treitz is included with the specimen. This maneuver clearly exposes the inferior mesenteric vein which is ligated in continuity and then divided. Changing contours of the aorta leads to localization of the inferior mesenteric artery which is ligated in continuity and divided. The site of transection of the colon is selected. This is usually at the junction of sigmoid and descending colon. A linear cutting stapler is used (Ethicon, Cincinnati, OH). The mesentery of the distal descending colon is transected perpendicular to the course of the colon so that there is no ischemia of the bowel. The branches of the sigmoid vessels on the left colic vessel are divided so that their normal Y configuration is converted to a V. This preservation of the intermediate blood supply of the colon helps prevent ischemia of the distal descending colon (Fig. 13.**15**).

A surgical towel is used to surround all small bowel and descending colon. These structures are preserved in the abdomen and retraction maintained by a second tier of wide malleable self-retaining retractor blades. The wide exposure allows clear perirectal dissection and a safe release of the specimen.

Centripetal dissection begins in the plane of the mesorectal envelope. An extension on the ball electrosurgical tip may greatly facilitate the exposure by keeping the surgeon's hand from obscuring the plane of deep dissection. Branches of the middle hemorrhoidal vessels are electrocoagulated and strong upward traction on the specimen allows the rectal wall to be cleared of perirectal fat. The perirectal tissue should be separated circumferentially from the muscular wall

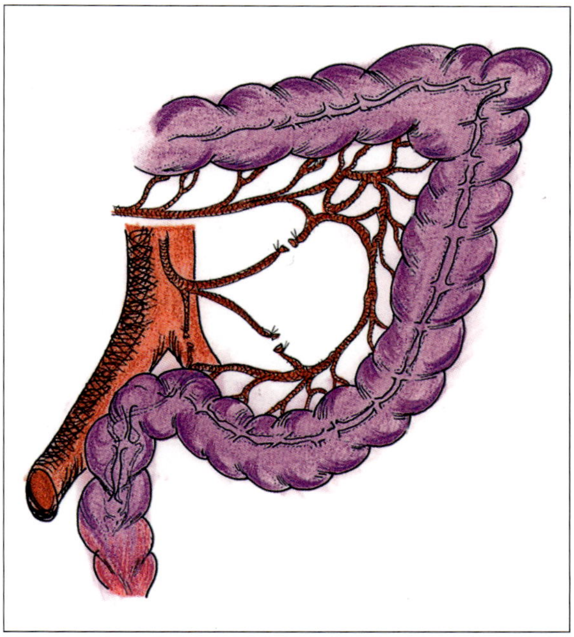

Fig. 13.**15** Release of the left colon for a tension-free colorectal anastomosis. There is a Y to V conversion of the intermediate vascular arcade of the descending colon to release this structure from the inferior mesenteric artery and vein.

of the rectum so that a stapler divides the rectum beneath the peritoneal reflection at approximately the junction of middle and upper one-third of this structure (Roticulator, Autosuture, Norwalk, CT; Fig. 13.**16**).

After transection of the rectum above the stapler the specimen can be removed. The pelvis is copiously irrigated to mechanically remove cancer cells as much as possible. The vaginal cuff is closed with zero Vicryl suture (Ethicon, Cincinnati, OH). The sutures are tied and left long so that they are available for traction to expose the rectal stump during the circular stapling of the descending colon to the stump of the rectum.

Pelvic Peritonectomy with Resection of the Rectosigmoid and Colon in Patients Having Prior Hysterectomy

Surprisingly, prior hysterectomy simplifies complete pelvic peritonectomy. The scar tissue along the ureters caused by prior dissection is not difficult to release if electroevaporative surgery is used. In almost all patients the uterine arteries and veins have atrophied as a result of prior hysterectomy so that electrocoagulation can be used to gain hemostasis along the complete course of the ureter. The round ligaments are electrosurgically divided as they exit the internal inguinal ring, the obliterated umbilical arteries are transected just lateral to the ureter and the ovarian vessels are ligated at the lower pole of the kidney.

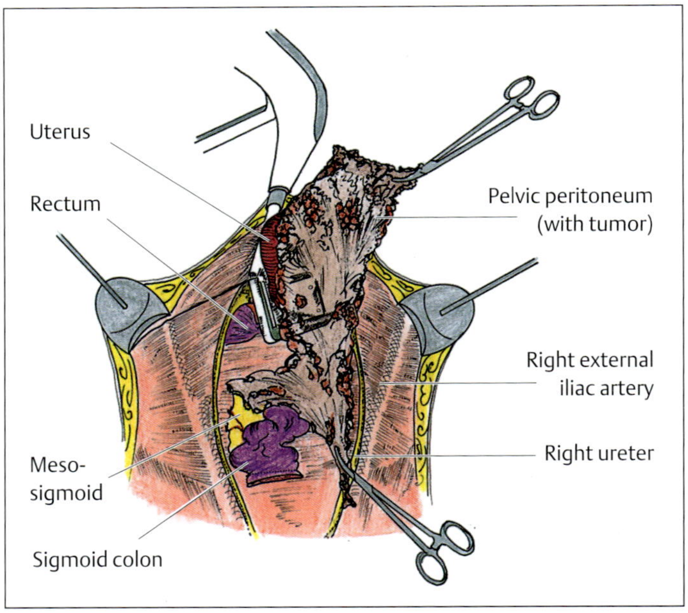

Fig. 13.**16** Pelvic peritonectomy. Resection of the rectosigmoid colon beneath the peritoneal reflection.

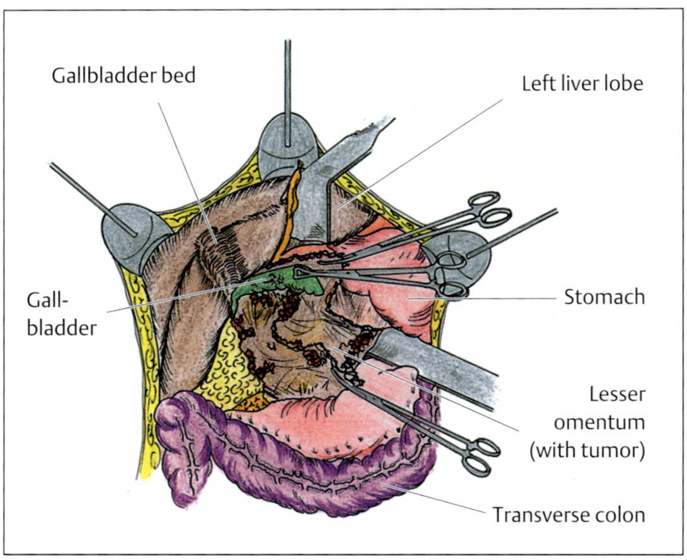

Fig. 13.**17** Lesser omentectomy and cholecystectomy.

One caveat in complete pelvic peritonectomy after prior hysterectomy involves dissection of the bladder. The prior hysterectomy involved a separation of the bladder from the lower uterus and cervix. Tumor will be seeded on exposed bladder muscle and may focally invade the bladder in the area of the old "bladder flap." Achieving a clear margin will require careful dissection through bladder muscle deep to the progressive tumor. Normally the bladder mucosa can be preserved. The muscle is reapproximated over the mucosa to prevent a bladder fistula from occurring postoperatively.

Cholecystectomy, Lesser Omentectomy, and Stripping of the Omental Bursa with Stomach Preservation

The gallbladder is removed from its fundus towards the common hepatic duct (Fig. 13.**17**). The peritoneum covering the porta hepatis is usually heavily involved by tumor. Dissection of this tissue is facilitated by blunt dissection along the porta hepatis just medial to the cystic duct and artery.

The resection of the lesser omentum is begun in the fissure of the gastrohepatic ligament that divides liver segments two and three from segment one. Great care is necessary not to damage the caudate process of the liver and its portal blood supply located on the anterior surface of this liver segment. Moreover, part (accessory left hepatic) or all (replaced left hepatic) of the left

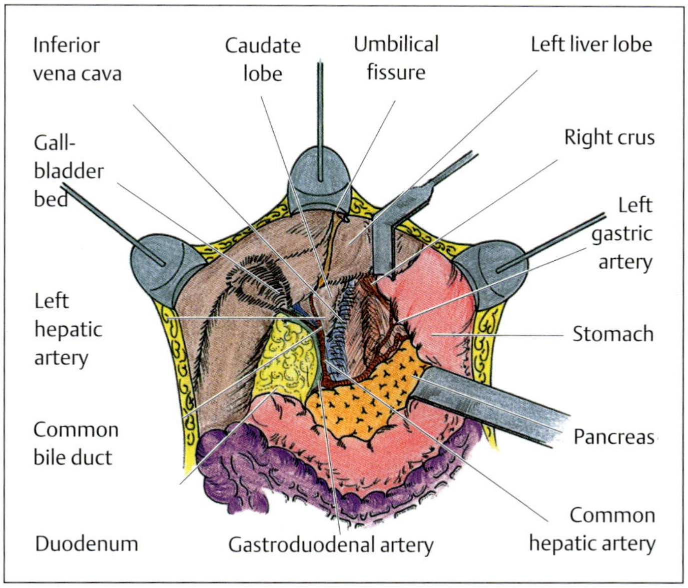

Fig. 13.**18** Stripping of the floor of the omental bursa completed.

hepatic artery may arise from the left gastric artery and cross the hepatogastric ligament towards the left lobe of the liver. Usually this arterial structure is ligated at its entrance to the liver and as it arises from the left gastric artery.

The stripping of the omental bursa starts from the divided phrenoesophageal ligament and continues along the inferior vena cava visualized directly beneath the caudate lobe of the liver. With strong traction tumor and peritoneum above the vena cava and the crus of the right hemidiaphragm are stripped away (Fig. 13.**18**). Lymph nodes along the common hepatic artery are preserved as far as is possible. Dissection of the lesser omental fat is in a clockwise direction along the lesser curvature of the stomach. Care is taken to preserve the left gastric artery and its branches to the stomach, the anterior vagus nerve, and the right gastric artery. A pyloroplasty or a gastrojejunostomy is indicated only if the pylorus is firm and tight.

Lesser Omentectomy with Total Gastrectomy

In approximately 10% of patients with mucinous appendiceal carcinomatosis the progression of mucinous tumor is such that the lesser curvature of the stomach cannot be separated from the stomach or from the left gastric vessels. Total gastrectomy will be required in order to complete the cytoreduction. A centripetal approach greatly facilitates the dissection. Branches of the right gastric artery are ligated as they arise from the hepatic artery and again as they enter the duodenum. This dissection requires a stripping of mucinous tumor from the posterior aspect of the duodenum within the subpyloric space. Effort is made to preserve some branches of the right gastroepiploic vessels to the duodenum. When the duodenum is freed up a linear stapler/cutter is used to transect the duodenum just below the pylorus.

In order to divide the esophagus the phrenoesophageal ligament is stripped away from the crus of the right hemidiaphragm and the peritoneum is stripped away from the vena cava starting beneath the caudate process of the liver. Multiple vessels from esophagus to stomach along the gastroesophageal junction are individually electrocoagulated to preserve a small portion of the proximal stomach. A linear/cutter divides the upper stomach 3 or 4 cm from the gastroesophageal junction. Centripetal surgery going around the left gastric artery and vein beneath the peritoneum overlying the pancreas completes the dissection. The left gastric artery and vein are ligated and then suture ligated to release the specimen.

☐ Tubes and Drains for Intraperitoneal Chemotherapy

Tubes and drains have a dual purpose. They remove physiologic fluid postoperatively and administer and drain the chemotherapy solution. These drains are positioned in the most dependent areas, the right subhepatic space, the left subdiaphragmatic space, and the pelvis. A Tenckhoff catheter (Quinton Spiral Peritoneal Catheter, Quinton, Inc., Seattle, WA) is placed to deliver the perioperative intraperitoneal chemotherapy. A chest tube is positioned if a left and/or right upper quadrant peritonectomy is performed in order to prevent fluid accumulation in the pleural space as a result of intraperitoneal chemotherapy and inflammatory reaction to diaphragm stripping (Fig. 13.**19**). All tubes and

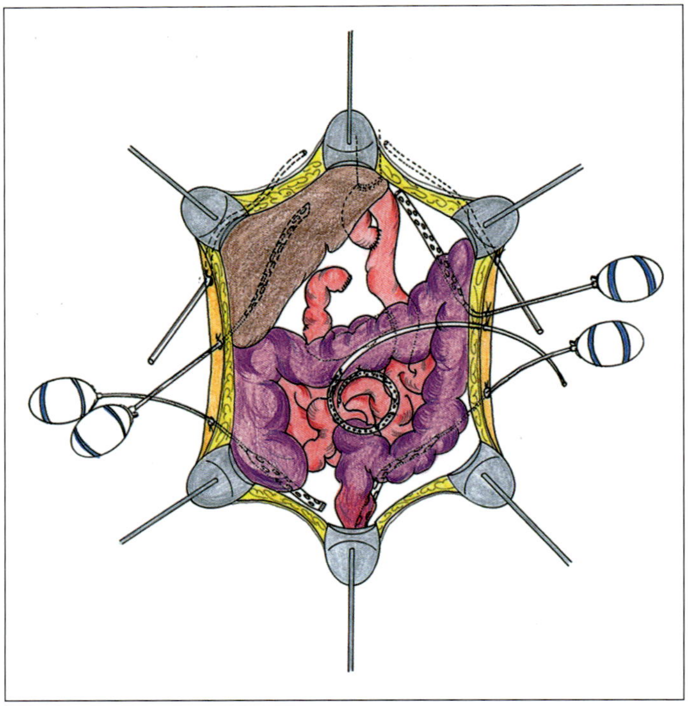

Fig. 13.**19** Tubes and drains after an extended cytoreductive surgery and hyperthermic intraperitoneal intraoperative chemotherapy.

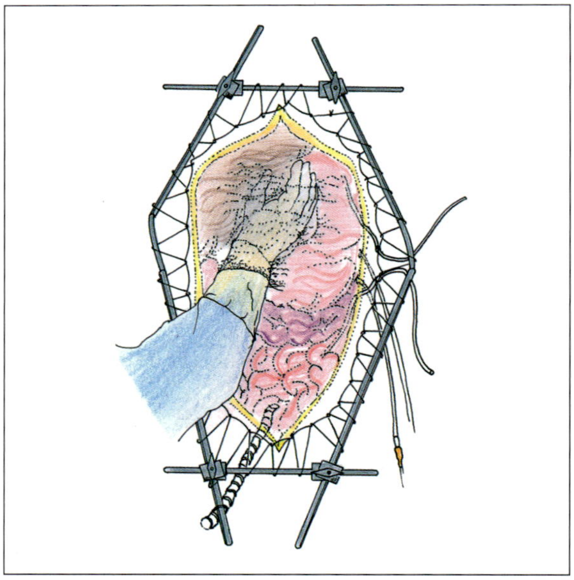

Fig. 13.**20** Intraoperative intraperitoneal chemotherapy by the Coliseum Technique. Suspension of the edges of the abdominal incision on the self-retaining retractor allows chemotherapy solution to be retained in the abdomen and pelvis. Continuous manipulation of the viscera causes uniform distribution of heat and chemotherapy to all peritoneal surfaces.

drains through the abdominal wall are secured with a purse-string suture at the skin.

Heated intraoperative intraperitoneal chemotherapy is performed at this time. All visible tumor should have been removed from the abdomen and from the pelvis and no suture lines are as yet performed except those required to close the ends of bowel loops or to close the vagina. Temperature probes are placed over the edge of the abdominal wall and secured with sutures. The skin edges are elevated on a self-retaining retractor with a sheet of plastic incorporated. A smoke-evacuation system is used to eliminate possible chemotherapy aerosols from the operating room environment. Chemotherapy treatment is administered as shown in Figure 13.**20**.[5,6]

☐ Reconstructive Surgery

Reconstructive surgery is performed to reestablish the gastrointestinal function and to prevent gastrointestinal fistula formation at a suture line or on the electroevaporized bowel surfaces. Intestinal suturing or stapling is performed after the administration of the intraperitoneal chemotherapy. The absence of tension is essential to performing a safe colorectal anastomosis. As described earlier the inferior mesenteric artery and veins are ligated and divided and its branches transected (Y to V) so as to preserve the intermediate vascular arcade. To gain complete mobility of the descending colon its attachments to the upper portion of the ureter, gonadal vessels, and perirenal fat need to be divided. These maneuvers are usually sufficient to allow a tension-free colorectal anastomosis. The anastomosis is performed with a circular stapler (Ethicon ILS-33, Cincinnati, OH). The stapler anvil is automatically secured in the proximal colon with a purse-string suture applier (Autosuture, Norwalk, CT). The circular stapling device is passed into the rectum and the stapler trochar is made to penetrate the middle of the rectal staple line. The two portions of the stapler carrying the bowel are then mated and the anastomosis completed by stapler firing. After completion of the anastomosis it is important to verify its safety. First, the completeness of the proximal and distal tissue rings are examined; then with the pelvis filled by saline irrigation, air is insufflated into the rectum. There should be no air bubbles noted despite air pressure within the distal colon. A digital rectal exploration is performed to discover bleeding from the staple-line at the anastomotic site.

In a majority of patients a right colectomy with resection of the terminal ileum containing mucinous tumor is required. A hand-sutured ileocolic anastomosis is recommended. To overcome the size discrepancy of terminal ileum and colon, the proximal colon is sutured to the antimesenteric border of the distal ileum. The end of the ileum is stapled off and oversewn with interrupted sutures (Fig. 13.**21**).

After a total gastrectomy the gastrointestinal tract continuity is reestablished performing an anastomosis between the end of the esophagus and the side of the jejunum. Before reconstruction of the esophagojejunal anastomosis is begun, proper exposure of the esophageal hiatus is necessary. The self-retaining retractor blades are maintained on the edges of the costal margin and the lower abdomen. The left lateral segment of the liver is elevated to the right and the blade of a malleable retractor is placed beneath the caudate process of the liver. This "second tier" of retractors holding viscera out of the operative site makes esophagojejunal anastomosis easy and safe for it is performed under direct vision.

The jejunum is divided with a linear stapler/cutter 20 cm below the Treitz ligament. Using a purse-string applier the anvil of a 29-mm circular stapler is positioned in the distal esophagus and secured by a purse-string suture. The staple line on the distal jejunum is removed so that a circular stapler is passed into the distal jejunum for 7 to 10 cm. The stapler trochar is passed through the small bowel wall and the two portions of the stapler are connected and the anastomosis completed. The open proximal jejunum is closed with a stapler (TA60, Ethicon, Cincinnati, OH) and the suture line inverted with interrupted sutures. An end ostomy with the proximal portion of the jejunum is performed in order to divert bile and digestive enzymes from the gastrointestinal tract (Fig. 13.**22**). The temporary duodenal exteriorization is performed to protect the esophagojejunal anastomosis and to decrease the incidence of small bowel fistula formation. The jejunostomy is closed at approximately six months as part of a second-look procedure.

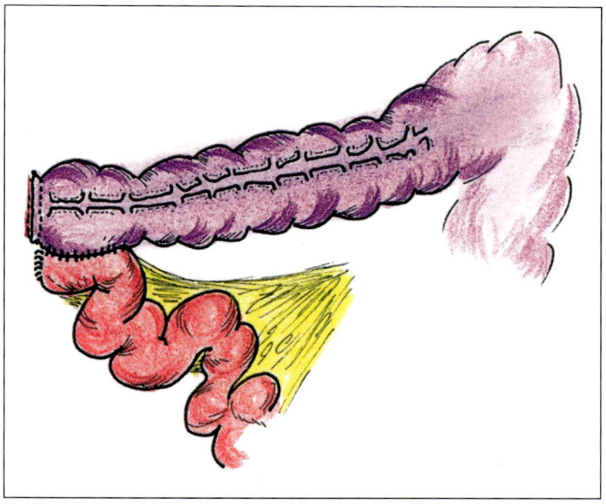

Fig. 13.**21** Anastomosis of end colon to antimesenteric portion of distal ileum.

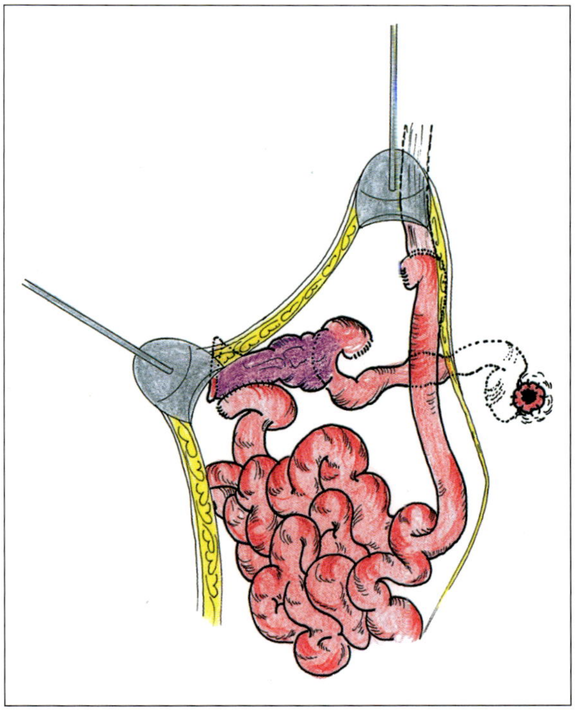

Fig. 13.**22** Reconstruction after total gastrectomy.

Discussion

The goal of cytoreductive surgery for peritoneal carcinomatosis, sarcomatosis, and mesothelioma is removal of all visible peritoneal surface malignancy.[5–8] The fundamental surgical technologies in cytoreductive surgery to treat peritoneal surface malignancy are the peritonectomy procedures.[2] The six above-mentioned peritonectomy procedures are available in order to resect all visible tumor from parietal or visceral peritoneal

5

Table 13.**1** Stop signals for surgical cytoreduction with curative intent. If the patient manifests any of these features a debulking with palliative intent should occur

1. Poor operative risk so that the patient is unlikely to survive the operation
2. Liver metastasis or clinical evidence of distant disease
3. Inability to clear the primary tumor mass
4. Inability to reestablish gastrointestinal function because of extensive peritoneal seeding

Stop signals 1 and 2 are established preoperatively. Stop signals 3 and 4 are determined after the abdomen has been explored.

surfaces. One or all six procedures may be required depending on the distribution and volume of peritoneal carcinomatosis. Only peritoneum visibly involved by cancer seeding is resected. The six procedures are: (1) greater omentectomy and splenectomy; (2) left subphrenic peritonectomy; (3) right subphrenic peritonectomy; (4) pelvic peritonectomy with rectosigmoid resection; (5) cholecystectomy, lesser omentectomy with stripping of the omental bursa and when peritoneal seeding has progressed to extensively involve the stomach; (6) associated total gastrectomy. Also, the frequent layering of mucinous tumor on the visceral peritoneum of the right colon and terminal ileum frequently requires extended right colectomy. Tumor nodules on small bowel mesentery are eradicated by electroevaporation but tumor on small bowel or mesenteric borders of the small bowel present a difficult and high morbidity resection.

5

Frequently the failure of prior surgery in the treatment of abdominal or pelvic tumors is the indication for peritonectomy procedures and so they are often performed in a reoperative setting. There are four principles in reoperative cancer surgery that the cancer surgeon should follow:

1. Optimal exposure of the operative field and complete hemostasis are necessary especially if the procedure is of significant duration.
2. Centripetal surgery is continuously employed to avoid costly errors in dissection.
3. Proper patient selection and a thorough knowledge of the natural history of the disease are necessary for adequate surgical judgement.
4. Carefully performed reconstructive procedure with intestinal diversion when indicated will keep morbidity and mortality to a minimum.

The centripetal approach is necessary for optimal cytoreduction. The surgeon proceeds from the periphery where the peritonectomy starts to the center where the tumor and the major vessels are located. He proceeds in a circular fashion around and around the malignancy. If there is the risk of hemorrhage, risk of damage to vital structures, or compromised margins of resection, it is necessary to move the dissection to another anatomic site. Centripetal surgery often begins to combine all six peritonectomy procedures into a single coordinated effort in peritonectomy. Deep dissection with poor visualization of the operative site should not be pursued.

Success in the management of peritoneal surface malignancy depends on the patient's physical and mental status, the biologic aggressiveness (invasive capabilities) of the tumor, its abdominal and pelvic distribution, and its volume. Extensive cytoreductive surgery with perioperative chemotherapy that does not result in a significant prolongation of a good quality of life is to be avoided. Selective factors are available and should be followed in planning the treatment of individual patients. These selection factors can be summarized as "stop signals" for cytoreduction (Table 13.**1**). If patients manifest any of these features, the goal of surgery should change from the cytoreductive approach with curative intent to debulking with palliative intent.

Low performance status, distant metastasis, high likelihood of incomplete cytoreduction, and inability to restore adequate gastrointestinal function are the most important stop signals in patients with peritoneal surface malignancy. In these instances the role of the oncologic surgeon is to treat surgical emergencies and provide palliation.[9] In these patients aggressive elective cytoreduction is contraindicated.

After extensive cytoreductive surgery and perioperative intraperitoneal chemotherapy return of gastrointestinal tract function may be prolonged. The surgery may last 10–14 hours and is associated with extensive bowel trauma, prolonged ileus, and retention of intestinal contents. Distention of intestinal loops will occur as a result of poor peristalsis. Delay in the wound healing process of traumatized bowel loops will occur because of treatment with cytotoxic drugs. All these conditions are predisposing to a high incidence of anastomotic leakage or fistulas. Bowel rest through nasogastric suctioning, ileostomy to decompress the small bowel contents or jejunostomy to divert it, may be necessary. With an ostomy, discharge of bowel content is easier and quicker and distension of bowel loops is decreased reducing the risk of fistulization. If there is extensive small bowel trauma, ostomy construction should be considered.

In the plan of treatment of many patients with peritoneal surface malignancy, a second-look procedure is mandatory. During second-look ostomies are closed, the abdominal cavity is explored looking for recurrent disease, and repeat cytoreduction and intraperitoneal chemotherapy are carried out.

The perioperative intraperitoneal chemotherapy is designed to prevent implantation of cancer cells and destruction of microscopic foci of residual cancer that the surgeon cannot see and therefore does not remove.

The intraoperative heated chemotherapy is administered after cytoreduction and prior to performance of intestinal anastomosis. Early postoperative intraperitoneal chemotherapy is delivered from the first through the fifth postoperative day. The chemotherapy solution is administered in the abdominal cavity through a Tenckhoff catheter. Dwell is for 23 hours and drainage is for 1 hour prior to the next instillation. With this perioperative administration of the drug the route and timing of chemotherapy directed at peritoneal surface malignancy is different from the traditional approach. First, the route of administration is intraperitoneal and not intravenous. The systemic absorption of the drug from the peritoneal cavity is low and the contact between the viscera and the chemotherapy solution is high. Second, the timing of intraperitoneal chemotherapy is with the surgery and/or the few days immediately thereafter rather than weeks or months later in an adjuvant setting.

In the past peritoneal surface malignancy was accepted as a terminal condition in which surgery was indicated only for palliation. The development of cytoreductive surgery and perioperative intraperitoneal chemotherapy has modified the surgical judgments for this condition. Also, changes in concepts of tumor biology suggest that peritoneal carcinomatosis, sarcomatosis, and mesothelioma may exist as an isolated form of disease without systemic dissemination. The technical details regarding peritonectomy presented here are of great importance in the treatment of peritoneal surface malignancy because a curative treatment for these diseases requires a complete cytoreduction. Selection of patients for a complete cytoreduction remains a crucial component of management so that patients with no chance for cure receive proper palliation but not an aggressive and disappointing cytoreduction that was not indicated. Perioperative intraperitoneal chemotherapy is essential to minimize the implantation of residual cancer cells and destroy microscopic foci of disease.

Conclusion

In spite of new developments in multimodality treatments, complete resection remains as an absolute requirement for cure of gastrointestinal cancer. Eradication of the last cancer cell is still the proper goal of cancer surgery within the abdomen and pelvis. Success in management of peritoneal surface malignancy depends on the surgeon's knowledge, skill, and proper utilization of electrosurgical technology. This chapter describes the current strategy that the surgeon should pursue in the treatment of patients with peritoneal carcinomatosis, sarcomatosis, and mesothelioma. Technical details required for this surgery include patient position and incision, complete lysis of adhesions, retraction, electroevaporative dissection, irrigation and suction, peritonectomy procedures, reconstructive surgery, and proper placement of tubes and drains for intraperitoneal chemotherapy. Fulfillment of the surgical requirements for treatment of peritoneal surface spread of cancer demands a working knowledge of this new technology for successful peritonectomy. It is possible to add these procedures to the armamentarium of the cancer surgeon.

References

1. Fortner JG. Inadvertent spread of cancer at surgery. *J Surg Oncol.* 1993;53:191–196.
2. Sugarbaker PH. Peritonectomy procedures. *Ann Surg.* 1995;221:29–42.
3. Zoetmulder FAN, Sugarbaker PH. Patterns of failure following treatment of pseudomyxoma peritonei of appendiceal origin. *Eur J Cancer.* 1996;32A:1727–1733.
4. Sugarbaker PH. Laser-mode electrosurgery. In: Sugarbaker PH, ed. *Peritoneal Carcinomatosis: Principles of Management.* Boston: Kluwer Academic Publishers; 1996:375–385.
5. Sugarbaker PH. *Management of Peritoneal Surface Malignancy using Intraperitoneal Chemotherapy and Cytoreductive Surgery: a Manual for Physician and Nurses.* 3rd ed. Grand Rapids, Michigan: The Ludann Company; 1998.
6. Sugarbaker PH. Cytoreductive Surgery and Intraperitoneal Chemotherapy for Peritoneal Surface Malignancies. In: Markman M, ed. *Regional Chemotherapy.* Totowa: Humana Press; 2000:225–248.
7. Sugarbaker PH. Management of peritoneal surface malignancy: the surgeon's role. *Langenbeck's Arch Surg.* 1999; 384:576–587.
8. Sugarbaker PH. Successful management of microscopic residual disease in large bowel cancer. *Cancer Chemother Pharmacol.* 1999;43:15–25.
9. Esquivel J, Sugarbaker PH. Elective surgery in recurrent colon cancer with peritoneal seeding (when to and when not to proceed). *Cancer Therapeutics.* 1998;1:321–325.

Retroperitoneum 6

14 Retroperitoneal Resections for Sarcomas Invading Adjacent Organs

Constantine P. Karakousis

Retroperitoneal sarcomas are uncommon. In the United States, there are approximately 5000 new cases of soft tissue sarcomas diagnosed annually, of which about 500 are retroperitoneal sarcomas. Nevertheless, in the course of time, every general surgeon will encounter several of these cases throughout his or her career. These tumors are encountered more often in referral centers. In general, they provide few symptoms and often they are diagnosed by the patients or their physician by palpation of a mass in the abdomen. Infrequently, vague pain or other symptoms from the gastrointestinal tract (e. g., obstructive symptoms or bleeding) may antedate the diagnosis. To this generalization of lack or paucity of symptoms, a notable exception is soft tissue sarcomas of the iliac fossa as well as those of the lesser pelvis abutting against the greater sciatic notch which may cause symptoms from compression of the femoral and sciatic nerves, respectively, referred in the distribution of these nerves. Retroperitoneal sarcomas are notorious for the difficulty they provide the surgeon for complete resection due to their relative inaccessibility and large size. However, with experience, the majority of these tumors can be resected if one takes full advantage of the position of the patient on the operating room table so that gravity is in favor of the surgeon and one uses adequate incisions to provide exposure and appropriate strategy in mobilizing and resecting these tumors. In the following, these tumors have been classified into: (1) those of upper quadrants of the abdomen; (2) flank tumors; (3) midline sarcomas; and (4) pelvic sarcomas. We describe here the operative technique in detail.

Upper Quadrant Sarcomas

For upper quadrant retroperitoneal sarcomas, the patient is placed in a lateral or semi-lateral position with the affected side up. An incision from about the mid distance between the xiphoid and umbilicus is extended obliquely to the costal margin. This incision is carried through the subcutaneous fat, the anterior rectus sheath, rectus abdominis, posterior rectus sheath and peritoneum and, more laterally, toward the costal margin through the external oblique, the internal oblique, transversus abdominis muscles, transversalis fascia, and peritoneum. This incision from the midline to the costal margin provides sufficient exposure for the surgeon to

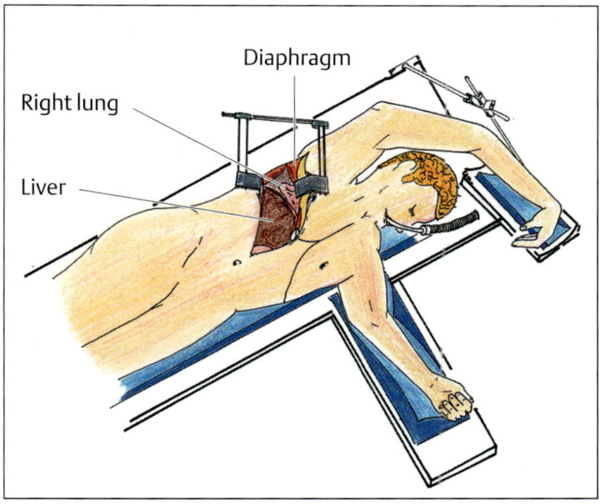

Fig. 14.**1** Thoracoabdominal approach to an upper (right) quadrant sarcoma. The oblique incision starts above the umbilicus and is extended through the 9th intercostal space. The diaphragm is opened. The right lobe of the liver and right lung are exposed.

explore the abdomen with regards to possible metastatic disease that might militate against or alter the course of resection of the tumor. Even in the presence of modest metastatic disease, however, in general, it is best to resect a primary retroperitoneal sarcoma and, if possible, to resect all other metastatic foci which provides good palliation and prolongation of life.[1] This incision provides an ample opportunity to assess the location of the tumor and, therefore, more accurately guide the direction of the incision into the lower chest which, depending on the exact location of the tumor, may be extended into the 9th, 10th, or 11th intercostal space. The costal margin is divided and a small segment of the costal margin is removed. The diaphragm is incised for 3 cm and this allows the insertion of a self-retaining retractor between the ribs (Fig. 14.**1**). One can then estimate how far posteriorly one may have to expand the thoracic portion of the incision in order to have the necessary exposure. The diaphragm is incised, as necessary for sufficient exposure, close to its insertion to the ribs so that the bulk of the diaphragm in the central area is not denervated. If there is, however, actual involvement of the diaphragm, the incision into the diaphragm will have to accommodate and circumscribe the area of involvement around the tumor. Visceral attachments are evaluated and whatever viscera can be separated off the tumor surface without coming

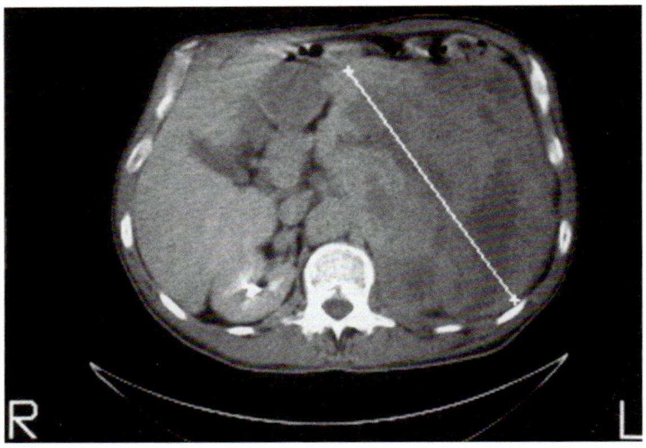

Fig. 14.**2** Soft tissue sarcoma of the left upper quadrant, resected through a left thoracoabdominal incision in combination with a midline abdominal incision.

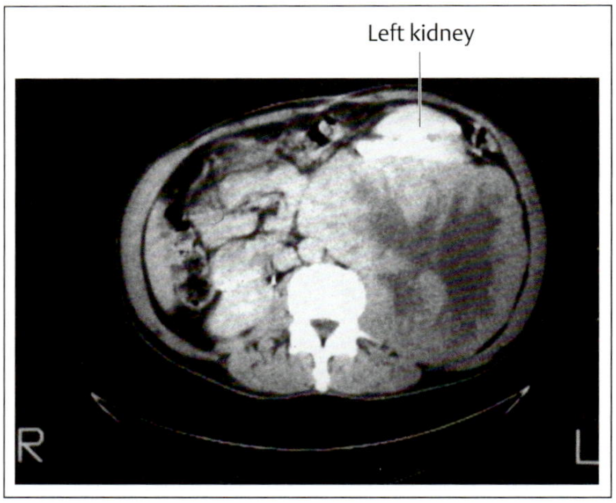

Fig. 14.**3** Left upper quadrant sarcoma showing the left kidney displaced anteriorly by tumor, also resected through a left thoracoabdominal incision.

too close to the tumor are dissected off the tumor. The splenic flexure of the colon and the hepatic flexure on the left and right sides, respectively, are structures to be assessed as to whether they are close to the tumor or not. In order to evaluate the visceral attachments to the tumor surface, however, it is generally desirable to mobilize the tumor posterolaterally to some extent and thus facilitate dissection between the tumor and other viscera. The peritoneum anterior and lateral to the tumor is incised around the mass and the retroperitoneal plane between the peritoneum and the lower chest and the upper abdominal wall is entered. If this plane appears to be uninvolved, one can continue on the same plane. Otherwise, one may have to enter the plane between the transversus abdominis and internal oblique or even that between the internal oblique and external oblique. In some situations, one may have to remove a portion of the lower chest or upper abdominal wall in its entire thickness. Usually, one can dissect between the tumor and transversus abdominis laterally and the tumor and quadratus lumborum posteriorly. There should be no hesitation, however, to remove either of these two muscles, should the tumor appear to be attached to either of them. If the respective flexure of the colon seems to be adherent to the tumor surface, then the bowel proximal and distal to the area of involvement is divided with a stapling device and the appropriate portion of the mesocolon, which is close to the tumor, is divided at its base so that this segment of large bowel, as well as its mesocolon, remain attached to the tumor to be removed en bloc with the latter. In the **left upper quadrant**, dissection through the lienorenal ligament allows the mobilization of the spleen and tail of the pancreas along with the tumor mass. Posterolateral to the spleen, the kidney is encountered and one has to decide whether it should be resected en bloc with the tumor or not, depending on its proximity to the tumor mass. The gastrocolic ligament is divided, entry into the lesser sac is gained and through this opening one can easily find the splenic artery coursing on the superior border of the pancreas and proceed to ligate and divide this artery. Immediately above and at the base of the mesocolon, the inferior border of the pancreas is identified. The inferior mesenteric vein, if close by, can be ligated and divided and then with a combination of blunt and sharp dissection, one circumferentially dissects and exposes both the anterior as well as the posterior surface of the pancreas medial to the area involved by the tumor. On the posterior surface of the pancreas, the splenic vein can be visualized, ligated, and divided at the same level as the splenic artery previously was divided. The pancreas itself can be divided either with a stapling device or by using mattress sutures to control any bleeding from the pancreatic parenchyma. Any attachment of the tumor to the greater curvature of the stomach can be dealt with by stapling that portion of the stomach so that the involved area remains on the surface of the tumor. With the thoracoabdominal incision used, one has good access to the esophagogastric junction and, therefore, one should be able to free both the posterior and anterior wall of the stomach medial to the area of involvement in the greater curvature for a left-sided retroperitoneal sarcoma. If the kidney appears to be involved, then it is dissected posteriorly and mobilized so that the renal artery may be identified, ligated, and divided. The renal vein is exposed from the anterior aspect of the kidney as it crosses transversely the abdominal aorta, it is dissected, vascular clamps are applied and it is divided, the two ends being oversewn with running vascular sutures. Because of the width of the renal vein, it is safer to do so than simply suture-ligate the stump of the renal vein (Figs. 14.**2**–14.**5**).

For sarcomas of the **right upper quadrant**, the patient is placed in a left lateral position with the right side up. The pleural space is entered and the diaphragm is incised sufficiently for exposure. Posterolateral mobilization of the tumor is then performed by dissecting behind the peritoneum and pleura so as to leave the peritoneum and lower portion of the pleura on the tumor surface. As on the left side, if there is invasion of the underlying muscular layer, then the dissection reverts to a more superficial plane between the muscles so as to maintain at least one muscle layer that appears grossly normal on the tumor surface. For involvement by the tumor of the diaphragm, the respective portion of the diaphragm is circumscribed around the area of involvement so that it can be left on the tumor surface. The right triangular ligament of the liver is incised peripherally. In case of liver involvement, which would be the right lobe in this case, the porta hepatis is exposed, the gallbladder is removed and the right hepatic duct, the right hepatic artery, and the right branch of the portal vein are sequentially dissected, ligated, and divided. For the right branch of the portal vein, because of its short length, it is best after this vessel is dissected out with a right-angled clamp to apply vascular clamps tightly before dividing it. It is wise to place a vascular suture on each side of this vein for extra control and safety. The venous trunk itself is then divided and the stump on each side is sutured with the vascular suture. If a vascular clamp is not applied tightly and holding sutures are not placed, the proximal stump may retract through the jaws of the vascular and disappear behind the hepatoduodenal ligament. If this perioperative complication occurs, the proximal stump of the right branch of the portal vein should be promptly compressed against the rest of the hepatoduodenal ligament from a posterior approach with the left index finger and brought closer to the lateral edge of the hepatoduodenal ligament where it can be sutured. This controls the bleeding. However, at the end of the procedure, after a right hepatic lobectomy, the choledochus must be opened in order to make sure that the vascular sutures do not involve any part of the main biliary duct. This type of mishap, however, can be avoided if the vascular clamps are applied tightly on each end of the short length of the right branch of the portal vein and vascular sutures are placed on either side (two on each side). Kocherization of the duodenum, incision of the gastrohepatic ligament, passage of a tape around the structures of the porta hepatis and then through a short segment of red rubber catheter

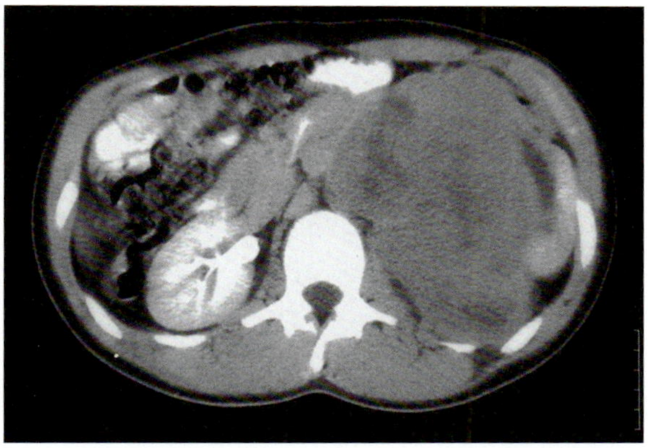

Fig. 14.**4** Sarcoma of the left upper quadrant resected with the left kidney, spleen, distal pancreas, and diaphragm.

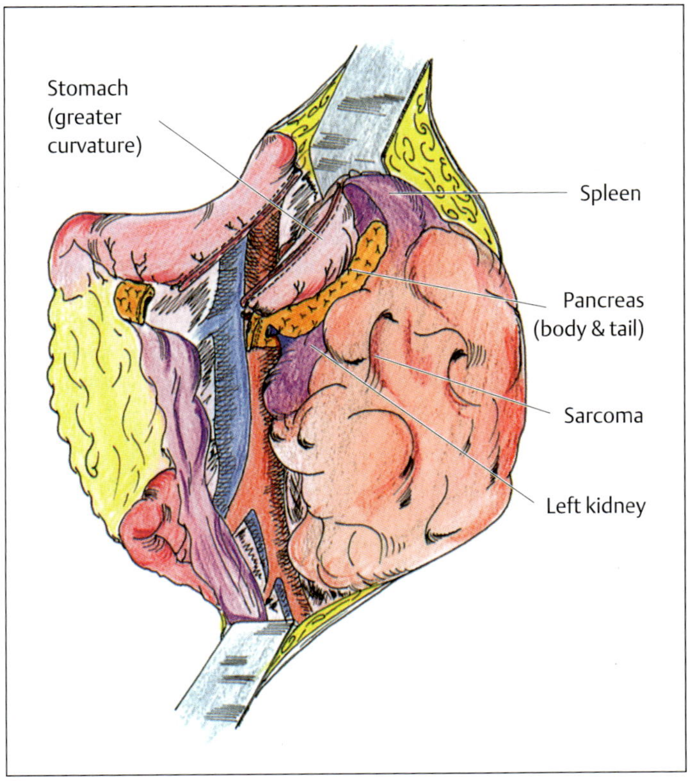

Fig. 14.**5** Left upper quadrant sarcoma after exposure and before removal. The tumor has invaded the greater curvature of the stomach, the spleen, the tail of the pancreas, and the left kidney. The stomach and pancreas are stapled; the renal and splenic vessels are ligated. The sarcoma is removed en bloc with these organs.

6

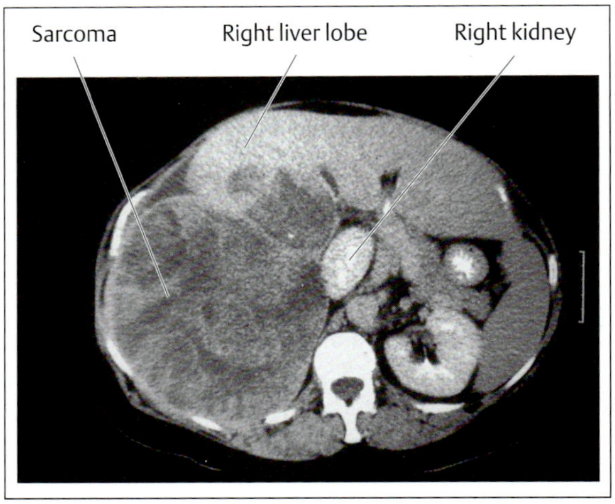

Fig. 14.**6** Sarcoma of the right upper quadrant involving the right lobe of the liver and right kidney displaced medially. It was resected through a right thoracoabdominal incision in combination with a midline incision.

(Rummel tourniquet) is an additional safety measure for control of potential bleeding (Pringle maneuver).

The right hepatic vein, if it is easy to be dissected, is ligated and divided. If not, later intraparenchymal ligation and division of this vein may be safest. One incises the Glisson's capsule from the gallbladder bed to the confluence of the hepatic veins and proceeds to cut through the hepatic parenchyma, being careful at all times so that the plane through the hepatic parenchyma is aiming to the right of the inferior vena cava. One member of the operative team should have a hand, therefore, on the lateral edge of the inferior vena cava so that it can be ascertained that the dissection proceeds in that direction through the hepatic parenchyma and does not veer to the other side, compromising blood supply to the remaining lobe of the liver.

On the right side, the hepatic flexure of the colon has to be dealt with and mobilized by dividing the peritoneal reflexion lateral to the colon and the colon itself dissected off if not too close to the tumor surface. If it is, then the appropriate segment of the colon is divided proximal and distal to the area of involvement and the corresponding mesocolon is left on the surface of the tumor for en bloc resection. The duodenum is Kocherized, the inferior cava is exposed clearly and the right renal vein is visualized. On this side, the right gonadal vein enters the inferior vena cava a few centimeters below the right renal vein and, if the tumor extends in front of the kidney, the gonadal vein is ligated and divided (on the left side, the gonadal vein drains directly into the left renal vein). If it appears that the tumor involves the kidney, the kidney is mobilized posterolaterally and the right renal artery is dissected, ligated, and divided from the posterior approach and then the renal vein is ligated and divided, preferably using vascular clamps through an anterior approach. If necessary, a cuff from the inferior vena cava is removed through the application of a lateral vascular clamp (Figs. 14.**6**–14.**9**). Thoracoabdominal incisions are well tolerated even by patients of advanced age.[2]

☐ Flank Retroperitoneal Sarcomas

These tumors are dissected with the patient in a lateral position with the affected side up. A flank incision is made over the protuberance of the tumor extending from the midline of the abdomen as far posteriorly as

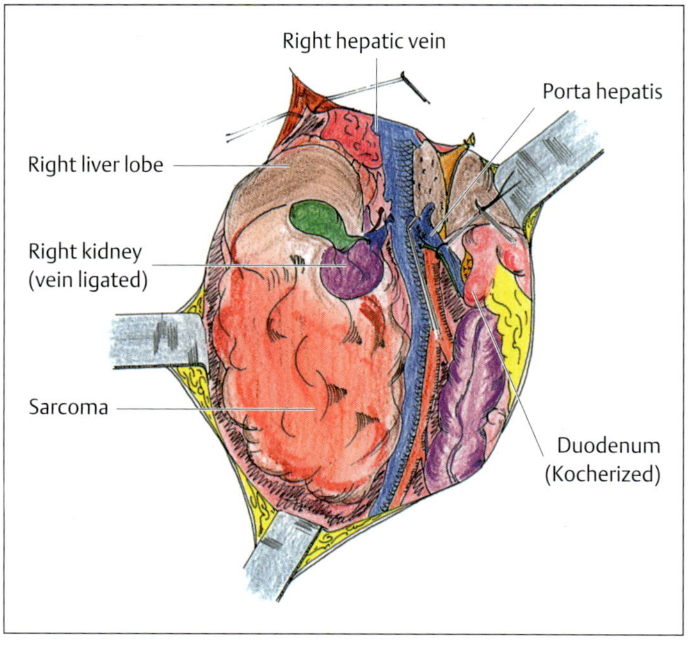

Fig. 14.**7** Right upper quadrant sarcoma after exposure and before resection. The duodenum is Kocherized. A Rummel tourniquet is applied to the porta hepatis. The tumor has invaded the right lobe of the liver and the right kidney. The right branch of the portal vein is clamped, the right hepatic vein is stapled, the cystic duct and the renal vessels are ligated. The exposure between the right side of the vena cava and the tumor is accomplished.

6

necessary in order to mobilize and dissect the tumor. This is combined usually with a midline incision. The approach again, as in the upper quadrants of the abdomen, is a combination of both transperitoneal as well as extraperitoneal dissection. Through the transperitoneal part of the incision, the respective colon is mobilized whenever that seems to be appropriate. Otherwise, the segment of colon that is attached to the tumor is divided proximal and distal to the area of involvement using a stapling device and the corresponding mesocolon is also divided so that the involved segment of colon and respective mesocolon are left with the tumor. Posterolaterally, the tumor is dissected off the lateral portion of the abdominal wall, removing any layers of muscle that may be too close to the tumor. Rarely, the tumor may be close to the femoral nerve which at this level is protected by the psoas muscle, and unless the psoas muscle is involved, it is not likely to be encountered in this location. As the mobilization of the tumor comes close to the midline on the right side, lumbar tributaries to the inferior vena cava are ligated and divided. The kidney may be involved and may have to be dissected and removed with the tumor mass. In the case of involvement of the inferior vena cava, this vein is dissected out proximal and distal to the tumor. The infrarenal portion of the inferior vena cava may be removed en bloc with the tumor without great difficulty. In this case, the inferior vena cava is exposed on its left side and the left renal vein and its insertion into the inferior vena cava behind the duodenum is exposed. In the case of a retroperitoneal **sarcoma of the flank on the right side** (Fig. 14.**10**) involving the inferior vena cava (Fig. 14.**11**) and kidney, one dissects the inferior vena cava above the level of the renal veins, both right and left, and below at the confluence of the right and left common iliac veins. At the lower end of the inferior vena cava above the confluence of the common iliac veins vascular clamps can be applied and the vein divided and oversewn, ligating and dividing any lumbar tributaries to this segment of the vein. Superiorly, two vascular clamps are applied obliquely on the inferior vena cava from below the entry point of the left renal vein to a point above the entry of the right renal vein to the inferior vena cava. In this fashion, one can remove the lower part of the infrarenal part of the inferior vena cava and preserve intact the continuity of the left renal vein into the inferior vena cava, while the tumor mass, the involved portion of the right colon, and the right kidney can be removed together with the mass (Figs. 14.**12**, 14.**13**).

For a retroperitoneal **sarcoma of the left flank**, the flank approach is again utilized with the patient in a lateral position with the affected side up (Fig. 14.**14**). A flank incision is made and this is extended to the midline. For both right-sided and left-sided flank tumors, it is necessary to perform this incision extending above

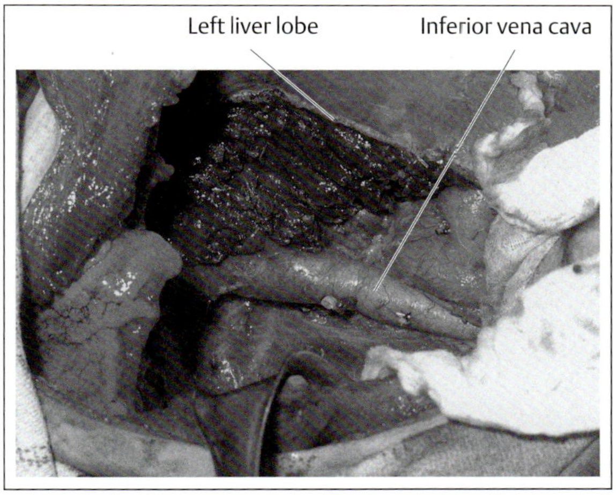

Fig. 14.**8** Operative field after resection of the sarcoma in Fig. 14.**6** showing the inferior vena cava and parenchyma of the remaining left lobe.

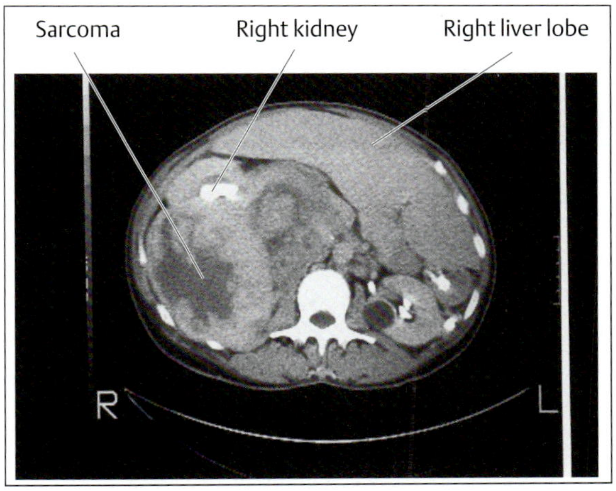

Fig. 14.**9** Sarcoma of the right upper quadrant displacing but not involving the right lobe of the liver. The right kidney is displaced anteriorly.

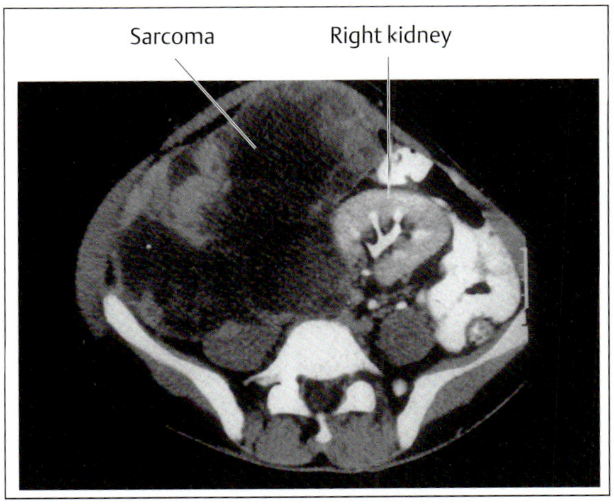

Fig. 14.**10** Sarcoma of the right flank displacing the right kidney to the left of midline. It was resected through a flank incision in combination with a midline abdominal incision.

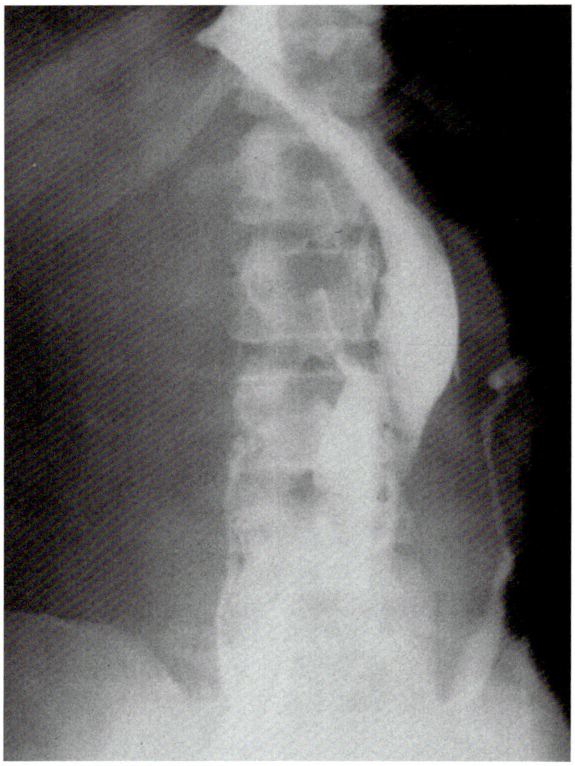

Fig. 14.**11** Same tumor as in Figure 14.**10** showing displacement of the inferior vena cava (IVC), which also had to be resected below the level of the left renal vein (the right renal vein and kidney were removed en bloc with the IVC).

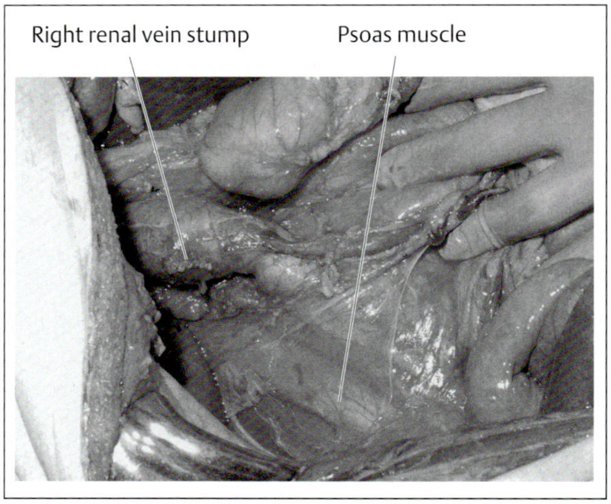

Fig. 14.**13** Operative field after resection of the tumor in Figure 14.**10** and 14.**11**.

Fig. 14.**14** Recurrent sarcoma in the left flank resected ▷ through a left flank incision in combination with an abdominal incision. The left colon and kidney were removed en bloc.

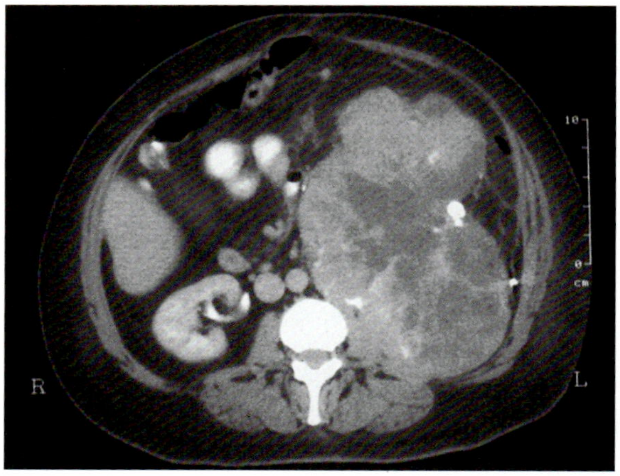

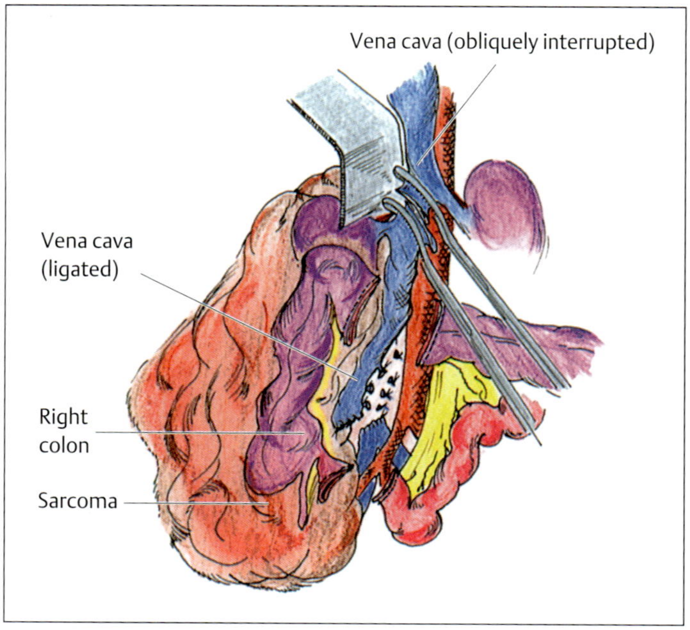

Fig. 14.**12** Right flank sarcoma after exposure and before resection. The vena cava, right kidney, and ascending colon are invaded. The distal ileum and transverse colon are stapled, the vena cava is stapled or sutured after iliac convergence, the lumbar tributaries are suture-ligated, a vascular clamp is applied obliquely below the left renal vein ostium. The tumor is resected en bloc with the ascending colon, right kidney, and infrarenal vena cava.

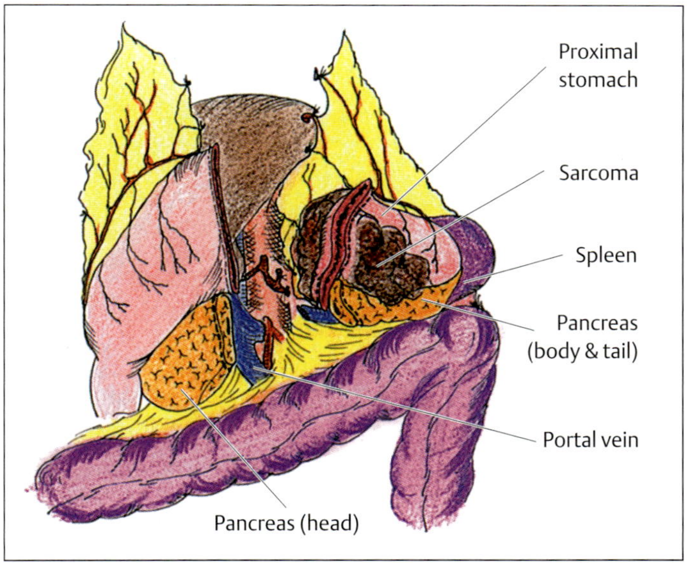

Fig. 14.**15** Lesser sac sarcoma after exposure and before removal. The tumor invades the proximal stomach, tail of the pancreas, and spleen. The proximal stomach and tail of the pancreas are stapled; the left gastric and splenic arteries are divided. The splenic vein is also ligated. The portal vein is exposed.

and below the area where the flank incision meets the midline and, therefore, create an angled "T" incision which provides adequate exposure for both the retroperitoneal as well as for the transperitoneal part of the dissection. Any visceral attachments to the tumor mass on the left side are dissected out if possible. Otherwise, the respective segment of large bowel and possibly small bowel is separated from its continuity and its respective mesentery is divided to be with the tumor mass. Posterolateral mobilization is again performed so that the tumor is mobilized first from its bed and then any connections with the aorta can be dealt with more effectively and safely.

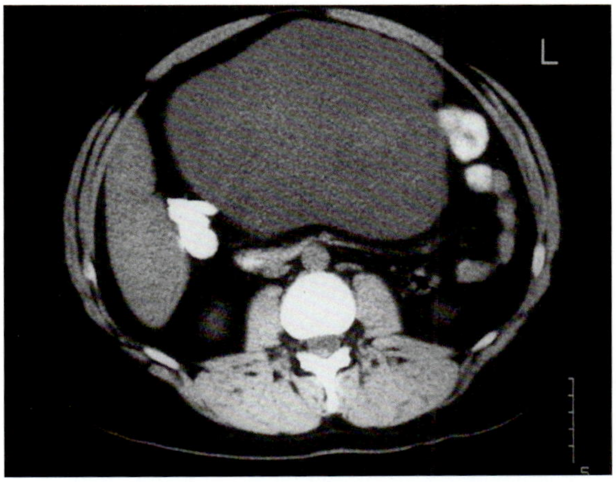

Fig. 14.**16** Liposarcoma involving the proximal mesentery of the bowel.

Midline Retroperitoneal Sarcomas

These are dealt with by having the patient in a supine position and using a long midline incision from the xiphoid to possibly the pubic symphysis. Retroperitoneal sarcomas in the lesser sac have to be dissected off the porta hepatis and the superior mesenteric vessels and, if this can be accomplished, the tumor becomes resectable even though part of the stomach and/or distal pancreas may have to be resected. It is easiest to identify the superior mesenteric vein by following the middle colic vein or another vein in the transverse colon down to its confluence to the superior mesenteric vein (Fig. 14.**15**). Soft tissue sarcomas, in contrast to adenocarcinomas or squamous cell carcinomas, can be dissected off adjacent structures and, although this is not the most desirable way of doing a resection, it should be possible for most retroperitoneal sarcomas in the area of the lesser sac to be macroscopically removed (R1 resection) by dissecting fairly close to the capsule of the tumor in the vicinity of critical structures. Adjacent organs (stomach, pancreas, transverse mesocolon) can be invaded. Whenever possible, their removal (total or partial) with safe margins is the state-of-art strategy. Retroperitoneal sarcomas in the area of the base of the mesentery of the small bowel should be assessed for their resectability by dissecting the superior mesenteric vessels. These tumors are usually large in size, often extending to the base of the mesentery. One has to first dissect out the loops of bowel that may be attached to the tumor and separate those whose vascular supply is not involved with the tumor. If the retroperitoneal sarcoma is close to the ileocecal area, the resection can be performed fairly easily by doing a modified right hemicolectomy with the involved distal ileum. In cases, however, where the mesentery is involved just below the mesocolon (Fig. 14.**16**), one may be able to free the first loop of jejunum (proximal to the mesenteric involvement). Then, one dissects the superior mesenteric vessels by following the mesentery immediately proximal to its involvement as well as just distal to it by the tumor. Visible mesenteric

6

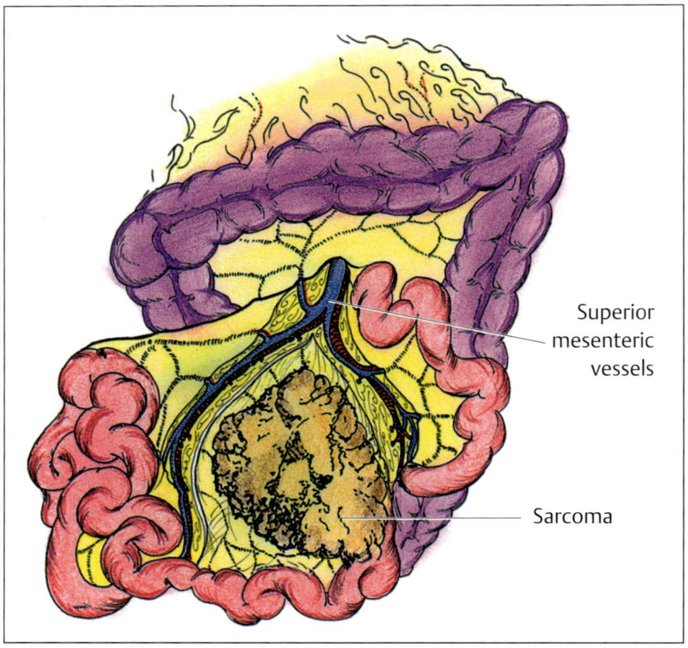

Fig. 14.17 Drawing illustrating the resection of the mesenteric tumor mass down to the surface of the superior mesenteric vessels.

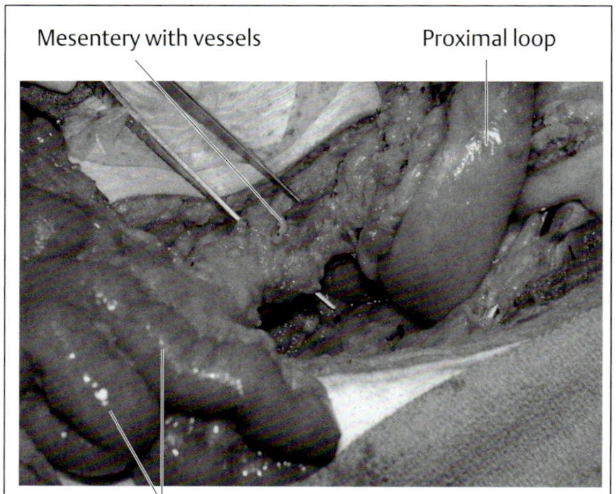

Fig. 14.18 Operative field after resection of the tumor of Figure 14.16. The forceps is showing a narrow piece of adipose tissue enclosing the superior mesenteric vessels and supplying the distal bowel.

branches are followed to the base of the mesentery by incising the mesenteric peritoneal leaf on either side. The trunk of the superior mesenteric vein is exposed and, if this is not involved, one proceeds to ligate and divide tributaries from the involved area of the mesentery. Immediately to the left and posterior to the vein, the superior mesenteric artery (SMA) is dissected and branches from the SMA to the involved area of the mesentery are ligated and divided (Figs. 14.**17**, 14.**18**). In this fashion, one can ascertain the resectability of a soft tissue sarcoma at the base of the mesentery, obtain the greatest margin that is technically feasible, and perform the dissection with full knowledge that the distal uninvolved bowel will have an adequate blood supply.[3]

A lower midline abdominal sarcoma (Fig. 14.**19**) may involve, in addition to bowel, a long segment of ureter that needs to be resected with the tumor while the kidney may be preserved. In this case, it should be possible to dissect a segment of distal ileum with its mesentery and separate it from the intestinal flow. By dividing this appropriate length of segment (generally 20 cm) with a stapling device proximally and distally, this segment of bowel is mobilized so that the distal end is sutured to the bladder in an end-to-side anastomosis and the proximal end near the staple line to the ureter using fine Vicryl interrupted or running sutures (Figs. 14.**20**, 14.**21**). It is not advisable to connect this segment of intestine to the distal end of the ureter if any

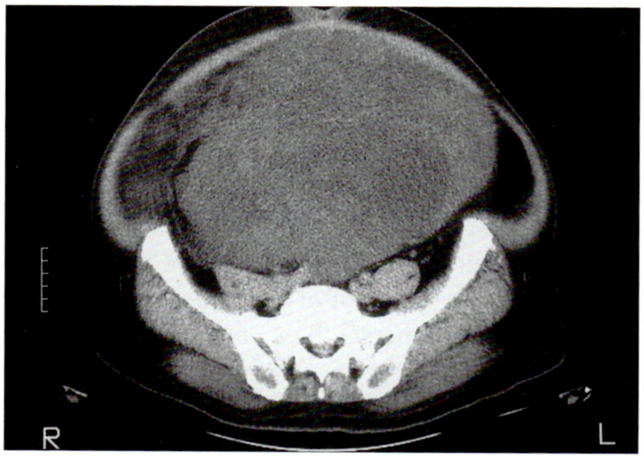

Fig. 14.19 Sarcoma of the midline of the lower abdomen, resected through a midline incision en bloc with the right colon and a segment of the right ureter.

6

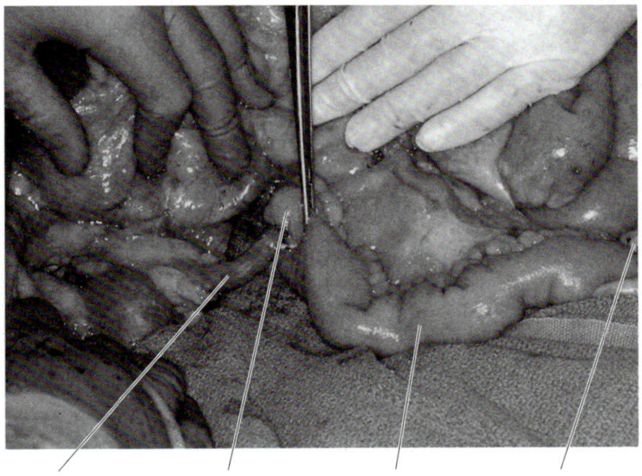

Fig. 14.**20** Operative field showing the ileal segment connecting the proximal ureter to the bladder. The forceps is pointing to the ureteroenteric anastomosis (to the right of the picture is the enterocystic anastomosis).

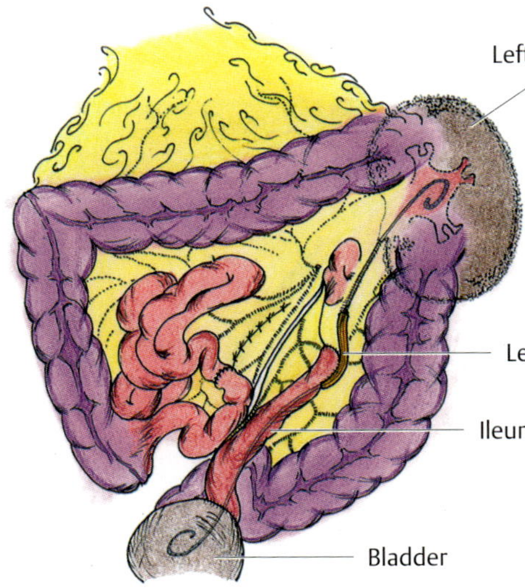

Fig. 14.**21** Drawing showing a segment of ileum, separated from the enteric circulation, connecting the proximal ureter on the left to the bladder in the case of resection of a long segment of ureter.

part of it is remaining because the thick secretions of the intestine may have difficulty going through the distal anastomosis between the defunctionalized ileal segment and the distal portion of the ureter.

☐ Sarcomas of the Pelvis

Sarcomas in the midline of the pelvis can usually be resected easily by dissecting around the tumor mass with adjacent normal tissues, i. e., a portion of the colon or bladder if these structures become involved. It is rare for a pelvic sarcoma to require a complete pelvic exenteration. Some of these pelvic sarcomas extend inferiorly and come close to the obturator foramen on both sides and, in this case, the lower midline incision, used for initial exploration, is extended bilaterally along the pubic crest to the pubic tubercle. The anterior rectus sheath and muscle are divided off the pubic crest. The peritoneum is incised lateral to the bladder on each side and, thus, the external iliac vein, as well as the obturator area and obturator foramen are exposed adequately. Incising the peritoneum at a point midway between the pubic symphysis and umbilicus in an inferolateral direction around the bladder is an important maneuver in facilitating exposure. Lateral extension substantially improves the exposure in this area (Fig. 14.**22**).[4] Unilateral extension of the transverse incision from the pubic symphysis can be employed when the tumor extends laterally only on one side.

For sarcomas in the lesser pelvis fixed to the wall of the lesser pelvis, extending into the obturator foramen or through the obturator foramen into the adductor group of muscles, it is possible to perform an adequate

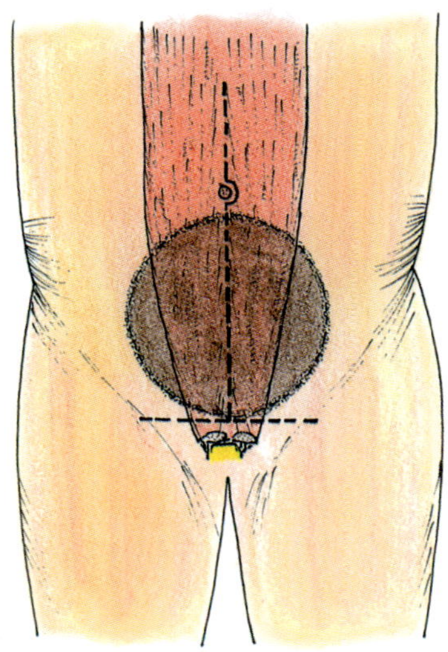

Fig. 14.**22** A reverse-T incision, transecting bilaterally the rectus abdominis off the pubic crest facilitating the resection of a midline pelvic sarcoma extending laterally to the obturator foramina.

resection by using the abdominoinguinal incision.[5,6] Chapter 10 of this book is devoted to this incision. This incision is indicated for pelvic sarcomas of the midline extending to one or both sides over the external iliac vessels to the iliac crest. Through the midline incision, there is no exposure to resect these tumors. This incision is also indicated for sarcomas of the iliac fossa, sarcomas involving the external iliac vessels, and those involving the wall of the lesser pelvis and pubic bone (also for matted, large, nodal masses in the external iliac or obturator area). The abdominoinguinal incision involves a lower abdominal midline incision with

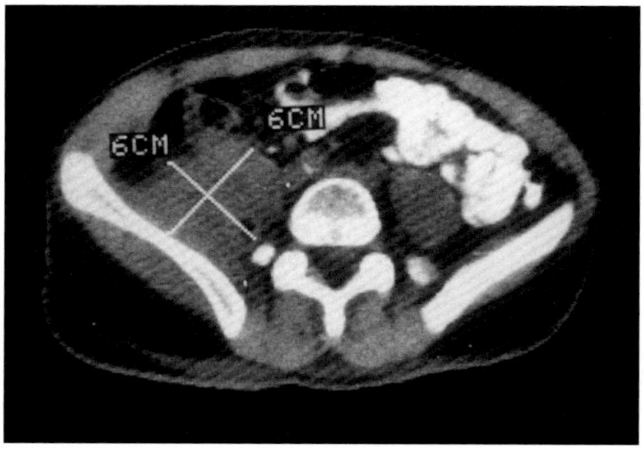

Fig. 14.**23** Mass in the right iliac fossa resected through a right abdominoinguinal incision.

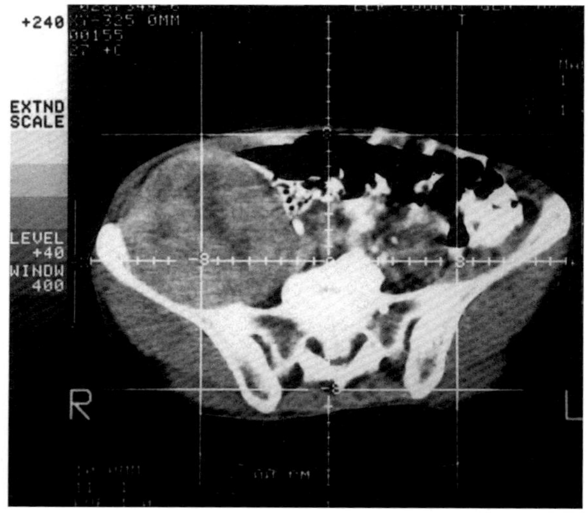

Fig. 14.**24** Mass in the right iliac fossa resected also through a right abdominoinguinal incision.

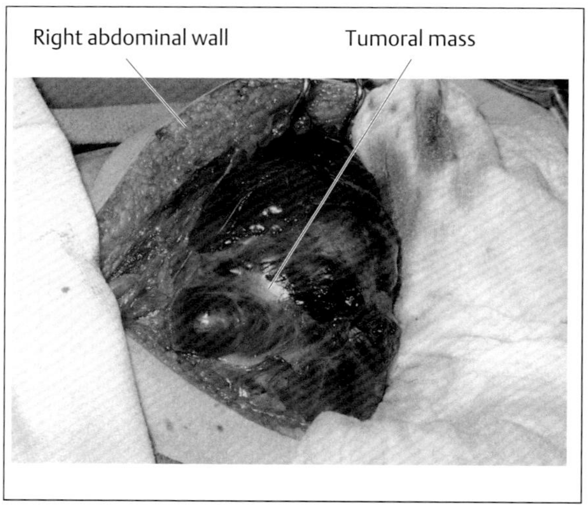

Fig. 14.**25** View of a lower abdominal mass as shown from a groin incision, removed through a right abdominoinguinal incision.

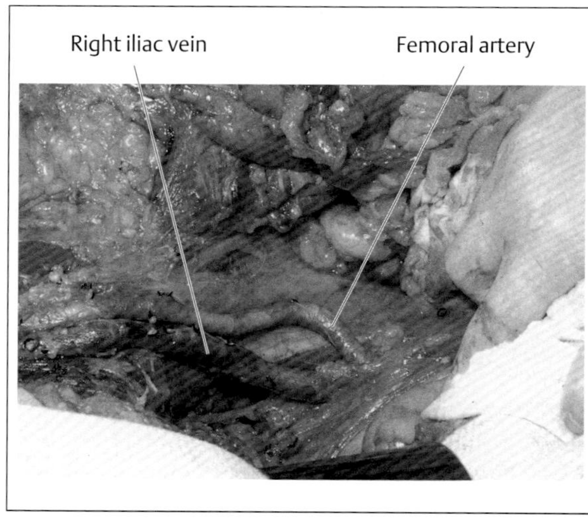

Fig. 14.**26** Operative field showing exposed right iliofemoral vessels following removal of the tumor shown in Figure 14.**25**.

the patient in a supine position, through which one can perform preliminary exploration and dissection of any midline structures off the tumor mass. The incision is then extended transversely toward the side of involvement from the pubic symphysis to the midinguinal point. From the midinguinal point, it is extended vertically for a few centimeters so that the common femoral vessels can be exposed (it is extended to the apex of the femoral triangle when a concomitant dissection of the inguinal nodes en bloc with large deep nodes is advisable). The ipsilateral rectus sheath and rectus abdominis are then divided off the pubic crest. The inguinal ligament is divided off the pubic tubercle and, as this part of the abdominal wall is lifted, the inferior epigastric vein and inferior epigastric artery more laterally are ligated and divided serially. This opens up the lower abdominal wall as the page of a book and in one continuous field the lower abdominal aorta, the common and external iliac vessels, and their continuity into the common femoral vessels become exposed without any interruption. For further exposure, the inguinal ligament is detached off the iliac fascia since the lateral part of the inguinal ligament is fused to this fascia.

For sarcomas of the iliac fossa (Figs. 14.**23**–14.**30**), the femoral nerve is dissected lateral to the common femoral artery by incising the iliac fascia. It is traced superiorly as it courses between the iliacus and psoas muscles. It is important for sarcomas in this location to have the ipsilateral extremity covered with a sterile stockinette so that it can be flexed at the knee and hip joints, a

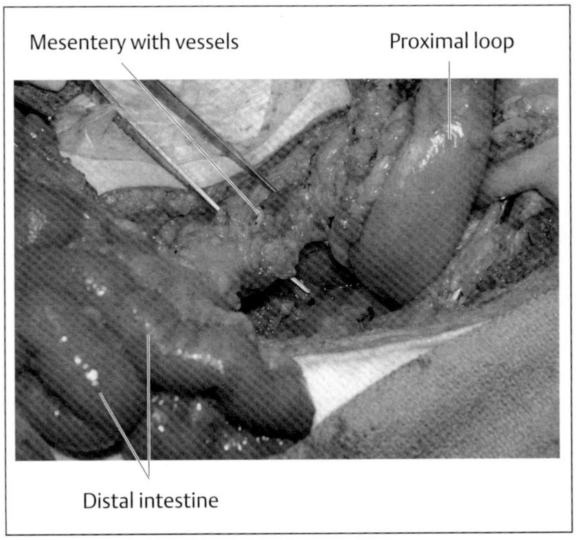

Fig. 14.**27** Mass in the right lower quadrant in the process of removal through a right abdominoinguinal incision. The epigastric vessels are surrounded by vessel loops.

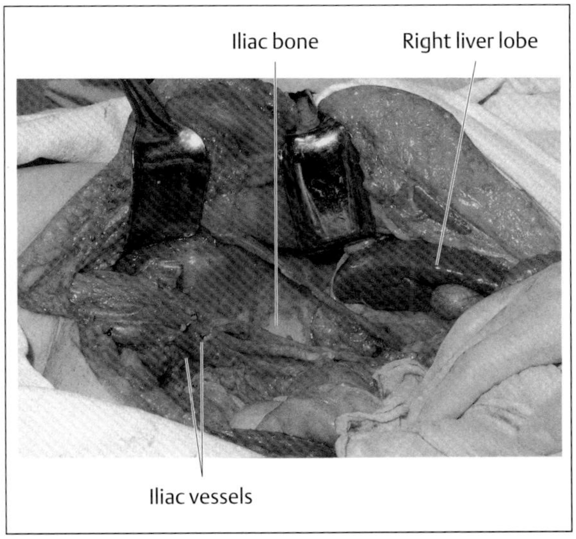

Fig. 14.**28** Operative field after resection of sarcoma of the right iliac fossa showing the exposed iliac bone.

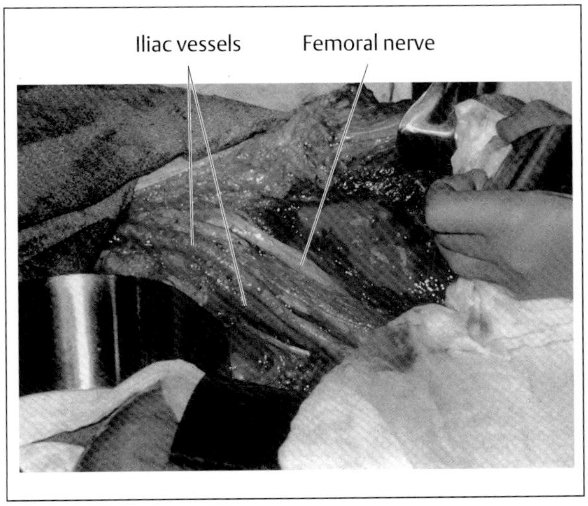

Fig. 14.**29** Operative field after resection of a sarcoma of the right iliac fossa with exposed iliofemoral vessels and femoral nerve.

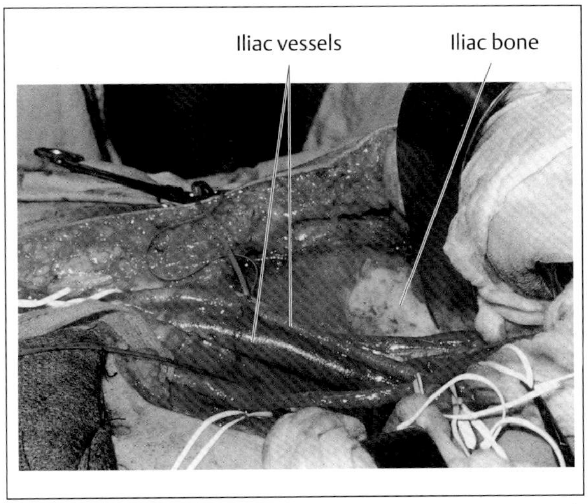

Fig. 14.**30** Operative field after resection of sarcoma of the right iliac fossa with exposed iliac bone.

6

maneuver which relaxes the femoral nerve as well as the iliofemoral vessels and allows their retraction and dissection off the tumor whenever that is feasible. In performing the abdominoinguinal incision, it is possible to preserve the spermatic cord in the male by incising the floor of the inguinal canal posteriorly, i. e., incising the transversalis fascia, extricating the spermatic cord off its inguinal canal and displacing the vas deferens medially. The spermatic vessels which proceed in a more direct cephalad direction as they issue from the internal inguinal ring can be preserved or sacrificed at this level, depending upon the proximity of the tumor. Ligation of the internal spermatic vessels above the internal inguinal ring is compatible with viability of the testis which is preserved, although it may atrophy, as long as it has not been simultaneously exteriorized off its scrotal bed, an eventuality which would interrupt the tenuous blood supply from the scrotum to the testis.

In sarcomas of the iliac fossa not involving the iliac bone, the iliacus muscle is detached off its origin from the iliac bone; the psoas may also have to be resected en bloc with the tumor. The femoral nerve, if it is not directly invaded by the tumor mass, can be preserved. If it is involved with the tumor mass, it can be sacrificed with a moderate functional disability. Patients in whom the femoral nerve has to be sacrificed are unable to extend the knee and may require external support for a while, but finally they are able to walk without using a cane, being able to extend the knee passively during ambulation. Occasionally, the segment of the external iliac and common femoral vessels may have to be re-

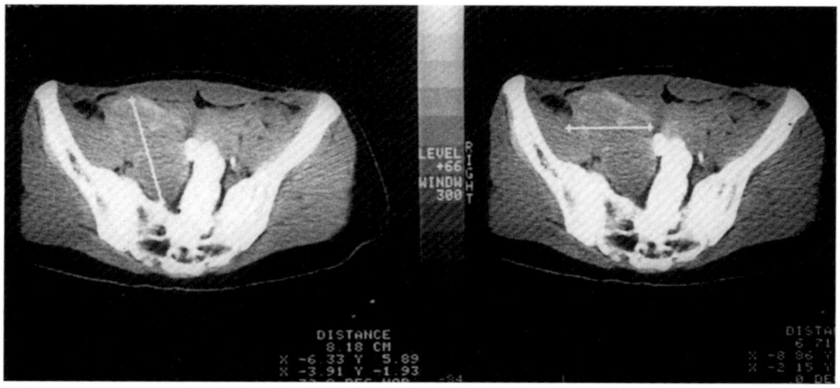

Fig. 14.**31** Fibrosarcoma of the right lower quadrant involving the right ureter and external iliac artery.

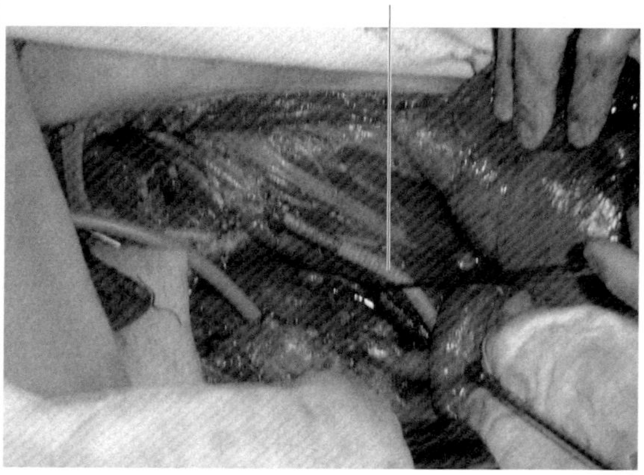

Fig. 14.**32** Operative field showing that the right external iliac artery has been resected and replaced with a graft and the distal ureter has been resected and the proximal end implanted in the bladder.

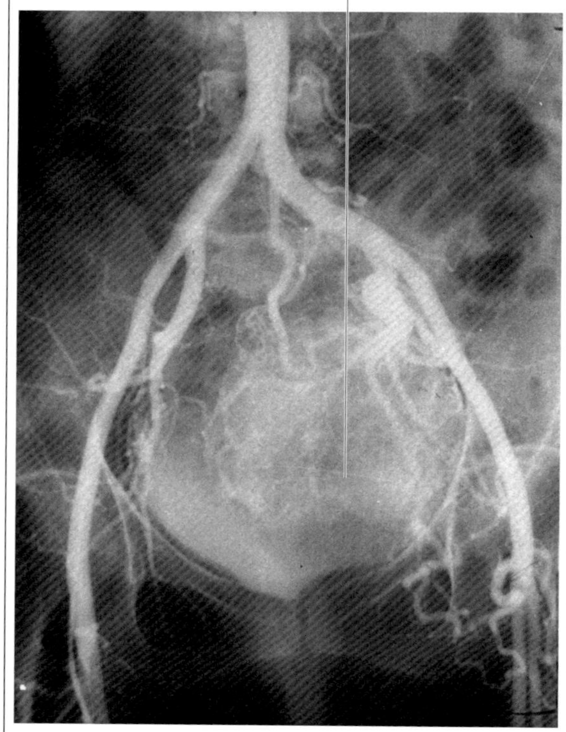

Fig. 14.**33** Hemangiosarcoma of the pelvis resected through a ▷ bilateral abdominoinguinal incision.

sected if involved by the tumor and replaced with a graft (Figs. 14.**31**, 14.**32**).[7] With the abdominoinguinal incision, it is easy to do so because the vessels are exposed in their continuity and one can have proximal and distal control.

The abdominoinguinal incision is also helpful for sarcomas involving the wall of the lesser pelvis (Figs. 14.**33**–14.**36**). The internal iliac artery is dissected and a vessel loop is passed around it. The tumor mass is separated from the bladder or a portion of it may have to be resected. On the lateral side, i. e., on the side of the wall of the lesser pelvis, the external iliac vein is retracted laterally and a tributary of the external iliac vein, i. e., the pubic vein, has to be ligated and divided. The fascia covering the obturator internus is incised and the plane is entered between the roof of the acetabulum and the obturator internus fibers. This plane, carried on the surface of the roof of the acetabulum, provides as a margin the obturator internus muscle when resecting a pelvic sarcoma in the lesser pelvis with lateral fixation. The uncomplicated abdominoinguinal incision is closed by approximating, with interrupted nonabsorbable sutures, the lateral portion of the inguinal ligament to the iliac fascia and the medial portion to Cooper's ligament. The rectus sheath and muscle are approximated to the pubic crest and the midline ab-

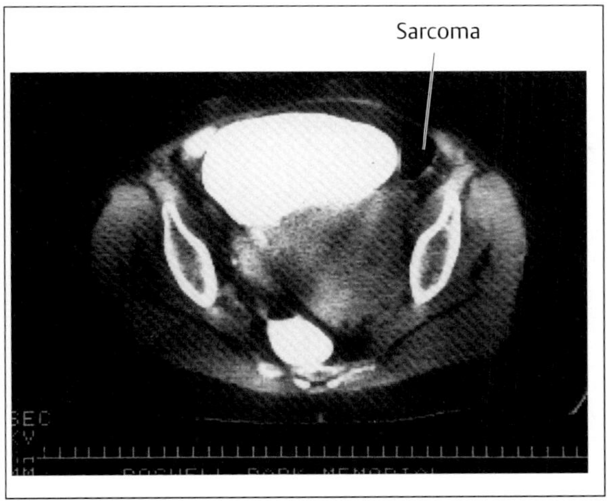

Fig. 14.**34** Sarcoma of the wall of the lesser pelvis on the left side.

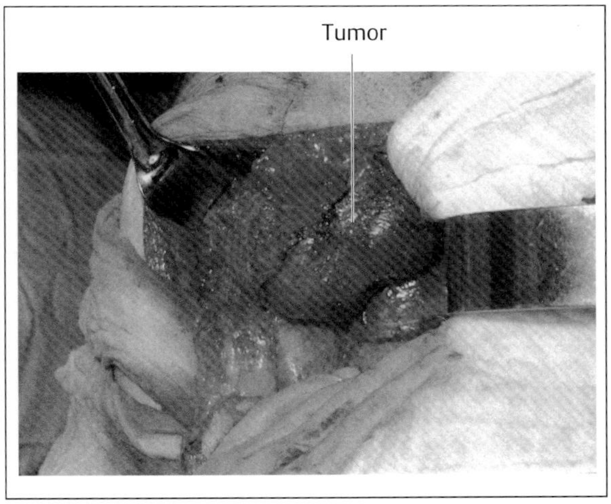

Fig. 14.**35** Through a lower midline abdominal incision, the tumor is medially exposed, but there is no visibility for exposure of the inferolateral aspect of the tumor.

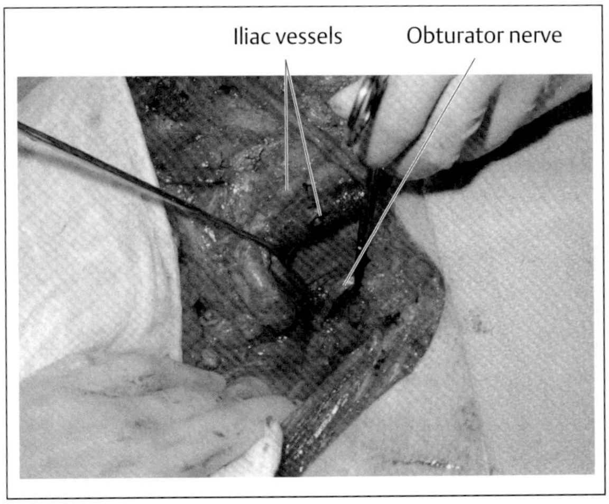

Fig. 14.**36** Operative field after resection of the tumor shown in Figure 14.**35** showing the external iliac vessels and obturator nerve.

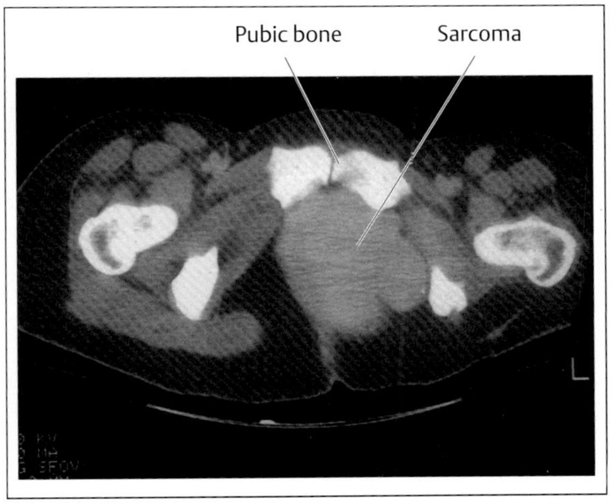

Fig. 14.**37** Soft tissue sarcoma of the pelvis involving the left pubic bone.

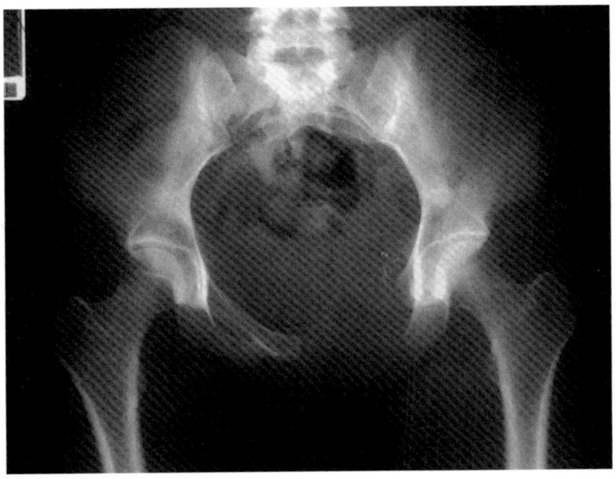

Fig. 14.**38** Postoperative X-ray showing the missing left pubic bone.

dominal incision is closed in a routine fashion. For pelvic tumors involving the pubic bone and/or by continuity the obturator foramen (Fig. 14.**37**) and the adductor group of muscles, through the abdominoinguinal incision, the pubic symphysis is exposed and dissected, both cephalad as well as caudally. A Gigli saw is passed around the pubic symphysis with which this is divided. A Gigli saw is passed around the anterior pubic ramus which is divided medial to the acetabulum and after division of the origin of the adductor group of muscles at a sufficient distance from any tumor involvement, the posterior pubic ramus is exposed close to the ischial tuberosity, surrounded with a right angle clamp and is divided with a Gigli saw (Fig. 14.**38**). The defect caused by removal of the pubic bone can be repaired with a mesh, being careful that the mesh does not abut directly against the iliac or femoral vessels. In cases of involvement by the soft tissue sarcoma of the inner

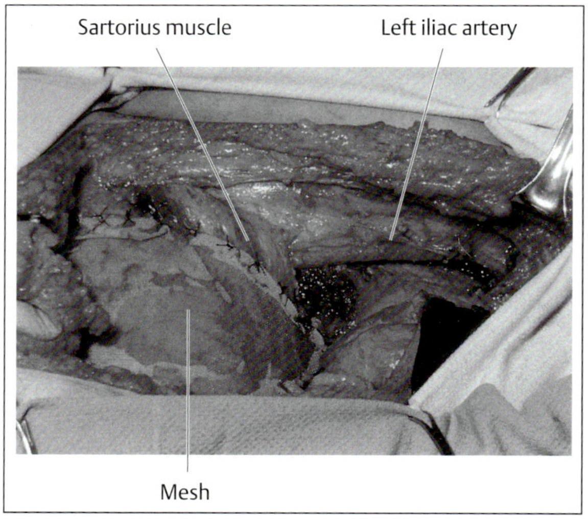

Fig. 14.**39** Operative field after resection of the left public bone and adjacent lower abdominal wall muscles due to soft tissue sarcoma, repaired with placement of mesh. The sartorius muscle has been mobilized to cover the femoral vessels.

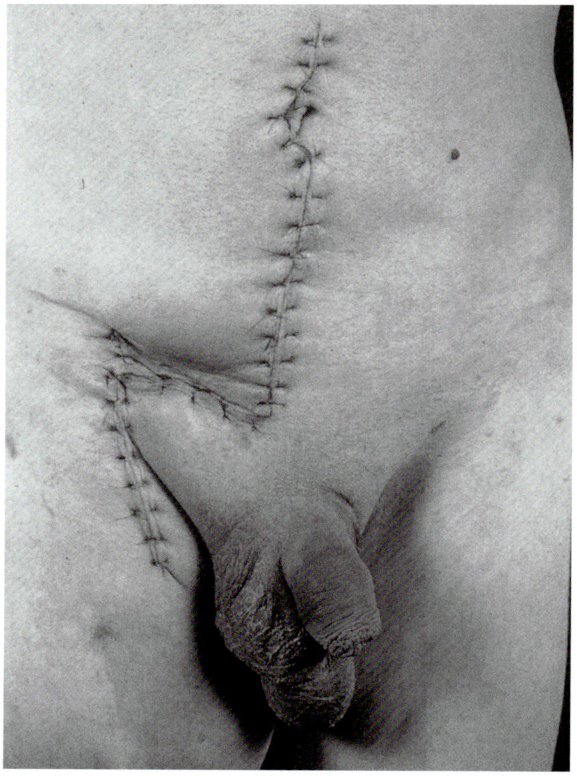

Fig. 14.**40** The abdominoinguinal incision heals well without any complications.

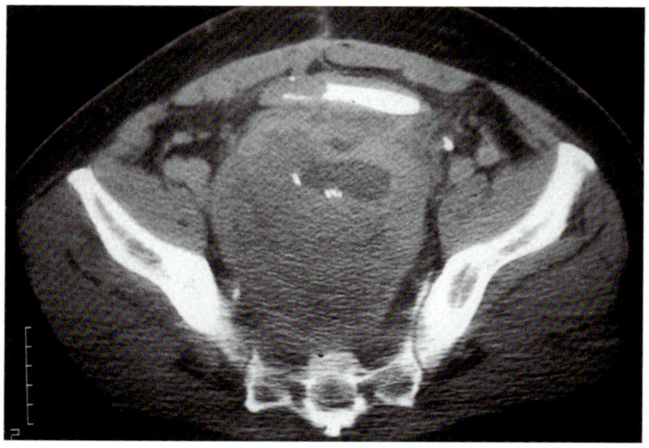

◁ Fig. 14.**41** Midline pelvic sarcoma which required a pelvic exenteration.

6

layers of the lower abdominal wall in the area of the iliac fossa, the abdominoinguinal incision is modified so that, at the level of the fascia, one can circumscribe the area of aponeurotic involvement. In some of these cases, one may end up removing the musculoaponeurotic layers of the entire thickness of the lower abdominal wall including the inguinal ligament. The repair in this case can be accomplished by using a mesh (Fig. 14.**39**), which is sutured lateral to the femoral artery and nerve to the iliac fascia, whenever the latter is available. If this fascia is unavailable due to its removal, the mesh is sutured to the ligaments of the anterior aspect of the capsule of the hip joint. Medially, the mesh can be sutured to Cooper's ligament. One, however, should provide, by rotating the sartorius or other tissue, coverage of the vessels so that the mesh will not be in direct contact with the vessels as it can erode through and cause hemorrhage of the artery. This is more likely to happen in the case of previous radiation.

In the experience of the author, it is actually preferable if one has to resect the lower part of the abdominal wall including the inguinal ligament, to reconstruct the defect by rotating a rectus abdominis flap from the contralateral side based on the inferior epigastric vessels and consisting of peritoneum, posterior sheath, and the muscle, the flap being divided at the costal margin so it can rotate laterally and reach all the way to the iliac crest. This flap is about 8-cm wide and can provide coverage for a defect in this area. The inferior part of the rotated muscle is sutured to the iliac fascia lateral to the vessels and to Cooper's ligament medial to the vessels. Superiorly, it is sutured to the defect in the musculoaponeurotic layers.

The abdominoinguinal incision in most cases heals well (Fig. 14.**40**). By using this incision or a simpler version when appropriate (reverse T-incision), the majority of pelvic sarcomas can be resected with preservation of organs not involved by the tumor. Rarely, a pelvic exenteration may be required (Figs. 14.**41**, 14.**42**).

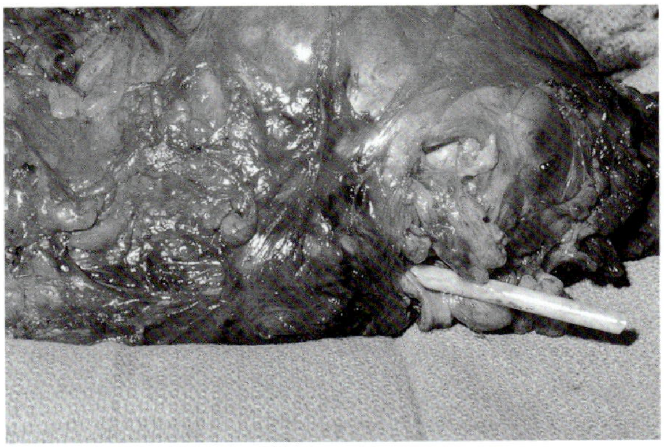

Fig. 14.**42** Specimen after pelvic exenteration showing the removed bladder and Foley catheter en bloc with the tumor.

Use of Prosthetic Material

Defects of the chest wall and diaphragm, upper abdominal wall, midabdominal wall, and lower abdominal wall may occur as the result of resection due to involvement by a retroperitoneal sarcoma. In this case, the full thickness of the muscular aponeurotic layer may have to be resected en bloc with the tumor mass. In the upper quadrant of the abdomen, following a resection involving the diaphragm, one starts by placing the mesh on the chest wall defect. It is joined then by another piece of mesh replacing the diaphragm. The mesh is kept taut at the center and it is folded to accommodate the circumferential defect. The suture is placed through the folded edge for greater strength. For abdominal wall resections requiring repair with a mesh, particularly in the lower part of the lower abdomen where loops of small bowel can abut against the mesh, it is extremely important to place autologous tissue between the mesh and the loops of bowel so as to prevent fistulization of the bowel which is apt to occur in 25% of the patients. This may occur postoperatively in a few days, but may also occur weeks or months following the repair. The most easily available material to cover the deep surface of the mesh is the greater omentum which can be elongated by releasing its attachments to the transverse colon. If further length is necessary the omentum is mobilized on the right gastroepiploic artery. On the opposite side, the omentum can be pediculated on the left gastroepiploic artery, thus reaching the pelvis. The greater omentum can thus reach all the way down to the groin and should be sutured underneath the defect so that the mesh is placed on top of the omentum to repair the musculoaponeurotic defect. In cases where the greater omentum is not available due to prior resection, one can mobilize the contralateral rectus abdominis whenever applicable to place underneath the defect or simply remove part of the peritoneum from another area of the abdominal cavity and suture it to the peritoneal defect and on top of that place the mesh to repair the fascial defect. This maneuver effectively prevents dense adhesion formation and fistulization. It appears that the free patch of peritoneum is able to survive within the low oxygen tension of the peritoneal cavity and prevents dense adhesion formation and fistulization which could eventually occur from direct contact of the deep surface of the mesh with the bowel loops.[8] With the availability currently of patches with a nonadhering surface, the concern for bowel adhesions or fistulization has been alleviated.

Technical Problems

An **iliac fossa tumor** involving the iliac bone or involving the gluteal muscles requires the inclusion of the internal hemipelvectomy.[9] In this case the patient has to be placed in a lateral or semilateral position exposing the ipsilateral abdominal wall and buttock. This incision extends from the posterior/inferior iliac spine along the iliac crest to the anterior superior iliac spine and then along the inguinal ligament to the pubic tubercle. The incision is deepened through the subcutaneous fat, external oblique aponeurosis, internal oblique, and transversus abdominis to enter the retroperitoneal space. The inguinal ligament is divided at the anterior superior iliac spine and then it is separated in its lateral third from the iliac fascia. In the retroperitoneal space the external iliac vessels are dissected and visualized. The ureter along with the peritoneum is displaced medially and the inferior epigastric artery and vein are serially ligated and divided. If the tumor only superficially involves the inner cortex of the left bone, one may then proceed with dissection on the lateral surface of the iliac bone using a cautery as well as a periosteal elevator exposing the lateral surface of the iliac bone, the sacroiliac joint posteriorly, and the greater sciatic notch more anteriorly. Some bleeding may be encountered close to the greater sciatic notch from the inferior or superior gluteal vessels but that can easily be controlled. The sartorius muscle is divided off its origin as well as the tensor fascia lata. The rectus femoris is divided off its origin. On the medial side, one divides the iliacus and psoas muscles below the level of the inguinal ligament and exposes the medial surface of the iliac bone immediately above the acetabulum. As the external iliac vessels are retracted, one can expose the greater sciatic notch on its medial aspect. Superiorly, the quadratus lumborum and the latissimus dorsi are divided off their attachment to the posterior part of the iliac crest and the sacroiliac joint is exposed on the medial side also by retracting the psoas muscle. The femoral nerve may be dissected and preserved, if possible. If one wishes to carry the bone dissection more proximally, i.e., through the sacral ala, one has to retract the lumbosacral trunk (L4, L5) coursing on the sacral ala en route to joining the sacral nerve roots in order to form the sciatic nerve. Having exposed the greater sciatic notch both medially and laterally, one then can pass a Gigli saw around the greater sciatic notch and saw through the bone to a point below the anterior inferior iliac spine. This will be the distal end of the resection and it is a centimeter or two above the roof of the acetabulum. Proximally, the bone is divided through the sacroiliac joint or sacral ala using osteotomes and, thus, the specimen can be removed. Whenever part of the gluteal muscles has to be resected, then an extension of the initially described incision from the anterior superior iliac spine toward the greater trochanter is performed and a flap is developed by dissecting on top of the fascia covering the gluteus medius and minimus in order to remove these muscles with the specimen. For removal of the entire hemipelvis the incision has to be carried out all the way to the pubic symphysis in order to divide the pubic symphysis with a Gigli saw, separate the adductor group of muscles off their origin from the pubic bone and divide the neck of the femur allowing removal of the specimen following division of the ipsilateral levator ani, sacrotuberous, and sacrospinous ligaments.

The case of a **pelvic sarcoma involving the lower sacrum**. The patient is placed in a right lateral position with the left side up and a lower midline incision is used to dissect whatever structures can be dissected off the anterior aspect of the tumor. Part of the rectosigmoid may have to be divided and left on the surface of the tumor. Through a posterior approach, one makes a longitudinal incision in the midline from the lumbosacral junction to the coccyx. Flaps are developed to the lateral edges of the sacrum and the origin of the gluteus maximus on each edge is divided, the anococcygeal raphe is divided and the precoccygeal space is entered. Then, by manual palpation of the tumor location, dissection continues on the side of the sacrum and around the tumor mass. If one can stay below the level of the S2 vertebra, then one can expect to preserve sphincteric control, both for the urinary bladder as well as the rectum. Ideally, one should expose the ischiorectal fossa, identify the pudendal nerve on each side at it courses on the obturator fascia and trace it superiorly so that when the posterior sacral plate is entered with neurosurgical rongeurs and the proximal sacral roots are displaced superiorly, one can preserve the continuity of the upper sacral roots to the pudendal nerve which courses around the ischial spine to the surface of the obturator internus.[10] Unilateral preservation of the pudendal nerve is sufficient to provide sphincteric control. The pudendal nerve is composed of the ventral S2 to S4 roots and is responsible not only for sphincteric control, but also for erection in men.

Sarcomas of the pelvis which extensively involve the pelvis in a way that they cannot be resected through a more conservative operation may require an (external) hemipelvectomy. For sarcomas which extensively involve not only the iliac fossa but also the wall of the lesser pelvis and infiltrate the bone, a posterior flap hemipelvectomy is used whenever the tumor does not extend to the buttock. The critical condition for viability of the posterior flap is the preservation of the gluteus maximus with the posterior flap. It has nothing to do with the level of ligation of the iliac vessels, i. e., whether at the common iliac or external iliac level.[11]

For tumors of the lesser pelvis which are extensive and involve the buttock, an anterior flap hemipelvectomy should be performed based on the quadriceps muscle which remains attached to the anterior flap and gets its blood supply primarily through the lateral circumflex branches of the profunda femoris vessels.[4]

☐ Discussion

In a collective review published in 1991 which covered all of the series of retroperitoneal sarcoma resections published in the United States, the overall complete resectability rate was 53%, with a range of 38–74%.[12] The five-year survival in this collective review was 34%, largely because nearly half the patients did not have their tumors resected. In this author's experience, the complete resectability rate of a group of primary and locally recurrent retroperitoneal sarcomas (n = 90) was 96% and the five-year survival for the primary retroperitoneal sarcomas was 66% (10-year survival was 57%).[13] Local recurrence is a major problem following complete resection of a retroperitoneal sarcoma. At 10-year follow-up, it was 91% in the collective review and 54% in our series. The 5-year survival varies according to the histologic grade. In the collective review, it was 74% for Grade I and 24% for Grades II and III tumors; in our series it was 88% for Grade I, 52% for Grade II and 45% for Grade III tumors ($p = 0.007$). In our series, the rate of local recurrence was 16% after wide resection and 56% after local excision (p 0.001). The 10-year survival was 61% after wide resection and 23% after local excision ($p = 0.01$), pointing to the need for wide resection of adjacent to the tumor viscera when that is feasible.[13] The complete resectability rate has remained the same in the last review of our series by using the techniques described above.[14]

The authors of the collective review discuss the issues related to operative technique. In their opinion, a patient with retroperitoneal sarcoma should be explored in a supine position through a midline abdominal incision from the xiphoid to the pubic symphysis and then following lysis of adhesions it should be determined whether the tumor mass can be separated from the aorta on the left side or the inferior vena cava on the right side. This certainly is a logical approach. It is, however, fraught with the risk of hemorrhage and may lead the surgeon to easily abandon the operation declaring the tumor unresectable. When the tumor extends right up against the aorta or inferior vena cava for an appreciable distance, it becomes impossible to find a plane and certainly impossible to do that with safety of surgical maneuvers in separating the tumor mass off the aorta or inferior vena cava. It is preferable for tumors of the upper quadrants of the abdomen, as well as the flank, to have the patient in a lateral position and through a combination of transperitoneal and extraperitoneal approach, mobilize the tumor off its bed and leave to last the handling of any attachments and connections between the tumor and the aorta or inferior vena cava. By mobilizing the tumor, it becomes possible to separate it off even only for a distance perhaps of a few millimeters from these major vascular structures and it becomes also easier to visualize any branches between these vascular structures and the tumor and to control any bleeding that may occur.

The position of the patient on the operating table should be selected so that gravity is on the side of the surgeon and not against the surgeon.

The second point of importance is the strategy to be followed in the removal of a retroperitoneal sarcoma and that may be summarized simply as a dissection which follows the path of least resistance. Since safety is a major consideration, it is always important to change the plane of dissection if the dissection no longer seems to be safe. By mobilizing the easily dissectible areas around the tumor, the tumor mass itself is further freed up and the areas which were previously difficult to dissect, become easier to do so. It is important for the surgeon to keep in mind the geometry of space and the objective to be accomplished, but there should be flexibility in alternating planes of dissection and areas of dissection, as needed and dictated by considerations of safety. It is important for the surgeon also to master the technique of safe dissection. A scalpel or cautery dissection is safer through compact tissues than a scissors dissection, the latter being appropriate and helpful when one incises transparent membranous tissues. For vascular tumors such as leiomyosarcomas, with a multitude of veins around the tumor mass, it is safer to perform a dissection away from the tumor not only in order to obtain a greater surgical margin but also because the blood supply to the tumor is carried out through stouter and fewer blood vessels away from the tumor surface. Ligating small veins around the tumor mass should be done carefully so that the point to be ligated is not placed under traction as the ties are being laid down and it is kept immobile. Otherwise, traction on a rather small or medium-sized vein may lead to its avulsion and bleeding. With the high rate of resection of retroperitoneal sarcomas that approaches that of extremity sarcomas, the five-year survival for retroperitoneal sarcomas approaches also the survival of extremity soft-tissue sarcomas.[15] Therefore, there is nothing mysterious about retroperitoneal sarcomas other than the difficulty they present in complete resection. With the use of appropriate positioning, adequate incisions, and the correct (but flexible) strategy in resection, these tumors are highly resectable in the vast majority of patients.

In the case of retroperitoneal sarcomas, wide resection (involving usually resection of adjacent organs), compared to local excision not only reduces the rate of local recurrence but also significantly improves survival.[14] The same phenomenon is not observed in extremity sarcomas where local recurrence does not appear to impact significantly on survival and can nearly always be resected, if necessary by amputation.[16] In retroperitoneal sarcomas, it is difficult to obtain local control and to resect satisfactorily local recurrences, while local recurrence may give rise to abdominal dissemination in the free peritoneal cavity.

The techniques elaborated in the resection of retroperitoneal sarcomas are applicable also to other histologic types. For example, the abdominoinguinal incision can be very useful in the resection of sigmoid or cecal carcinoma with posterior and/or anterior fixation in the iliac fossa[17] and in the surgical treatment of gynecologic tumors with lateral pelvic fixation.

References

1. Karakousis CP, Blumenson LE, Canavese G, Rao U. Surgery for disseminated abdominal sarcoma. *Am J Surg.* 1992;163: 560–564.
2. Karakousis CP, Pourshahmir M. Thoracoabdominal incisions and resection of upper retroperitoneal sarcomas. *J Surg Oncol.* 1999;72:150–155.
3. Karakousis CP, Lopez R, Holyoke ED. Technique of resection of mesenteric tumors. *Am J Surg.* 1979;137:693–695.
4. Karakousis CP. Surgery for Soft Tissue Sarcomas. In: Karakousis CP, Bland K, Copeland EM, eds. *Atlas of Surgical Oncology.* Philadelphia: WB Saunders; 1995: 283–400.
5. Karakousis CP. The abdominoinguinal incision in limb salvage and resection of pelvic tumors. *Cancer.* 1984;54: 2543–2548.
6. Karakousis CP. Abdominoinguinal incision in resection of pelvic tumors with lateral fixation. *Am J Surg.* 1992;164: 366–371.
7. Karakousis CP, Karmpaliotis C, Driscoll DL. Major vessel resection during limb-preserving surgery for soft tissue sarcomas. *World J Surg.* 1996;20:345–350.
8. Karakousis CP, Volpe C, Tanski J, Colby ED, Winston J, Driscoll DL. Use of a mesh for musculoaponeurotic defects of the abdominal wall in cancer surgery and the risk of bowel fistulas. *J Am Coll Surg.* 1995;181:11–16.
9. Karakousis CP. Internal hemipelvectomy. *Surg Gynecol Obstet.* 1984;158:279–282.

6

10. Karakousis CP. Sacral resection with preservation of continence. *Surg Gynecol Obstet*. 1986;163:270–273.
11. Karakousis CP, Emrich L, Driscoll D. Variants of hemipelvectomy and their complications. *Am J Surg*. 1989;158: 404–408.
12. Storm FK, Mahvi DM. Diagnosis and management of retroperitoneal soft-tissue sarcoma. *Ann Surg*. 1991;214:2–10.
13. Karakousis CP, Gerstenbluth R, Kontzoglou K, Driscoll DL. Retroperitoneal sarcomas and their management. *Arch Surg*. 1995;130:1104–1109.
14. Ferrario T, Karakousis CP. Retroperitoneal sarcomas: Grade and survival. *Arch Surg*. 2003;138:248–251.
15. Karakousis CP, Proimakis C, Walsh DL. Primary soft tissue sarcoma of the extremities in adults. *Br J Surg*. 1995;82: 1208–1212.
16. Karakousis CP, Proimakis C, Rao U, Velez AF, Driscoll DL. Local recurrence in soft-tissue sarcomas and survival. *Ann Surg Oncol*. 1996;3:255–260.
17. Karakousis CP, Cheng C, Udobi K, Lascola RJ. Abdominoinguinal incision in adenocarcinoma of the sigmoid or cecum. Report of two cases. *Dis Colon Rectum*. 1998;41: 1322–1327.

Index

Notes Page numbers followed by 'f' and 't' refer to figures and tables respectively.

I

J

K

L

M

N

O

P